The Invention of Madness

STUDIES OF
THE WEATHERHEAD EAST ASIAN INSTITUTE,
COLUMBIA UNIVERSITY

The studies of the Weatherhead East Asian Institute of Columbia University were inaugurated in 1962 to bring to a wider public the results of significant research on modern and contemporary East Asia.

The Invention of Madness

State, Society, and the Insane in Modern China

EMILY BAUM

The University of Chicago Press
Chicago and London

The University of Chicago Press, Chicago 60637
The University of Chicago Press, Ltd., London
© 2018 by The University of Chicago
Published 2018
Printed in the United States of America

27 26 25 24 23 22 21 20 19 18   1 2 3 4 5

ISBN-13: 978-0-226-58061-6 (cloth)
ISBN-13: 978-0-226-55824-0 (paper)
ISBN-13: 978-0-226-58075-3 (e-book)
DOI: https://doi.org/10.7208/chicago/9780226580753.001.0001

Library of Congress Cataloging-in-Publication Data

Names: Baum, Emily, author.
Title: The invention of madness : state, society, and the insane in modern China /
    Emily Baum.
Other titles: Studies of the Weatherhead East Asian Institute, Columbia University.
Description: Chicago ; London : The University of Chicago Press, 2018. |
    Series: Studies of the Weatherhead East Asian Institute, Columbia University
Identifiers: LCCN 2018017663 | ISBN 9780226580616 (cloth : alk. paper) |
    ISBN 9780226558240 (pbk. : alk. paper) | ISBN 9780226580753 (e-book)
Subjects: LCSH: Mental illness—China—History—20th century. | Mental health
    services—China—History—20th century.
Classification: LCC RC339.C4 B395 2018 | DDC 362.20951—dc23
LC record available at https://lccn.loc.gov/2018017663

Contents

Acknowledgments

Madness, it is said, is the most solitary of afflictions. One could easily say the same about writing a book. I am fortunate, however, to have been surrounded by a supportive group of mentors, colleagues, and friends who made this process a much less solitary one.

This book would not have been possible without the unfaltering encouragement of Joseph Esherick and Paul Pickowicz. Their intellectual rigor, professional guidance, and (dare I say?) paternal support have shaped me into the scholar I am today. Andy Scull has the dubious honor of being the only person in the world to have read and commented on two entirely different iterations of this manuscript. When I was still poking around for a research project many years ago, he provided my first entryway into the seemingly impenetrable world of madness; since then, his humor, guidance, and incredible generosity have shaped this project in innumerable ways.

At the University of California, San Diego, Sarah Schneewind set a consistently high standard and challenged me to surpass it, and Suzanne Cahill, Lu Weijing, Cathy Gere, and Ari Heinrich were all formative influences. Throughout graduate school, I was lucky to be surrounded by an incredible group of fellow Sinologists, including David Chang Cheng, Maggie Greene, Miriam Gross, Brent Haas, Jenny Huangfu Day, Justin Jacobs, Judd Kinzley, Jeremy Murray, Amy O'Keefe, Jomo Smith, and Xiaowei Zheng. Today, they continue to provide a network of personal and professional support across the United States and overseas.

In Beijing, Yang Nianqun sponsored my research and provided a university affiliation. Zhang Daqing facilitated my return to Beijing for additional research. I am extremely grateful to Chen Qi for her assistance on several occasions. The staff at the Beijing Municipal Archives, in particular Liu Yanchen, offered a welcoming place to set up shop, and Janet Upton and Nathan Keltner made Beijing feel more like home. Yvon Yiwen Wang was not only a fellow researcher, runner, and roommate but also a dear friend. In Taiwan, Sean Hsiang-lin Lei gave helpful feedback when my project was still in its infancy, and Wang Wen-ji brought useful references to my attention and pointed out errors in interpretation. In New York, Lee Hiltzik and the rest of the staff at the Rockefeller Archive Center provided a comfortable place to conduct research.

I was fortunate to land at the History Department at the University of California, Irvine, where my colleagues have, without complaint, helped me to navigate the strange and entwined worlds of academia and Southern California. I'd especially like to thank Jeff Wasserstrom, Laura Mitchell, Anne Walthall, and David Fedman. Jennifer Munger offered assistance in countless ways, and I'm exceptionally grateful for her constant optimism, reassurance, and editorial eye.

The idea for this book first took shape during a conversation with Andy Liu in a Taiwanese cat café. Throughout, he has provided a sympathetic ear to my frustrations, both academic and existential. Philip Thai read every word of my early drafts and gave insightful feedback. When we first began our scholarly exchange, we were little more than acquaintances; today, I am happy to consider him a close friend. Maggie Greene generously offered to read more versions of my introduction than I'd care to count, even when she did not necessarily have the time to do so. Y Thien Nguyen gave perceptive comments and unflagging support, reminding me numerous times that what I had to say was worth saying.

Over the past few years, I've presented several parts of this book in embarrassingly inchoate forms. I am grateful to have received encouraging and perceptive comments from Amy Borovoy, Marta Hanson, Yumi Kim, Zhiying Ma, Sonya Pritzker, Ruth Rogaski, Fabien Simonis, and Margaret Tillman. A University of California Humanities Research Initiative Junior Faculty Manuscript Workshop grant gave me the opportunity to bring together several gifted scholars from across the University of California system and beyond. I am indebted to Perry Link, Laura Mitchell, Jennifer Munger, Andy Scull, Jeff Wasserstrom, Theodore Jun Yoo, and Mei Zhan for their invaluable comments on everything from my theoretical grounding to my prose.

The research, writing, and publication of this book would not have been possible without the generous funding provided by a Fulbright Institute of International Education grant, a Social Science Research Council International Dissertation Research Fellowship, a Jacob K. Javits fellowship, the Rockefeller Foundation, a University of California Hellman fellowship, a National Endowment for the Humanities summer stipend, an American Council of Learned Societies Henry Luce Program in China Studies postdoctoral fellowship, several grants from UC San Diego, UC Irvine and its Medical Humanities Initiative, and a UC Irvine Humanities Commons subvention grant. I am additionally grateful to Amanda Swain and Julia Lupton for bringing funding opportunities to my attention and helping to hone my proposals.

At the University of Chicago Press, Karen Merikangas Darling seamlessly guided me through this daunting process. Priya Nelson convinced me that Chicago would be a fitting home for the book, and she was entirely correct. At the Columbia Weatherhead Center, Ross Yelsey has consistently been enthusiastic about the project and responsive to my queries. I would additionally like to thank Evan White and Susannah Engstrom for their editorial assistance, Julia Turner for her close reading of the manuscript, and two anonymous reviewers for their perspicacious feedback.

A version of chapter 6 appeared as "Healthy Minds, Compliant Citizens: The Politics of Mental Hygiene in Republican China, 1928–1937," *Twentieth-Century China* 42, no. 3 (October 2017): 215–233. It is republished here by permission of Twentieth Century China Journal Inc. Parts of chapter 7 were previously published in "Choosing Cures for Mental Ills: Psychiatry and Chinese Medicine in Early Twentieth-Century China," *Asian Review of World Histories* 6, no. 1 (January 2018): 8–32. They have been reproduced by permission of Brill.

On a personal note, I would like to thank Keith Murphy, for his aesthetic and editorial sensibilities, among many other things; John Moule, for supporting my endeavors with pride; the city and people of Rogers Park, Chicago; the trainers at Barry's Bootcamp; the numerous cat cafés of Beijing and Taipei, where most of my ideas were incubated; and my own cat, Lou, for reminding me that nothing is more important than punctual feedings and copious brushings.

Finally, my mother, Donna Hansen, has, in one way or another, sustained and supported everything that has gone into this book, as well as everything that has come before it. I dedicate this to her.

Introduction

In the fall of 1921, thirty-five-year-old Wang Fengming suddenly went mad. The madness came and went at first, but as the Beijing winter approached and the days became shorter, his condition gradually became much worse. He refused to eat or drink, would not go to sleep, and created an endless disturbance for his wife and adolescent child. On the morning of December 1, Fengming's elderly father, Wang Fu, brought his son to the local police precinct hoping to have him placed within the municipal asylum. As he explained to the functionaries on duty, his family was exceptionally poor and therefore could not manage to look after Fengming any longer. In fact, he continued, it was due to their abject poverty that Fengming had gone mad in the first place; distressed over his recent unemployment, he had one day (and without warning) "caught a mad illness" (*huan fengbing*) that refused to be pacified. The police, accustomed to cases such as this, approved the transfer to the asylum and took Fengming into their custody. A mere three weeks later, however, Fengming was found dead. As the manager of the asylum noted in his report to the chief of police, Fengming's mad condition had quickly degenerated into an illness of "overabundant mucous fire." At four o'clock in the morning on December 22, phlegm had filled his throat, his vital energy (*qi*) refused to circulate, and his clothes became soaked with sweat. The physicians could do nothing to revive him.[1]

On its own, the story of Wang Fengming is not particularly noteworthy. At the municipal archives in Beijing, one can easily find hundreds of records almost identical to this one, all of which took place in the short interval between the overthrow of the Qing dynasty in 1911 and the onset of war with Japan in 1937. But the case of Wang Fengming, ordinary though it might have been, is also historically peculiar. Situated roughly at the midpoint of this book's narrative, Fengming's brief account captures a unique confluence of actors, strategies, and attitudes toward madness that would have been unheard of two decades earlier—and irrelevant only two decades hence. On the one hand, the asylum where Fengming met his untimely end was an undeniably modern import; prior to its establishment in 1908, mad people were generally kept within the home or, if not violent, allowed to wander at will. On the other hand, the asylum would cease to exist in Beijing by the mid-1930s. Succeeded by a newer institution—the psychopathic hospital—the asylum was ultimately removed from the care of the police and turned over to the hands of the psychiatric expert. Fengming's story, in short, represents a transitional moment in the ongoing "invention" of madness in Beijing. In order to understand why these transitions occurred at the times that they did, it is necessary to place this story within a much longer chronology, one that stretches both backward and forward in time.

✳

This book traces a genealogy of madness across the temporal and human geographies of early twentieth-century Beijing. In particular, it charts the process by which individuals who had "caught a mad illness" were slowly remade into individuals who were considered "mentally ill" (*jingshen bing*). Prior to the waning years of the Qing dynasty (1644–1911) and the early years of the Chinese Republic (1911–1949), madness was not necessarily perceived as a discrete pathology. Although the Chinese of the late imperial period certainly recognized the existence of mad acts and mad people, madness itself was interpreted more as a transitory symptom than a higher-order category of disease; as such, physicians and institutions for the specialized management of the insane were never considered necessary (if they were even considered at all). By the onset of the Second Sino-Japanese War in 1937, however, these earlier attitudes had largely changed. People who displayed strange behaviors or psychological irregularities were increasingly categorized as "mentally ill," placed under the jurisdiction of the psychiatric specialist, surveilled by the overlapping mechanisms of the police and the physician, assessed by the gaze of the forensic psychologist, and compelled to undergo new therapeutic procedures that were centered within the psychopathic hospital. Over the course of just four decades, the mentally ill person in Beijing had become, to borrow Michel Foucault's words, "gradually, progressively, really and materially constituted."[2]

This process, of course, did not occur in quite so straightforward or linear a fashion as the one I have outlined above. As the story of Wang Fengming can attest, the path from "mad" illnesses to "mental" ones had to first traverse a lengthy and uncertain terrain that belonged neither strictly to the world of Chinese medicine nor to that of contemporary neuropsychiatry. In Fengming's case, physicians at the municipal asylum framed his madness in a distinctly Chinese vocabulary yet did so in a therapeutic space that had no antecedent in Chinese culture. Moreover, once the mentally ill body had been "materially constituted" in the 1930s, the Beijing people did not just relinquish their pre-existing views of madness for those that had been imported from the West. Quite the opposite, individuals continued to subvert, appropriate, or simply ignore different aspects of psychiatric epistemology in ways that conformed to their personal worldviews and immediate needs. In other words, psychiatric ideas and practices did not emerge in Beijing fully formed, nor were they entirely successful at subverting old practices and conceptual systems. Instead, the amorphous disorder of madness—as well as its provision—was continuously invented and reinvented over the first half of the twentieth century. Why, and by what process, did this reinvention occur? And what, more generally, does this process reveal about the relationship between China and the West or state and society in the adoption and evolution of new epistemological norms?

When historians have sought to explain the shifting material and intellectual conditions of early twentieth-century China, they have clung tightly to the telos of "modernity" as an explanatory device. As many scholars have shown, the members of the Chinese intelligentsia were deeply moved by the desire to join the ranks of "modern" civilization, and it was in the service of this goal that they paved the way for Western learning (chemistry, sociology, psychiatry) to take root.[3] To the iconoclastic intelligentsia, the modern ethos was synonymous with historical progress and, hence, antithetical to the apparent backwardness of their own scholarly traditions; in Leo Ou-fan Lee's words, modernity was "closely associated with a new linear consciousness of time and history," in which "present and past became polarized as contrasting values."[4] Against the backdrop of foreign imperialism and domestic instability, the values of modernity—science, rationality, and the progressive dissociation from religion and superstition—appeared as a panacea to the innumerable problems facing the Chinese nation.[5] For historians who study Republican China, it was this striving for modernity—the unquenchable thirst to "leap into the time of the modern," as Shu-mei Shih has put it[6]—that compelled the intelligentsia and political elite to advocate for the adoption of Western forms of scientific knowledge.

That the discourse of modernity indelibly altered the intellectual landscape of early twentieth-century China is undeniable. But the abstract desire for modernity, I would suggest, is only the beginning of the story, not its end. More specifically, if members of the iconoclastic elite simply wished to mimic the structures of psychiatric modernity they had encountered in the West and Japan, how can we explain the convoluted, indirect, and lengthy process by which these structures were ultimately realized in China? And what, moreover, accounts for the incomplete and contested nature of psychiatric modernity when it was, at least partially, achieved in the 1930s? A narrow focus on the ideological quest for the "modern" is insufficient to fully address these questions because it leaves off at the very point at which they appear. If we wish to understand why madness evolved in Beijing in the particular ways it did, it is necessary to reorient our thinking about the role modernity played in broader processes of historical change—and, more importantly, to interrogate the very nature of Chinese modernity itself.

In asking these questions, I diverge somewhat from previous scholarship on the history of medicine in the late Qing and early Republican periods. In Chinese historiography, medicine has been treated as a predominantly ideological concern, one that mainly appealed to the modernizing agendas of the intellectual and political elite. As earlier studies have shown, the progressive intelligentsia embraced scientific biomedicine as a constituent part of the "national struggle for progress and modernity," a struggle that appeared to play out within the pathological body itself.[7] Convinced that the health of the individual was tantamount to the health of the nation, intellectuals glorified the ameliorative powers of Western medicine while denigrating the supposed backwardness of their own traditional regimens. As Bridie Andrews has recently argued, the reformist elite did not view biomedicine as a mere set of dispassionate practices but, more crucially, as a symbolic element of the "shared striving towards the ideals of modernity."[8] Meanwhile, conservative intellectuals defended "traditional" Chinese medicine out of an interest in an alternative form of modern subjectivity, one that would allow for the preservation of their own cultural identity.[9] In both cases, medicine has been theorized as another facet in the broader intellectual imperative to enter the ontological universe of the modern.

For historians, the battle over medical practice was not just an ideological project but also a political one. Throughout the early twentieth century, successive government regimes undertook the process of medical modernization out of a legitimate fear that the imperialist powers would further erode their sovereignty if they did not.[10] Much like in other colonized parts of the world, poor sanitary conditions in China were upheld as justification for Western intervention.[11] To Western and Japanese observers, China was swarming with pathogens and disease, and the Chinese themselves—the "sick men of Asia," as they were then referred—appeared to embody the very nadir of deficiency and deprivation.[12] Public health thus became a prerequisite for national autonomy, as well as a tool by which the state could better discipline the bodies of its citizenry. By taking measures to contain the spread of plague, sanitize the urban landscape, and more effectively monitor and optimize the health of its own populations, the Chinese state became far more involved in the pursuit of public health—including the policing of madness—than it had ever been at any point in the past.[13]

Although intellectual and political histories are certainly critical for understanding the advancement of new scholarly paradigms, they shed less light on how these ideas were applied, experienced, and ultimately remade on a more quotidian level. In this book, accordingly, I argue that the abstract striving for psychiatric modernity simply marked a starting point for what would prove to be a far more complex and enduring trajectory. Once introduced, psychiatric institutions and discourses took on a life of their own, and their uses and meanings were continually transformed by a variety of people—from government functionaries to the urban poor—who implemented or encountered them in the midst of pursuing their own material, practical, and political ends. New meanings and practices of madness, in other words, were not just imposed onto the Beijing public from above or without but instead "invented" by a range of actors in ways unique to, and determined by, the specific needs and conditions of Beijing society itself.

My use of the term *invention* is intentional. To invent means to create or devise, and I specifically employ this term to emphasize the agential quality of local knowledge production in early twentieth-century China. I do not mean to imply, however, that madness either did not exist in imperial China or was not recognized as such. As other scholars have shown, mad people attracted both the attention and the intervention of families, communities, and the imperial state far in advance of the Republican period.[14] At the same time, though, the vocabularies and technologies of control that were used on the insane during the preceding dynasties had little in common with those of the early twentieth century. Madness was therefore not invented in the sense that it was suddenly "thought up" out of thin air, but the morphology of the condition (alongside its related institutions) was so thoroughly transformed during the Republican period as to no longer be recognizable to its imperial antecedents.

By using the concept of invention as a heuristic device, moreover, I aim to draw attention to alternative possibilities for conceptualizing the nature of Chinese modernity. In many studies of the colonial or semicolonial world, modernity is often framed as a transferable condition that originated in the West and was subsequently appropriated by non-Western populations, though often in incomplete or unconventional ways. This approach, as critics have pointed out, has perpetuated the impression that colonized peoples were only "consumers" of modernity rather than producers.[15] Throughout this study, by contrast, I treat modernity not as a ready-made set of ideas and practices but instead as an ongoing, dynamic, and negotiable process, one that was only given meaning through the act of ordinary people going about their lives. In the case of psychiatry, it was *through*—rather than prior to—the quotidian engagement with foreign structures, vocabularies, and systems of knowledge that new meanings of madness ultimately coalesced and took shape. Thus China was not merely "awakened" to the possibility of psychiatric modernity but actively and continuously created that modernity in its own likeness.[16]

Madness and the Modern

What is it about madness, though, that enables us to shed light on the modern condition? For the Chinese, the significance of madness had much to do with its power as a tool of cultural critique. It was not purely coincidental that the first Western-style vernacular short story to appear in print—and one of the most famous pieces of twentieth-century Chinese writing in general—was Lu Xun's (1881–1936) "Diary of a Madman" (Kuangren riji), published in 1918.[17] Modeled on Nikolai Gogol's work of the same name, "Diary of a Madman" follows an unnamed protagonist's descent into lunacy as he convinces himself that the people around him are harboring a secret desire to "eat men"—that is, that they are complicit in a feudal cannibalistic tradition. As a "modernist text" that forcefully expresses its "unmistakable aspirations for modernity," Lu Xun's fictional account at once criticizes the barbarism of his fellow countrymen while evoking hope for a more humane future.[18] Following Lu Xun's lead, contemporary authors like Lao She (1899–1966) and Xu Zhuodai (1880–1958) similarly deployed madness to critique the Chinese delusion of national and moral superiority; in each case, madness appeared less as a material pathology than as a metaphorical signifier of a stultifying, man-eat-man tradition.[19]

That the trope of madness found ready usage among the modernizing intelligentsia was not just because it effectively underscored the deficiencies of Chinese culture but, more importantly, because it served to illuminate the very nature of Chinese-ness itself. Similar to the allegorical uses of madness in Western literature, the insane in Chinese fiction—by dint of their marginality—elucidated the values of their social order even as they renounced them.[20] In Lu Xun's writing, the madman is the only character to offer a sober analysis of his family's deeply engrained moral failings—and the only character, furthermore, to extend a prescription for their redemption. By acting as a foil to the benighted masses, mad people in the literary imagination have routinely functioned to expose the rotten marrow of their political and cultural institutions.[21] This function became particularly salient in the Republican period; as intellectuals wrestled with the need to devise a distinctly Chinese-cum-modern subjectivity, the madman's expository role as "monster yet mirror" was all the more crucial for their articulation of what it meant to be Chinese.[22]

Madness, however, was more than a symbolic marker of "moral illness."[23] At the same time that the literati were invoking the mad condition in a figurative fashion, other social actors considered madness problematic because of how *concretely* it implicated—and disrupted—so many aspects of everyday life. As a psychosomatic affliction, the disorder was alternately appropriated by physicians, faith healers, and families, each of whom jostled for unique jurisdiction over the governance of the maladapted body. In the realm of the law, mad people continuously traversed the uncertain boundary between social deviance and criminal transgression. And in the hands of Western missionaries, madness was additionally used to reinscribe racial and cultural difference; particularly in the colonial context of the late nineteenth and early twentieth centuries, Western regimes deployed the language of psychiatry as a rationale for establishing a biopolitics of control over native populations.[24] To the political elite, each of these aspects served as a cruel reminder that the Chinese had neither determined a precise technology for healing the insane nor an effective method by which to manage them; even worse, perhaps, was the confusion over which agency should be held responsible for such functions in the first place.

It was precisely because madness occupied such a ubiquitous (and ambiguous) position within various realms of governance and knowledge that the disorder became so vitally important to the modernizing sensibilities of the late Qing and early Republican regimes. By nature of its polysemic quality, madness called attention to the pervasive bankruptcy of native managerial, reformative, and therapeutic modalities. Indeed, while the vagrant insane had long incited the condemnatory gaze of local and foreign observers alike, no centralized mechanism had hitherto been developed for their suppression and control; while imperial jails had occasionally confined the bodies of the murderous mad, no effort had been undertaken to remold them, either through labor or moral suasion, into productive citizens; and while Chinese medicine had certainly endeavored to heal the corrupted faculties of the manic and the morose, it was only biomedicine (or so it seemed) that had developed an authoritative taxonomy of the elusive disorder. If, intellectuals realized, they wished to solve *all* the problems associated with the insane—to control as well as cure, to rehabilitate as well as repurpose—then this would require a *complete and total entry* into the ontological world of scientific modernity.

The centrality of madness to the modern experience thus stemmed from several causes: its ability to lay bare, in all its unsightliness, the essence of Chinese culture; the way it both cut across and bound together multiple facets of social, political, and intellectual life, highlighting in the process their cumulative defects; and its testament to the ineffectiveness (if not total absence) of native regimens for the regulation, disciplining, and optimization of errant bodies. As both symbol and substance, madness was inexorably being interwoven into the medical, moral, legal, political, and spiritual fabric of Chinese life—emphasizing, as it did so, the conspicuous inadequacies of each. All of these facets resonated with different segments of the Beijing elite, who, at various points during the early twentieth century, prescribed various remedies for their resolution. Convinced that China's entry into the hallowed world of the modern required the prior enhancement of—and control over—the functioning of Chinese minds, intellectuals and political agents ventured, with increasing confidence, into the new world of psychiatric epistemology and practice.

This is not to say, however, that psychiatric modernity was strictly an elite concern. Much the opposite, as subsequent regimes introduced new ideas and institutions for the care and confinement of the insane, ordinary people were the ones to apply them and put them into practice. In the process of doing so, they demoted the "modern" from an exalted abstraction to a lived reality, thereby changing its utility and meaning. A major goal of this book, then, is to go beyond the lofty declarations of political and intellectual tracts in order to unearth the more quotidian activities buried beneath them; following Michel de Certeau, I aim to excavate the "innumerable practices by means of which users reappropriate the space organized by techniques of sociocultural production."[25] In other words, while taking into consideration the modernist aspirations of the fin-de-siècle elite, I also consider how ordinary people "used" new disciplinary and medical technologies to suit their own ends—and in so doing, transformed the very nature of psychiatric modernity itself.

Writing the History of Madness

Given the importance of madness to Chinese modernity, it is puzzling that the subject has received so little attention in the historiography of early twentieth-century China.[26] Its absence has likely stemmed from several causes. While scholars of madness in the Western world have made ample use of historical materials like hospital records and patient diaries, such sources are arguably harder to come by in the Chinese context.[27] China's relatively late entry into the world of institutional psychotherapeutics, even in comparison to the rest of East Asia, has additionally made it a less obvious site of inquiry.[28] But more than this, the enigmatic quality of madness itself has perhaps inspired a certain degree of intellectual trepidation. To write about madness is to write about a subject in a constant state of metamorphosis—once we believe we have our finger on it, it mutates into something else. The same could be said for psychiatry. Throughout the late nineteenth and early twentieth centuries, the discipline expanded and contracted and jostled for professional turf, seeking to define itself at the same time as it endeavored to define the object of its inquiry. With no steady ground to stand on, madness has loomed as a daunting topic indeed.

Considering the uncertainty of our starting point, how do we go about demarcating the boundaries of a condition that has, for so many years and in so many cultures, appeared to defy definition? To put this differently, how do we write a genealogy of a disorder that has been at once omnipresent and constantly in flux? To begin, it is useful to situate ourselves within the terrain of medical anthropology, where scholars have long distinguished between the technical issue of *disease* and the embodied experience of *illness*. While the former is typically defined as "an alteration in biological structure or functioning," the latter encompasses a much broader spectrum: from the interpretation and expression of pain to the various modalities by which individuals seek relief from suffering.[29] Without denying the utility of biomedical models, which have attempted to isolate the source of mental disorders within the materiality of the brain and nerves, anthropologists have simultaneously suggested that disorders of psyche and soma transcend the "paradigmatically biological" and must also be considered part of the "cultural domain."[30]

For historians of madness, the distinction between illness and disease has proven essential for interpreting the vicissitudes of psychiatric disorders across time and space. Irrespective of whether psychopathic *diseases* manifest as stable, biological entities,[31] historians have viewed the *illness* of madness—how it has been named, identified, experienced, treated, and popularly imagined—as entirely contingent. As the historian Michael MacDonald has claimed, interpretations of madness, as well as the reactions it has provoked, are "determined by the material conditions, social organization, and systems of thought that characterize a particular culture and age."[32] To seek out what it means to be "mad," therefore, we must position ourselves within the specific temporality of the society in question—keeping in mind that "attitudes towards madness [are] never an island" but are instead enmeshed within, and conditioned by, the material and intellectual circumstances of the era.[33]

That conceptions of madness are subject to change does not mean, however, that the disorder is simply a figment of our collective cultural imaginary. In contrast to the social theorist Thomas Szasz, who views mental illness as a "myth" and psychiatry as a tool of social control, I do not deny the reality of mental distress or the tangible effects that it has inflicted on the patient and her society.[34] Rather, I am more inclined to agree with the perspective of anthropologists like Arthur Kleinman and Janis Jenkins, who conceive of the disorder as an intricate web conjoining physiological processes, social structures, cultural norms, and personal subjectivities. In Kleinman's view, "[T]he forms and functions of mental illness are not 'givens' in the natural world" but are instead "embedded in *social systems*" that imbue the disorder with symbolic meaning.[35] In the absence of a cultural context that demarcates normal from abnormal behavior, the disease of madness might still exist—but it might not be interpreted as an illness, per se. Throughout this book, accordingly, I treat mental illness as a very real affliction, but one that is simultaneously shaped by the boundaries of individual and cultural perception.

As etiologies of madness have shifted over time—from humoral imbalance to hormonal imbalance, from demonic possession to neurological malfunction—so too have the therapeutic strategies that have aimed to contain it. Although madness was considered a primarily familial concern throughout most of human history, the rise of scientific psychiatry in nineteenth-century Europe progressively shifted the onus of care from the family to the medical expert. In Western historiography, the reason for psychiatry's success has been the topic of prolonged academic debate.[36] Early scholarship on the subject claimed that psychiatry naturally triumphed over prior forms of managerial care because it was able to combine "humanitarianism" with a "more scientific understanding of insanity."[37] This contention, however, has long since been called into question.[38] Beginning with Michel Foucault's *Madness and Civilization,* which argued in part that psychiatry merely replaced earlier modes of physical restraint with an equally pernicious form of psychological coercion, scholars like Andrew Scull and David Rothman have challenged psychiatry's pretense toward "rationality" and "disinterested benevolence."[39] Emphasizing, moreover, the profound limits of psychiatric therapeutics— most early alienists were little more than "caretakers of custodial dumping institutions," as Scull has put it[40]—historians have also debunked the notion that psychiatry's success could be attributed to its superior efficacy.

The cause for psychiatry's growth, scholars have instead suggested, must be sought within the particular intellectual and socioeconomic conditions of the countries in which it flourished. In eighteenth- and nineteenth-century England, France, and the United States, urbanization undermined community cohesion, thereby necessitating the rise of public institutions for the poor, indigent, and insane.[41] The growth of market capitalism witnessed the advent of the so-called trade in lunacy, in which entrepreneurs and medical men erected private madhouses for the purpose of financial gain.[42] Meanwhile, the advance of rational secularism and the decline in demonological thought was linked to a more naturalistic understanding of madness; appealing to the cachet of scientific materialism, psychiatric experts maneuvered to claim a jurisdictional monopoly over the mentally ill.[43] By the early twentieth century, psychiatry was able to gain a widespread degree of cultural credence, despite its inability to cure. It did so, according to the sociologist Andrew Abbott, by "attaching [its] expertise to values with general cultural legitimacy," such as "rationality, efficiency, and science."[44] The rise of scientific psychiatry, in other words, was not historically inevitable but rather contextually specific.

The preceding points are especially critical to keep in mind for the Chinese case, since the writings of Western missionaries could easily lead us to believe that psychiatry was far more advanced—and Chinese medicine far more impoverished—than they were in reality. Though clothing itself in the guise of a dispassionate empiricism, psychiatry at the turn of the twentieth century was hardly more coherent, systematic, or effective than the "traditional" regimens that biomedical physicians denounced; and the psychiatric expert, though couching his diagnoses in the rhetoric of an impartial science, was undeniably influenced by the gendered, racial, and religious stereotypes that were common to his culture.[45] Nor was treatment of the insane a wholly standardized field of practice. While neurologists searched for the roots of the disorder within the material lesions of the brain, psychoanalysts sought to "forge a science of inner life" by plumbing the depths of the unconscious mind.[46] Within the far-flung regions of the colonized world, moreover, medical missionaries linked madness to religious idolatry—and its cure to Christian salvation. For these men and women, madness was a disorder of neither the brain nor the mind but rather a sickness of the soul.[47]

Despite this panoply of therapeutic approaches, what each of these factions shared was a profound inability to cure the amorphous disorder. Just as neurologists failed to identify (much less resuscitate) the diseased matter of the lunatic's brain, psychoanalysis was rebuffed as mere fantasy, located somewhere on the spectrum between bombast and bunk. Within the overrun asylums and crowded lunatic wards of the Western world, meanwhile, the chronic insane were dismissed as degenerative and thereby unsalvageable; if science could not cure them, then they could not be cured.[48] Though loath to admit it, psychiatrists at the turn of the century were little closer to unveiling the truths of mental illness than they had been over one hundred years earlier, when the profession of "mad doctoring" had just begun to emerge in the madhouses and lunatic asylums of London and Paris.[49] On the eve of the Chinese Republic, insanity remained "a veritable Proteus," as Roy Porter once put it: elusive in its origins, inconstant in its manifestations, and ultimately intractable in its cure.[50]

The deepening influence of psychiatry in Beijing (as elsewhere in the developed and developing world) thus had very little to do with the forward march of historical "progress" or the clinical superiority of biomedical expertise. In contrast to the Whiggish optimism of earlier historians, psychiatry in the early twentieth century had few empirical benefits to offer the Chinese public. If we wish to understand the source of its appeal—as well as the ways that it was understood, appropriated, and applied in everyday Beijing life—we must look not to the discipline itself but instead to the society in which it took root.

The Setting

Throughout the first half of the twentieth century, urban China bore witness to an extraordinary, and in many ways unprecedented, amount of political, intellectual, demographic, and institutional change. Following the forced "opening" of China to Western colonialism during the mid-nineteenth century, several cities along the eastern seaboard were transformed into major centers of trade called treaty ports. Within these treaty ports, foreigners established banks and businesses, remade the urban landscape with paved roads and electric lights, and governed independent settlements called concessions, which were entirely exempt from Chinese laws. As a result of the shifting material and administrative conditions of the treaty ports, coastal cities quickly morphed from low-populated government centers to bustling hubs of commercial and cultural activity.[51] Migrants left their natal homes en masse in search of opportunity, thereby disrupting the cohesion of community networks in the countryside and contributing to rising rates of homelessness and vagrancy in the cities. Businessmen broke free of government oversight to establish huge, capital-driven industries that could compete with foreign conglomerates. And for the literate Chinese, the bourgeoning world of print media enabled new forms of mass communication and popular critique.

Although the above conditions were generalizable to much of urban China, Beijing nevertheless differed from the treaty ports in one important way. After the Qing dynasty's loss to the foreign powers during the Second Opium War (1856–1860), several Western nations were allowed for the first time to establish permanent diplomatic legations in the capital city. But unlike other metropolises such as Shanghai and Tianjin, which were cleaved into separate administrative zones for foreign and Chinese settlements, Beijing was never reduced to the status of a semicolonial concession. Consequently, while Western and Japanese residents may have exerted an increasingly marked influence on the rhythms of Beijing life, the capital retained its sovereignty well into the 1930s.[52]

Due to Beijing's political autonomy, the effects of foreign imperialism were experienced differently in the capital than elsewhere along China's eastern periphery. Even as the city's infrastructure shifted to accommodate new bureaucratic, demographic, and technological needs, these changes, as David Strand has argued, were "less decisive" than in directly colonized locations like Shanghai.[53] At the same time, lack of foreign investment meant that Beijing saw comparatively little industrial development over the course of the Republican period, and the city's inland location further rendered it, according to Madeleine Yue Dong, a "peripheral player in the new world economic system." Beijing's economically disadvantaged status vis-à-vis its littoral counterparts had severe repercussions for the local population. Particularly after the Chinese capital was relocated to Nanjing in 1928, poverty became an almost ubiquitous experience for the city's residents; as sociological data show, close to three-fourths of the Beijing people suffered from economic insecurity, while over a quarter lived in conditions of abject destitution.[54]

Beijing's specific niche in the global reticulations of imperialism and industrial capitalism has several important implications for this study. First, while poverty was nothing new in the early twentieth century, the poor themselves were progressively thrust into the spotlight as targets of social control and moral reform. Influenced by globally circulating discourses that linked poverty to national weakness, the Beijing municipality made it a priority to contain and rehabilitate its poor and indigent populations—among whom the insane figured prominently.[55] The segregationist impulse that accompanied the turn to disciplinary governance was most clearly manifested in the erection of the Beijing Municipal Asylum, the first public asylum in China and an institution whose history underlies much of this book's longer narrative. Second, because Beijing never lost its political autonomy during the period in question, records from local facilities like the asylum are composed in an entirely Chinese (rather than Western) voice. These documents, which include oral testimonies from the insane and their families, offer a rare, albeit fragmented, glimpse into the lives of historically marginalized actors. While such testimonies were necessarily mediated by the functionaries who transcribed them, they nevertheless provide a window onto the activities and survival strategies of ordinary people, particularly as they navigated the bureaucratic machinery of Beijing's early policing networks.[56]

By concentrating on one particular site (with occasional excursions out-side it) over a relatively short period of time, this book not only traces major changes in the knowledge and practice of madness but also seeks to excavate the buried logics behind which these paradigmatic shifts took place. To do so, it proceeds both horizontally across time and vertically across class. Focusing on intellectual and political elites alongside low-level municipal functionaries, policemen, petty businessmen, and poor urban residents, this book aims to show how new meanings and practices of madness were forged through a dy-namic and dialogical interaction between foreign and Chinese, elite and subal-tern, state and society. Even as new terminologies, ideologies, and institutions were initiated from above, their deployment, legitimation, and ultimate inte-gration into preexistent epistemologies and therapeutic strategies—that is to say, their *use in practice*—depended to a significant extent on individuals who might otherwise appear insignificant to the historical record.

*

Chapter 1 examines how madness was conceptualized in late imperial China prior to the introduction of psychiatric medicine, and shows how the "mad illness" straddled medical, religious, supernatural, legal, and social realms of knowledge. Due to the heterogeneous ways in which madness was framed in the popular imaginary, mad people were never considered the unique pur-view of a single expert profession. Conceptions of the insane began to change around the turn of the twentieth century, in tandem with the establishment of the Beijing Municipal Asylum in 1908. As chapter 2 describes, the police who administered the asylum proactively arrested vagrant, sojourning, and dis-placed lunatics in the interest of preserving public order. In the act of doing so, they imbued mad people (*fengzi*) with a deviant identity, one that justified their preemptive institutionalization even in the absence of criminal activity.

Chapter 3 builds on this narrative by describing how poor urban fami-lies exploited municipal services to relieve themselves of the financial and emotional burdens of madness. Using the insane as a pretext for municipal involvement, urban publics legitimized the increasingly intrusive activities of the local police by affirming the relationship between insanity, poverty, deviance, and disruption. While mad bodies were being policed, madness itself was also being imbued with new medical meanings. In the mid-1920s, as chapter 4 shows, "psychiatric entrepreneurs" began to market specialized proprietary medicines and private psychopathic hospitals to the middle and upper classes. Introducing new forms of madness such as neurasthenia, these entrepreneurs expanded the taxonomy of the disorder as a way to attract the financial interests of Beijing's moneyed consumers.

Chapters 5 and 6 turn their attention to the relationship between political power and control over the insane. Chapter 5 discusses the belated incorporation of neuropsychiatry into the municipal apparatus in the mid-1930s, which occurred as a result of a partnership between the Guomindang (Nationalist Party) and an American medical school, the Peking Union Medical College (PUMC). As this chapter argues, municipal functionaries pursued this collaboration to meet their immediate financial and political interests; by turning the asylum over to the care of the PUMC, the municipality both relieved itself of a significant economic burden and bolstered its own political legitimacy. Chapter 6, which momentarily departs from Beijing, explores the short-lived mental hygiene movement, a national campaign that gained momentum shortly before the outbreak of war with Japan in 1937. The movement, which sought to inspire social conformity and obedience to Guomindang rule, did so by classifying nonconformist behaviors—including support of communism—as a form of mental illness.

By the end of the 1930s, madness looked very little like it had at the dawn of the century. This is not to say, however, that new conceptions of mental illness had fully subverted preexistent conceptions of what it meant to be "mad." To the contrary, Chinese medicine proved incredibly resilient and elastic, able to assimilate competing paradigms without relinquishing its own epistemic authority. Chapter 7 explores four ways that Chinese medicine and neuropsychiatry had merged by the onset of the Second Sino-Japanese War. Focusing on issues of translation, medical theory, and therapeutic practice, it shows how the two conceptual systems ultimately coalesced in a mutually symbiotic fashion.

Before proceeding, a note on terminology is in order. Despite the derogatory nature of terms like *madness* and *madman*, I use these words throughout this book out of an interest in historical and linguistic authenticity. Prior to the advent of psychiatric medicine in Beijing, madness was not conceptualized as an inherently "mental" disorder, and it would be anachronistic to translate it otherwise. I employ words like madness and lunacy, moreover, to more easily differentiate between Chinese terms like *diankuang* or *fengdian* (madness) and psychiatric neologisms like *jingshen bing* or *shenjing bing* (mental illness or nervous disorder). The latter only came into common use in the 1920s and 1930s, though they did not necessarily replace earlier conventions. In order to convey the intended semantics of these words, I retain the distinction between *madness* and *mental illness* where applicable.

Contracting the "Mad Illness"

In 1866, the governor general of Zhili province, Liu Changyou (1818–1887), became embroiled in a particularly bothersome investigation. During the summer of that year, it had come to Liu's attention that a local peasant named Zhang Luodai had plotted to burn a French priest to death in the reading room of a nearby temple. Aware of the already tense relations between locals and French missionaries, and wishing to avoid an unnecessary scandal in his province, Liu quickly dispatched an official to bring Zhang to the provincial seat for questioning.

Liu soon realized that the case was far more complicated than he had originally been led to believe. In the middle of the eighth month of the previous year, Zhang's son, the fifteen-year-old Zhang Shuqin, had suddenly and unexpectedly "contracted symptoms of a mad illness" (*huhuan fengdian bingzheng*) in the midst of his studies.[1] He raved and hallucinated, yelled and cursed, but despite copious treatments, he could not be brought to reason. Zhang's family was soon at its wit's end. Although they had engaged several physicians to visit the boy and had prayed to the gods and ancestors to relieve the child of his suffering, their efforts had all come to naught. It was only after many weeks of disturbance that Zhang learned of a healer who might be able to treat his son. Li Luolai, Zhang's neighbor and a recent convert to Catholicism, approached Zhang with the proposition. Revealing that he knew of a Catholic priest who was adept at "harassing spirits" and "expelling evil" through his close reading of the scriptures, Li proposed enlisting the cleric to relieve the boy of his mad symptoms.

At first, Zhang demurred. But as his son's entanglement with evil (*xie*) became increasingly severe, he ultimately found no choice but to relent.[2] "I troubled Li Luolai and his son to quickly travel to a Catholic church about six *li* away from our village," Zhang confessed. Once there, Li invited the priest, Father Ai, along with four other clergymen to go with him to the local temple, where they would read the scripture and pray. "The priest had instructed that he didn't want idlers to spy on them while they completed their business," Zhang related, "so I had left the doors [to the temple] unlocked. I noticed, though, that the reading room had been slightly rearranged. Others must have entered it beforehand and not closed it up again." When the Catholics arrived, they soon set about their business, aided by a torch that Father Ai had carried with him to light the way. After only an hour of prayer, however, an intense fire enveloped them, causing their clothes to be set ablaze. Although everyone survived, they were unable to determine who had set the fire and why.

Throughout his interrogation, the elder Zhang insisted that he had not been engaged in a quarrel with the priest or plotted to kill him. Quite the opposite—he had invited the missionaries to his village with the sincere hope that they could "expel his son's illness" (*chubing*). Zhang's son, Shuqin, was also brought to the provincial seat and questioned under torture. But because the young boy "was only sometimes lucid," his testimony proved useless. In the end, the investigators concluded that the fire must have been caused by fireworks that had been stowed in the temple. It was even proposed that the mad boy, in his absurd and unknowing state, was likely the one to have stashed them there. But because of Shuqin's "severe confusion" and "lack of recollection" about the event, there would be no way to know for certain. At the end of their lengthy interrogation, the two men were released to return home. Although Zhang Luodai was likely made to confine his son lest a similar incident occur in the future, the historical record does not reveal any charges or penalties being lodged against either man.[3]

The case of the mad Shuqin reveals much about how madness was articulated, interpreted, and managed in an era before institutionalization had become common practice. More specifically, the various ways that Zhang Luodai sought to rid his son of the "symptoms of a mad illness," coupled with the governor general's decision to allow both men to return home without penalty, attest to the diverse and decentralized means by which madness was confronted in the late Qing. In this chapter, I read the aforementioned case not simply as an example of late imperial jurisprudence or state-society relations, but also as an entryway into understanding the ontological world of the mad person on the eve of the Republican period.

In late nineteenth-century China, madness had not yet become a discrete object of professional knowledge. Straddled between multiple realms of human inquiry, it blurred the already indistinct boundaries between medicine and religion, cosmology and the occult. The apparent vagaries of the condition, combined with the imprecision of its origin, meant that no expert profession or institutional arrangement had risen up to claim unique jurisdiction over the management of the mad body. Instead, the treatment of madness remained an ad hoc business, subjected to a constellation of etiological explanations and therapeutic strategies and unbeholden to the claims of a specialized psychiatric authority. Throughout the late imperial period, in other words, madness was seen as plural, rather than monolithic, and the responses it provoked reflected this perceived heterogeneity.

Managing Madness

The mid-nineteenth century was a period of both extreme turbulence and intensive reform. At the time that the incident involving Zhang Shuqin was taking place, the Qing state was floundering to right itself after a series of wars—both civil and international—had nearly forced the dynasty to its knees. The massively destructive Taiping Rebellion (1850–1864) had only been quelled a few years earlier, the humiliation of the Opium Wars was still fresh in the memory, and the Qing state, confronted with the superior military technologies of the Western world, was struggling to find its place in a new international system while still retaining faith in the superiority of its traditions. In the face of such political and existential tumult, madness might not have seemed the most pressing of concerns. But for the Qing dynasty, the question of how to handle mad people—particularly the criminally insane—was both a highly important and ongoing legal issue.

Throughout the many years and changing conditions of Qing rule, the dynasty typically handled the problem of madness by decentralizing responsibility for the insane onto families, neighbors, and mutual aid groups. As early as 1689, the Qing had mandated that families preventively keep watch over "people with a mad illness" (*fengbing zhiren*), lest they commit a serious crime such as homicide. In 1732, the Yongzheng emperor increased the terms of this legal substatute, insisting on the mandatory registration of the insane and their confinement within the home. If the unfortunate individual somehow managed to escape his protective custody and commit murder, the penal code relieved him from physical punishment;[4] instead, his family was held legally responsible for the crime and punished monetarily (with compensation to the relatives of the victim) and physically (with as many as one hundred strokes from a heavy rod).[5] The 1689 and 1732 rulings thus served to formalize a family-centered approach to the management of madness. While officials could easily intervene in the presence of mad behaviors, the brunt of the supervisory responsibility fell to the family or local community.

Although the 1732 substatute remained on the books until 1908, it was neither consistently enforced nor regularly observed. Unless the madman proved dangerous or committed a serious crime, many local officials were content to turn a blind eye to the problem.[6] Families, too, were often reluctant to abide by the legislation and devised ways to skirt their registration responsibilities by emphasizing the intermittent nature of the condition. Claiming that madness was only a temporary disorder—one marked by prolonged periods of lucidity and clarity of purpose—relatives of the insane remained optimistic that the affliction could be managed and eventually cured without resort to compulsory confinement.[7] Aside from the violent insane who were kept locked within the home or inside a county jail, many madmen and madwomen continued to wander freely, flagrantly flouting the orders for their urgent imprisonment.

Medical missionaries who traveled to China in the late nineteenth century were aghast to observe this very phenomenon. Charles Selden (1861–1938), an American physician who managed a refuge for the insane in Guangzhou, noted that among his Chinese medical students, "there was not one who had not seen insane persons" roaming the streets, and some had seen as many as ten. "There are no restrictions put upon [the insane] by the government," he wrote in the *China Medical Missionary Journal.* "So long as they are not found stealing or suspected of such, or doing anything violent, they may go about at will."[8] Robert Fortune (1812–1880), a Scottish botanist who traveled to Beijing in 1861, made a similar observation. Within the city gate, he remarked, beggars crowded around fruit vendors and market peddlers in the hopes of receiving a spare copper. They were "ragged, filthy," Fortune wrote, "and in many instances apparently insane."[9] Charles Selden attempted to find official justification for this leniency by writing a letter to the viceroy of Guangdong and Guangxi provinces, inquiring about governmental provisions for the mentally unwell. The response was exactly as he had suspected. "If the patient is found quiet," the viceroy wrote, "he will be allowed the liberty of going anywhere, and no one is appointed to have authority over such." It was only on occasions when the lunatic proved violent that he would be "imprisoned by the authorities or by his father or family relative."[10]

The decision to allow mad people to wander at will reflected the widespread sentiment that the insane did not necessarily pose a threat to individual or communal safety. Throughout the nineteenth century, families frequently justified their noncompliance with the Qing code by claiming that that the mad person never incited trouble and, accordingly, did not need to be incarcerated. In 1892, for instance, a case was brought before the governor general of Sichuan province concerning a lunatic named Huang Zhixing. Huang was well known within the community, and his transitory madness had never been interpreted as particularly dangerous until the day on which he stabbed a French priest through the palm of the hand. When authorities questioned the local community about why the man had not been registered or confined, they received the same response from several neighbors: "He never stirred up trouble before, so we never reported him or took him into custody."[11] As long as the man did not prove bothersome, most were content to overlook both his mad disorder and the dictates of the law.

In some ways, the Qing code itself contributed to this communal laxity. Since families were only penalized for noncompliance if their mad relative committed a crime, many decided that the risk of punishment was insufficient to justify the cost and logistics involved in confining the insane.[12] In other instances, the uncertain juridical status of the mad person enabled families and local authorities alike to skirt their legal responsibilities. Although the Qing code had identified the penal denomination of "homicide due to madness" (*fengbing sharen*) from as early as the seventeenth century, the code did not explicitly mention other forms of criminality that should be handled differently due to the existence of mad behaviors.[13] When the governor general of Sichuan was forced to prosecute the case of Huang Zhixing, therefore, he was necessarily unsure of how to proceed. "We've looked for a legal precedent," he wrote to the Qing general office, "but haven't found anything relating to 'an injury being caused due to madness' [*yinfeng shangren*]." The law was clear on what to do when a mad person committed homicide, the memorial continued: the criminal should be locked up and his family and neighbors flogged one hundred blows apiece. But Huang hadn't *killed* the priest; he had merely injured him. "How should we punish him in accordance with the law?" the governor general anxiously inquired. "Should we lock him up? Should we wait until his illness is better and then determine what to do? Should we abide by the homicide statute but make a discretionary reduction?"[14] The ambiguous place of madness in the late Qing code contributed not only to the improvisational nature of legal action but also to the ad hoc ways in which mad people were managed in society at large.

I do not wish to appear overly sanguine in this regard, however. While the mad person may have been permitted certain liberties in some situations, in other instances he was treated like the very antithesis of humanity itself. Medical missionaries soberly observed how Chinese families kept their mad relatives confined within pig baskets, troughs, and chicken coops, thereby eliminating the distinction between human and animal (see figure 1.1). Some households, moved more by practical necessity than existential commiseration, further adopted violent solutions to the troublesome insane. "Many bear the marks of the whippings or poundings they have received or of the fetters

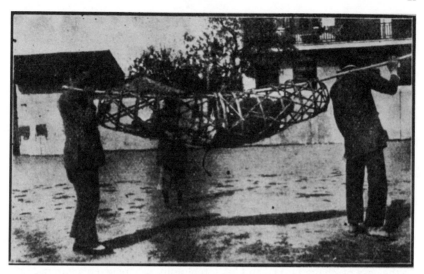

FIGURE 1.1. An insane person restrained in a basket intended for transporting pigs (John G. Kerr Hospital for the Insane, Reports for 1916–1917)

that have been on hands or feet," Charles Selden remarked. "The common custom is to chain the person to a post or a heavy stone in the house, so that he or she may not be able to go out into the street or do violence to men or things."[15] The physician J. H. Ingram (1858–1934) similarly heard rumors of a father who drowned his mad son in a river and a mother who "hired ruffians to break a leg and an arm of her son, in order that he might not be able to terrorize the neighborhood."[16] Such actions, missionaries conceded, were by no means commonplace, but they were also not outside the realm of possibility.[17]

Despite individual measures such as these, though, the practice of confining or abusing the insane was hardly universal. While families may have chosen to lock up their mad relatives if they had gotten into trouble or provoked the unwanted attention of local officials, the generally tolerated presence of mad people in public spaces proved that not all families were persuaded to adopt such stringent measures. Even Charles Selden, though normally disdainful of Chinese approaches to handling madness, was moved to admit that "true affection on the part of the family for their insane" was not altogether atypical. At the facility where he worked, Selden observed numerous instances in which families showed deep sympathy and concern for their loved ones, visiting them frequently and bringing whatever delicacies they could afford.[18]

Given the general laxity with which families of the insane adhered to Qing laws, it is necessary to distinguish between the legal code itself and the context in which it was enacted. Throughout the nineteenth century, families routinely ignored imperial commands to register and confine their insane relatives within the home. Believing that mad people were not inherently dangerous, and hopeful that their relatives would quickly recover their wits, they often found ways to circumvent the letter of the law. Mad people consequently continued to populate the landscape, attracting official sanction only after they had committed a crime. That the mad boy Zhang Shuqin was allowed to travel freely outside of the house—even going so far as to stash fireworks in the local temple—could hardly be considered an exceptional incident.

Treating the Mad Illness

It was not just the management of mad people that generated diverse responses throughout the late Qing. In matters of treatment, too, families employed a variety of methods to rid their relatives of the so-called mad illness. In the case of Zhang Luodai and his son Shuqin, we are given a glimpse into the constellation of ways that a late imperial family might have interpreted and treated mad behaviors. During his interrogation, the elder Zhang insisted that he had exhausted all options of treatment before being moved, out of sheer desperation, to call for a French priest to come to his village. "Medicine and prayers both came to naught [yidao jiebu jianxiao]," he affirmed before the imposing figure of his interrogator. Indeed, if the former strategies had worked, the entire incident might have been avoided altogether.

Families in the late Qing considered madness a simultaneously biological, emotional, supernatural, and moral issue, and it was therefore not uncommon to concurrently "send for a doctor and entreat the spirits" (yanyi qiushen) without cognitive dissonance.[19] In much the same way as madness was treated in late sixteenth- and early seventeenth-century England, Qing families experimented with a range of somatic therapies alongside mystical and astrological ones—though they did not always differentiate between the various typologies of treatment in such a clear-cut way.[20] Because of the perceived heterogeneity of the disorder, madness in late imperial China was never considered the unique purview of a particular medical specialist, such as a psychiatrist or psychologist. Instead, families may have enjoined the help of literati physicians, herbalists, shamans, faith healers, and fortune-tellers in tandem; concerned less about the domain of each respective healer than the success of his or her treatments, relatives of the insane pursued a variety of therapies concurrently and in different combinations.

Those who treated the insane, meanwhile, did not necessarily view "madness" as a discrete or self-contained condition. Physicians and healers used a variety of expressions to describe different behaviors and disease patterns, and there was no single, unified term that they employed to encompass all variations of mad symptoms. By the late nineteenth century, three general "types" of madness had coalesced: *kuang* (excited or violent madness), *dian* (apathetic or withdrawn madness), and *xian* (epilepsy or falling madness).[21] It should be noted, though, that the etiological boundaries between these terms were not always clearly delineated; hence, different authors invoked them in different ways and in different combinations, and their symptomatic referents were neither static nor fixed.[22] Some physicians did not even refer to "madness" at all but instead to underlying illness patterns that could induce mad behaviors, such as "heart sickness" (*xinji*), "liver *qi*" (*ganqi*), or "mucous confusion" (*tanmi*), which will be discussed below. The term *fengbing* (mad illness), meanwhile, was typically used only in a juridical context and was rarely invoked by physicians.

Madness, in short, was considered a variegated affliction. It manifested in multiple forms, exhibited a variety of psychosomatic symptoms, and was induced by a congeries of biological, emotional, moral, and cosmological phenomena.[23] Because the disorder crossed so many etiological lines, healers and patients alike tended to view mad behaviors as primarily symptomatic, rather than taxonomic. That is to say, madness was typically interpreted as the psychosomatic *expression* of a biological, emotional, or moral problem but was not consistently construed as a higher-order problem itself.[24] Consequently, mad patients continued to be treated by general practitioners and faith healers who assumed that the underlying source of the affliction was no different than any other disorder they might be called on to treat.

SENDING FOR DOCTORS

When faced with the onset of mad behaviors, Chinese families frequently entrusted the treatment of their relatives to the care of local physicians. In the late nineteenth century, Chinese medicine had not yet been standardized into a uniform system of knowledge. Individual physicians instead employed treatments that derived from, and were unique to, the diverse medical lineages from which they had apprenticed.[25] As Bridie Andrews has noted, the medical "profession" itself was not even considered a singular entity during this time, as healers alternately took the form of drug peddlers (*lingyi*), female midwives, vulgar quacks (*yongyi*), and literati Confucian physicians (*ruyi*), the latter of which often maintained detailed notes about their patients' conditions in medical case records (*yi'an*).[26] Despite their diversity in approach, however, most medical practitioners of the late Qing shared common assumptions about the basic causes of the mad condition.

Previous works have gone into much detail to describe the etiological vicissitudes of madness between the Han dynasty (206 BC–AD 220)—when textual references to mad disorders first appeared in the classical text *Huangdi neijing* (Yellow emperor's inner canon)—and the fall of the Qing dynasty in the early twentieth century.[27] From roughly the third to tenth centuries AD, mad behaviors were typically attributed to the pathogenic influence of wind. Wind, believed at the time to be the most harmful of the six major pathogens (the others being cold, summer heat, dampness, dryness, and fire), was popularly considered the "origin of the one hundred diseases."[28] As Shigehisa Kuriyama notes, because winds "arose unexpectedly, suddenly, [and] irregularly," they were typically associated with disorders of movement and delirium, including epilepsy and mania.[29]

Starting in the eleventh and twelfth centuries, physicians began to question the inherent relationship between madness and wind, asserting instead that mad behaviors were likely caused by pathogenic fire accompanied by an accretion of mucous in the chest. The famous Yuan dynasty physician Zhu Zhenheng (also known as Zhu Danxi, 1282–1358), writing in the fourteenth century, synthesized recent developments in medical theory when he tersely noted, "Mucous in the chest makes people mad."[30] The solution to the problem—now known by names as suggestive as "mucous confuses the openings of the heart" (*tanmi xinqiao*) and the illness of "mucous fire" (*tanhuo*)—was not to expel the invasive wind but rather to attack the accumulation of mucous through purgatives and emetics. By the beginning of the Qing dynasty, the mucous etiology of madness had gained the most widespread currency among literate physicians, having almost entirely defeated competing schools of thought.

In medical case records of the late Qing, mucous and madness remain closely linked. The eminent practitioner Ma Peizhi (1820–1903), who gained renown for having acted as court physician to the Empress Dowager Cixi (1835–1908), noted in several instances how a "mad sickness" (*dianji*) had occurred after mucous fire had risen into the chest and disturbed the mental faculties (*shenzhi*). The remedy, he wrote, involved "transforming the mucous" (*huatan*) and inducing it to descend below the chest so as to "render the mental faculties clear."[31] The Qing practitioner Chao Weifang (1869–1929) similarly observed how a patient plagued by insomnia, lack of appetite, and general anxiousness suffered from mucous fire, which took advantage of the "insufficient *qi* in his heart."[32] And Wang Shixiong (also called Wang Mengying, 1808–1867) described the case of a young man whose "mad epilepsy" (*dianxian*) had begun when "an excess of mucous" had caused his "chest and diaphragm to become full and stuffy."[33]

The close association between mucous and madness derived from widely shared assumptions about the structure and morphology of the human body. Physicians of the late Qing believed that mental processes, emotions, and metaphysical attributes (such as the "essence" and "soul" of the individual) were dispersed evenly across the five *zang* and six *fu* organs, each of which governed different cognitive and emotional faculties.[34] The kidneys, for instance, were affiliated with the emotion of fear along with the person's essence and will (*jingzhi*), the spleen governed worry as well as intention and wisdom (*yizhi*), and the liver and lungs housed the earthly (*hun*) and ethereal (*po*) souls, respectively.[35] Within this envisioned corporeal bureaucracy, the heart emerged as the "ruler" (*zhu*) of the organs, capable of dispatching orders to other parts of the body and responsible for maintaining normal somatic functioning. The reason the heart was imbued with such power was due to the belief that the heart housed the person's spirit or mind (*shen*) and was therefore the organ associated with thinking and knowing; the brain, in Chinese medicine, played little or no role in mental activity.[36]

Because of the intimate relationship between cognition and the heart, physicians typically attributed disordered thoughts and behaviors to an obstruction, malfunction, or imbalance of the vital fluids within the region of the chest, which could then affect the normal activities of the spirit-mind (*shen*). When mucous accumulated in the chest, for instance, it could choke off the internal organs and obstruct the efficacy of *shen*, which then resulted in mental, physical, and behavioral disturbances. The renowned physician Ding Ganren (1865–1926), who belonged to the famous Menghe lineage of Chinese medicine,[37] attested to this phenomenon in his description of a patient afflicted with *dian* (apathetic or withdrawn madness): "When mucous gathers in the midsection, it clouds up the clear orifices and blocks the path on which the spirit-mind comes and goes. The upper body, which is usually clear and spacious, then becomes like a village of cloud and mist. As a result, the spirit mechanism [*shenji*] is rendered ineffective." Mucous, in other words, stifled the normal functioning of the spirit-mind by blocking its regular channels of communication. For Ding Ganren, the only recourse in such a situation was to eliminate the accumulation of mucous and liberate the *shen*. "I have drawn up seven 'attackers' and three 'replenishers,'" Ding concluded, "so as to dispel the stubborn mucous and save the vital fluids."[38]

Medical missionaries were both perplexed and frustrated by their patients' insistence on the pathological role of mucous. Although Western physicians had similarly attributed madness to mucous and humoral imbalance for over two millennia,[39] this view had largely been discredited, at least among university-educated practitioners, by the turn of the twentieth century.[40] "[The

Chinese] are entirely ignorant of the fact that the seat of the disease is in the brain," Charles Selden haughtily wrote in 1905.[41] To his chagrin, Selden's patients and their families insisted that the cause of madness lay in the copious amount of mucous "choking up" the organs within the chest; so ingrained was this idea that even patients with some knowledge of their own condition spoke of "having overmuch 'phlegm.'" The problem with this belief, as Selden explained, was not simply that it was incorrect but, more importantly, that it was harmful. At the missionary hospital where he worked, families, attendants, and even local officials frequently smuggled in native remedies for eliminating mucous. Most of these, such as oil of *Aleurites cordata* or croton oil, were nothing more than powerful emetics and purgatives. By inducing such severe and violent vomiting as to leave the patient incapacitated, these medicines might have temporarily quieted the symptoms of agitated mania but offered no long-term cure.[42]

Regardless of the central role played by mucous in Qing etiologies of madness, explanations for the origins of mad behaviors were far more complex than a reductive focus on mucous alone. As Nathan Sivin has written, the body in Chinese medical theory was conceived as a "congeries of vital processes," wherein health required the attainment of a "physiological, emotional, and moral balance."[43] To physicians of the late Qing, it was necessary to move beyond a purely biological vision of psychosomatic malfunction in order to understand the multiple origins of the mad condition. Looking both inward and outward, they endeavored to isolate the source of the pathology.

Cognition

Some physicians focused on the role that cognition played in the onset of mad behaviors. Because Chinese medicine viewed mental and physical processes as inextricably connected, the relationship between mind and body was more dialectically structured than bifurcated in the Cartesian sense. That is, although Chinese medicine could and did differentiate between mind and body, the two were considered so mutually constitutive that it would not have been possible to treat them as fully independent entities.[44]

Medical case records frequently emphasize the correlation between mental overexertion and biological malfunction. The Qing physician Ma Peizhi, for instance, distinguished between somatic and psychic events but described them as developing dialectically within the integrated space of the afflicted body. In the case of a certain Mr. Zhu, Ma traced the cause of the patient's withdrawn madness to the fact that he "thinks too much," which had led to a physical deficiency within the heart and spleen. In another case, similarly, Ma observed that the patient's falling madness had occurred as a result of excessive contemplation. To treat the latter patient, Ma recommended a therapeutic regimen that straddled both mental and physical spheres. On the one hand, he noted, "We must free the patient from worry and cherish him. He must be good to himself, and regulate and conserve his health." On the other hand, Ma also recognized the need to address the physical manifestations of the disorder. Drafting a prescription that would "harmonize the heart and spleen, transform the mucous, and comfort the lungs," Ma underscored the mutually inseparable relationship between psychological and somatic processes.[45]

Other practitioners adopted a similar approach. In the spring of 1906, the physician Zhou Xiaonong (1876–1942) described the case of a painter from Ningbo who was suffering from an illness of liver *qi* (a disorder characterized by explosive anger, among other symptoms). Zhou inquired if the man "thought too much." In addition to prescribing a medicinal treatment, he counseled the painter "not to become vexed so as to avoid arousing the liver, and not to contemplate too much so as to avoid obstructing the spleen."[46] Ding Ganren also observed that excessive use of the mental faculties had a direct bearing on the health of the physical body. In one case file, he noted that a patient afflicted by withdrawn madness had been "contemplating excessively. [Because he was] thinking deeply, the heart had been exhausted."[47]

In sum, the belief that psyche and soma were seamlessly interconnected meant that mental processes within Chinese medicine never approached the dualist model of the mind-body split. The very act of psychological overexertion could thus cause a biological malfunction—one that could easily lead to the onset of mad behaviors and emotional distress.

Emotions

In addition to contemplation, emotions could also induce—as well as counteract—mad acts and disordered thoughts. Just as cognition was viewed as inextricable from the physical body, emotions were treated as agents that could both cause and cure somatic malfunction. Popular tales circulated of famous doctors who successfully manipulated the emotions in order to neutralize mad behaviors. In the case of a scholar who "went mad from happiness" after passing the imperial exams, a talented doctor corrected the madness by convincing the scholar that he was on the verge of death. Believing that he would not make it home in time to bid a final farewell to his parents, the scholar became so frightened that his madness was immediately cured. The physician justified his actions by invoking the classical medical text *Huangdi neijing*, which states that "fear overcomes happiness." In order to counteract the patient's mania, the physician explained, fear could serve as an antidote to excessive joy.[48]

Although physicians acknowledged the indivisible relationship between emotions and madness, they were often more concerned about the physical manifestations of excessive emotionality than the cause of the emotion itself.[49] For example, the physician Ma Peizhi described an incident in which a patient had become sick with the symptoms of withdrawn madness after having experienced "fright and fear." In Ma's analysis, the "fright" had caused the patient's qi to become chaotic, which had injured his heart, while the "fear" had caused his qi to descend, which had injured his kidneys. The injury to his internal organs had subsequently led to an accumulation of mucous in his chest, which had resulted in distorted thoughts, irregular sleep, and abnormal emotions ("he sings and laughs or cries and weeps"). Ma's treatment for the affliction, which involved "draining [the mucous] around the heart and warming the gallbladder," did not address the original source of the "fright and fear" but focused instead on the patient's bodily symptoms.[50] The physician Zhou Xiaonong similarly detailed a case in which a forty-year-old man named Ye Meicun contracted a mad illness after having experienced a severe fright. Like physician Ma, Zhou fixated on the patient's physical disorders rather than on the emotional trauma itself. Drafting a prescription, he declared that he would need to settle the patient's liver, reduce his mucous, and manage his internal dampness.[51] In this way, doctors like Ma and Zhou recognized the injurious effects of the emotions but treated the resulting disorders through somatic, rather than psychological, means.

Environment

While some physicians looked inward to discover the source of mad behaviors, other physicians looked to the patient's external environment. To the literate physician of the late Qing, a patient's inner constitution and outer comportment were intimately related to the environment in which he or she had become ill. The individual possessed a "microcosmic body," as Shigehisa Kuriyama so eloquently put it,[52] which both mimicked in form and responded in kind to the macrocosmic universe surrounding it. Thus, meteorological events such as wind, rain, and heat were not interpreted as divorced from the pathological body, but were often assumed to be the very source of illness itself.

The connection between external pathogens and internal disorders was reflected in the ways that the sick body tended to replicate the natural environment in which it had fallen ill. In the case of a peasant named Chen Xiaoyuan, the physician Wang Shixiong observed, "It had rained excessively for the whole month, to the point that everything was flooded. The summer was scorching hot, and many people fell sick with heat illnesses." Patient Chen, Wang continued, likewise harbored "excessive wetness that had transformed into heat," which had ultimately resulted in "vigorous heat and confused madness" (*zhuangre hunkuang*). After being treated with cooling agents such as gypsum and rhubarb, the man was healed.[53] The physician made a similar determination in the case of Wang Yuechu's daughter-in-law, who "flailed her arms and spoke crazy words." Although it was only spring, Wang noted that the temperature had been "oppressively hot"; consequently, the woman's internal fire had been raised, which had led to an accumulation of mucous in the chest. Wang prescribed a concoction of mucous-rolling pills three times a day and confidently declared that if the woman followed his directives, "the mucous will descend and the spirit will be cleared."[54] In both cases, Wang Shixiong captured the essence of late Qing medical practice. Drawing a direct parallel between the pathogenic influence of heat, the accumulation of mucous in the chest, and the onset of mad illnesses, Wang gave full expression to the epistemological trends of his time.

Gender

In most medical case records, madness was presented as an ungendered disorder. The treatments described above, though just a small sample of a much larger clinical reality, reveal that madness manifested similarly in men and women. Because the body in Chinese medicine was conceptualized as "androgynous," to use Charlotte Furth's term, doctors were not theoretically expected to devise alternative treatments for their male and female patients. Instead, etiologies of madness crossed gendered lines, and therapies given to men were typically considered appropriate for women as well—just in different doses and concentrations.[55]

Nevertheless, certain forms of madness had obviously gendered connotations, particularly those resulting from pregnancy and parturition. The month that followed childbirth was considered an acutely dangerous time for the mother, as her blood and vital fluids had been gravely depleted. Given her vulnerable condition, it was not uncommon for the woman to develop postpartum madness (*chanhou diankuang*), a disorder marked by mental confusion and ghostly visions.[56] As Hsiu-fen Chen has shown, furthermore, late imperial case records periodically attributed women's madness to sexual frustration and emotional trauma. Nuns and widows who refrained from sex, as well as young women who were disappointed in love, were particularly susceptible to bouts of mania. The "flower madness" (*huadian*) they experienced was characterized by an intense, yet unfulfilled, yearning for men, which sometimes caused them to "strip off their clothes" and "have heterodox thoughts."[57] Thus, even if men and women inhabited an androgynous body in theory, social constructions of gender routinely informed the application of medicine in practice.

The diversity of the above cases—and the wide variety of stimuli that could trigger mad behaviors—highlights a critical point about the perceived nature of madness in late imperial medical theory. In nineteenth-century case records, madness was not consistently described as a higher-order or self-contained condition, but rather as the symptomatic and behavioral *expression* of imbalance, malfunction, excess, and deficiency. The etiological disunity of madness prevented its crystallization into an autonomous object of medical knowledge. In most cases, madness was understood more as the transitory manifestation of an ulterior disease pattern than a discrete disease category.[58]

Since mad behaviors were typically considered a temporary aberration rather than a permanent condition, late imperial physicians did not refer to their patients as "madmen" (*kuangren* or *fengzi*).[59] While these terms may have been used colloquially, they were never invoked officially; instead, physicians tended to highlight the illness pattern rather than the patient's personality type. Just as an English speaker might say that she had "caught a cold" without condemning herself to the fate of a stigmatized identity, madness in Qing medicine did not necessarily demand that the afflicted individual be branded with the designation of a particular ontological status. Indeed, practitioners of Chinese medicine premised their treatments on the assumption that mad illnesses were transient conditions. If the dynamism of the pathological body matched the dynamism of the external universe, then illnesses could be cured simply by harnessing and deploying the underlying principles of the natural world.

ENTREATING THE SPIRITS

Even when families trusted the expertise of local physicians, they often experimented with treatments that lay outside the realm of natural healing. In the case of Zhang Shuqin, the boy's father mentioned in his interrogation that he had prayed to spirits and communed with otherworldly forces in addition to employing medical practitioners. In the everyday treatment of mad illnesses, natural and supernatural approaches were not seen as mutually exclusive. To the contrary, families employed both approaches concurrently in order to achieve the most expedient remedy.

In late imperial China, shamanism, prayers, and offerings to the gods were common tactics for counteracting madness. Families who employed supernatural methods of healing did not necessarily interpret them as wholly distinct from the naturalistic approaches described above. In the words of the psychiatrist Keh-ming Lin, the individual in Chinese medicine was conceptualized as an "integrated organism," positioned "within the context of his cosmological, natural, and social environments."[60] The body and its surroundings were therefore envisioned as existing on a continuum, and the same supernatural forces that were believed to induce headache, fever, and mad behaviors were also assumed to cause environmental and political anomalies like drought, eclipse, and dynastic decline. When alternative explanations for such phenomena were unavailable, the Chinese attributed psychosomatic, environmental, and sociopolitical aberrations to displeased spirits or malevolent gods.[61]

Belief in demonic possession was interwoven into religious and medical practice. Families presumed that depraved spirits could take the form of animals like foxes and snakes, and they customarily erected houses of worship to placate these bestial specters. A missionary in Beijing noted in 1885 how the worship of the fox had become so popular in the capital that "crowds of people" flocked to local shrines in its honor, "soliciting the cure of all manner of diseases."[62] Others left offerings at the tombs of deceased ancestors in order to obtain their celestial favor. A displeased ancestor, it was believed, could incite various types of bodily harm, not least of which included epileptic fits, loss of bodily control, or mad speech and mad acts. In the popular imaginary, temples and shrines were junctions of correspondence between this world and the next, and they were commonly depicted in periodicals as places where otherwise healthy people could unexpectedly "go mad."[63]

Often, families attributed the earthly interference of otherworldly spirits to moral transgression. If an individual neglected to pay proper respects to her deceased ancestors or committed some sort of moral offense, the implicated spirit might demand redress through punishments like madness, chronic illness, crop failure, or drought.[64] In Shandong province, for instance, a legal case arose involving two relatives, Sheng Yongtian and Sheng Yongcheng, who had pooled their money in order to purchase wood for the construction of a house. After the house was built, Yongcheng owed Yongtian a significant sum but continually reneged on his debts. Yongtian eventually brought the case to court, but Yongcheng, having earlier forged a receipt to prove that the debts had been cleared, swore under oath that he had paid back the loan in full. Soon after the suit was dismissed, Yongcheng "went crazy and died" (*fengdian ersi*). In no uncertain terms, the author of the tale concluded that Yongcheng had gone mad because he had "harmed heavenly principles. This was truly retribution."[65]

Because of the inherently moral implications of spirit possession, families were sometimes compelled to resort to extreme measures—including violence, imprisonment, and even death—in order to silence the compromised individual and keep her out of the public eye.[66] Yet, while severe actions such as these necessarily attracted the pen of the righteous missionary, they could hardly be considered the norm. Far more frequently, families appealed to more benign and salutary measures as a way to return the unfortunate victim to her normal state of productivity and health. Focusing their collective hopes on the power of the shaman or Daoist priest, families employed healers of faith to converse with the offending spirit, interpret the source of the disorder, and offer goods or prayers so as to mitigate the damage of the transgressive act.

Chinese periodicals from the late imperial period attest to the prevalence of shamanism and ritualistic faith healing in the therapeutic space of urban and rural China alike. The Shanghai newspaper *Shen bao* (Shanghai times) recounted the tale of a medium who cast spells and employed the Eight Trigrams (a geomantic and divinatory tool) in the hopes of treating a man who had "suddenly contracted a mad illness" (*hude dianji*).[67] Another article reported the case of a philanthropically minded temple patron, who donated money and prayed to the spirits after his eldest son had gone mad in the midst of an illness.[68] Missionary records also confirmed the widespread use of shamanic rituals, which included tactics like writing the character for "demon" on pieces of paper, burning these to ash, and convincing the mad victim to imbibe the ash mixed in water or tea.[69] If prayers and offerings proved ineffective, faith healers sometimes resorted to more invasive procedures. The missionary John Nevius (1829–1893), who was stationed in Shandong, observed that when mad people laughed erratically, rolled on the ground, leaped about, or contorted their arms and legs, families hired exorcists to puncture the victim's body with needles so as to allow the offending demon to escape—proof, perhaps, that acupuncture continued to straddle the boundary between medical and supernatural practice well into the nineteenth century.[70]

Frequently, a family's decision to patronize a shaman was informed by the behavior of the mad person himself. According to the American physician Andrew Woods (1872–1956), who practiced medicine in both Guangzhou and Beijing, his patients all "previously believed in the existence of demons and in the ability of demons to enter and control human beings." As a result, their enactment of madness was influenced by "ideas that had been previously held of demoniacal behavior," such as "frenzies, ecstasies, angers or violent attacks on onlookers."[71] In other words, Woods interpreted demonic possession as little more than a communally sanctioned performance inspired by a pre-existing belief in supernatural entities; because patients acted in accordance with popular repertoires, their families were naturally convinced of the supernatural origins of their condition.

Yet, while Woods remained skeptical of such behaviors, other missionaries pointed out that the extreme, and often self-injurious, nature of these beliefs transgressed the bounds of mere performance. The missionary John Dudgeon (1837–1901) described a man from Beijing who, believing himself possessed by a fox, cut a hole in his windpipe in an attempt to provide exit for the creature. A young boy, likewise, arrived at a missionary hospital with his belly split open, convinced beyond doubt that a spirit had accosted him at his bedside and compelled him to undertake the surgery. And there was the family of nine who each fell prey to an invasive snake spirit. Coiling itself around the legs of its victims, the snake tormented each member of the family until they "could not straighten [their] limbs," lost color, and died.[72] Was this madness, religious belief, or something wholly separate? Missionaries, themselves, were unable to distinguish insanity from superstition—so completely did the two run together.[73]

Although shamanistic rituals were certainly widespread, not everyone supported the logic that linked madness to possession. Literati physicians, in particular, were vocally averse to supernatural practices. Doctors like Zhou Xiaonong and Wang Shixiong both denounced the ways that families ignorantly coupled medical treatments with shamanism—often to the detriment of the patient himself. In the case of a thirty-year-old peasant named Wu Gaoming, who suffered from vigorous internal heat and excited madness, physician Zhou remarked that he had crafted an unusually efficacious prescription. He was frustrated to learn that the patient's family had supplemented his remedy by hiring a shaman, whom they enjoined to pray on their son's behalf. "Because Wu's family sent for a shaman," Zhou lamented, "his illness once again became worse."[74] Physician Wang also bemoaned the union of medical and supernatural practice. Called to the bedside of a woman whose illness "appeared to be mania," the doctor recounted how the woman's family had previously employed an assortment of faith healers. Each had charged enormous fees, yet had failed to treat the patient's worsening condition.[75]

While Chinese physicians decried the use of shamanistic rituals as a way to both monopolize patients and limit potentially harmful practices, medical missionaries derided shamanism as the inevitable result of non-Christian "heathenism." Charles Selden mocked the superstition of the "idol worshippers" and asserted that "many untaught peoples" attributed mad behaviors to "the indwelling of evil spirits in the man concerned."[76] Hugh White (1870–1940), a Presbyterian missionary in Shanghai, observed that demonism consistently displayed itself as "antagonism to the name Jesus" and should be considered "the natural, logical outcome of polytheism." Denouncing demon worship as "unscientific" and "abnormal," he concluded that such superstitious practices did not occur "where Christianity prevails."[77] And the Baptist reverend Timothy Richard (1845–1919), musing on the "spiritual benefits of Christianity," sneered that the Chinese attributed insanity to "possession by evil spirits, by foxes and such things." Writing from his mission post in Shandong, he declared that the only true cause of the sickness was the righteous hand of the Christian god.[78]

The irony of such statements was twofold. First, while missionaries claimed to be the spiritual salvation of the Chinese masses, often their very presence engendered the disordered behaviors that called for recourse to shamanism in the first place. It was not atypical, particularly in moments of crisis, for the Chinese to resort to displays of mad possession as a way to signal their resistance to the imposition of the intrusive foreigner. The historian Paul Cohen has previously described how poor peasants in northeast China conducted possession rituals to combat the "evil" presence of Christian missionaries in their town.[79] Similarly, Hugh White, the missionary noted above, recalled how a high-ranking Daoist acolyte went mad after a group of Christian evangelists arrived in her village. Although the woman had never displayed signs of madness before, the foreigners' invasive presence compelled her to behave so wildly that she was only mollified after having been forced into chains.[80] The appeal to spirit possession, in other words, can at least partially be interpreted as an expression of resistance against the foreign intrusion.

Second, although Christian missionaries derided shamanism as superstitious, they, too, practiced a form of religious healing that was no more "scientific" than its Chinese counterpart. John Nevius was known across the missionary community for having employed the "Scriptural plan" in the face of the Chinese lunatic, while John Dudgeon spoke of the "Biblical method of casting out devils" and the effectiveness of religious exorcisms.[81] By denigrating Chinese shamanism, missionaries were effectively doing little more than throwing stones in glass houses. Indeed, it should not be forgotten that the father of Zhang Shuqin—the mad boy who began our tale—had also exploited the services of a French priest in order to expel the evil influences that plagued his son.

MADNESS AS SOCIAL RESPONSE

In addition to ascribing madness to biological malfunction or moral transgression, Chinese families also attributed the onset of mad behaviors to more mundane causes. Social and economic pressures, grievances within the home or community, and marital and sexual relations were all considered reasons that a person could potentially go insane. Zhang Luodai, for instance, claimed that his son had gone mad in the midst of his studies. Although he does not specify how the two were related, it is likely that the boy was preparing to take his first round of civil examinations in the hopes of securing a place in the Qing bureaucracy. China's "examination hell," as the test has been called, was not only intellectually rigorous but also emotionally demanding. A man who passed the exams could ensure the increased social standing and economic prosperity of his lineage. A man who did not would have no recourse but to try again.[82]

The trope of the overworked scholar was regularly highlighted in late Qing periodicals. It was not uncommon for men, burdened by the weight of their family's collective aspirations, to suddenly "go mad" while preparing for the civil service exams. The leader of the disastrous Taiping Rebellion, Hong Xiuquan (1814–1864), is commonly said to have developed madness after having failed the test on several occasions; convinced that he was the Chinese brother of Jesus Christ, he led a millenarian uprising that killed at least twenty million people.[83] On a less extreme level, too, the examination system took its toll on the minds of young men. There was the scholar in Hong Kong who, as soon as the doors to the examination hall had been closed, abruptly grabbed his scroll and shredded it to pieces, causing the scraps to "fly like butterflies" around the room.[84] There was the man from Hunan who spent day and night shut away in his study, dreaming of becoming an official until the point at which he went mad.[85] And there was the popular tale of the famous physician, described earlier, who was called to treat a scholar who had gone insane from the happiness of his examination success. After having failed the imperial exams numerous times, the man only managed to obtain the rank of *juren* (provincial-level candidate) after having studied continuously for ten years. The relief of his success had been, evidently, too much to bear.[86]

The connection between madness and social pressures was frequently framed in gendered terms. Men went mad from the responsibilities attributed to their sex, such as economic matters and the emotional burdens associated with leading the household. An American physician named Benjamin Hobson (1816–1873) recalled a confrontation with an insane man in Guangzhou, whose wife and mother had chained him to a large piece of granite out of concern for their safety. The man, Dr. Hobson noted, muttered endlessly to himself about monetary concerns. When questioned, the lunatic was sporadically lucid. "It appeared," the physician concluded, "that his mind had been much depressed by losses in trade."[87] The American doctor Robert Ross similarly observed that the "heavy responsibility thrust upon youth by the death of his father" often led to a disordered mind. The sudden promotion in social position was frequently accompanied by delusions of grandeur, as the new patriarchs envisioned themselves to be kings, emperors, and rulers of nations. Their fears of inadequacy, meanwhile, "had been dispelled in their new mental world."[88]

While men went mad from the pressures that accompanied their status as paterfamilias, women's lunacy was thought to derive from problems related to marriage, childbirth, and unsatisfactory domestic relations. Women who failed to give birth to male offspring experienced delusions that they were pregnant or became haunted by the fear that their husbands had taken younger, more attractive, and more fertile mistresses. The abusive relationship between mothers-in-law and daughters-in-law was a common trope in the onset of madness, as was the inevitable rivalry between wives and concubines. And the loss of a child not infrequently led to madness in the unfortunate women forced to bury their offspring—a theme that would continue to haunt the minds of mothers well into the Republican period.[89] The gendered nature of madness served not only to provide a convenient explanation for the source of strange behaviors, but also to prescribe and delimit the boundaries of the woman's sanctioned social role. Just as the "hysterical" woman in Victorian England shouldered the expectations that had been placed on her as a function of her sex, the perceived source of madness in Qing China served to circumscribe the reasons for which a person could legitimately go insane.[90]

The ability for onlookers to trace the source of a person's madness to a communally understood adversity helped to relieve the victim of moral culpability. Unlike supernatural explanations for mad behaviors, which often centered on the imagined transaction between moral transgression and demonic retribution, madness that was conceptualized as socially derived was not nearly as laden with ethical implications. Although families might have still employed a physician or shaman regardless of the perceived source of the disorder, their belief that the madness originated from an understandable trauma helped to absolve the victim of blame. In such circumstances, the mad person was not seen as an object of disdain but rather as a potential source of collective sympathy.[91]

Late Qing pictorials reinforced the tendency toward collective sympathy by highlighting the pitiable origins of the mad condition—and the pitiable condition of the mad individual, as well. One pictorial described a group of young women, who, en route to a local temple to burn incense, were confronted at knifepoint by a band of thieves. After being stripped of their jewelry and silks, the women all went mad out of fright.[92] Another article told the story of the recently married Mrs. Yao, who was incessantly reprimanded and harassed by her mother-in-law. During an especially vehement dispute, the girl "suddenly broke into laughter, as if she had gone crazy."[93] And there was the particularly moving case of the elderly Mrs. Wang, who was described as an upright and virtuous woman. Her idling son, however, preferred to pass his days at the opium den while relying on his mother to eke out a living. Mrs. Wang's prolonged anxiety over her dishonorable offspring eventually caused her to go insane. "Of those who hear this tale," the author lamented, "who could not sympathize with such a plight?"[94] Stories such as these underscored the blamelessness of the mad person. Indeed, the fact that so many of these accounts featured exemplary women further served to emphasize this point.

When madness was presented as the logical outcome of a known misfortune, it was possible for the lunatic to be transformed into an object of empathy and commiseration. In depictions such as the ones above, madness was not construed as a disorder to be loathed and reviled but rather as an affliction that underscored the very fragility of the human condition. According to Robert Ross, the insane and their families almost always ascribed madness to universally experienced anxieties, fears, and pressures—issues that arose from the conditions of the social system itself. There was the recurring trope of the "domineering Chinese mother-in-law," as well as the visualization, typically experienced by men on the eve of their wedding, that headless "girl devils" had entered their chamber and disturbed their sleep. Problems relating to "friction in the household economy" were rife, as were "morbid apprehensions" resulting from anxieties about sex and marriage.[95] Although Ross's observations can easily be read as a critique of the Chinese social system, they are not without instructive merit. Both to those who experienced it and those who witnessed it, madness appeared as the pathological expression of universally known pressures and obligations. Consequently, outside observers could not only identify with the social conditions that had provoked the mad disorder but also recognize their indirect complicity in the system that had contributed to its inception.

The ability to look past the peculiar comportment of the mad person and identify with the essence of his or her affliction might have, at least partially, contributed to the leniency with which mad people were treated in late imperial China. Just as poverty was considered a "morally neutral concept, reflecting fate rather than individual failure,"[96] the insane were not necessarily held liable for their condition. Instead, late Qing pictorials depicted madness as the heightened expression of social discontent—an almost inevitable reaction to outside forces that one could otherwise not escape. The potential for public sympathy thus served to mitigate the otherness of the mad condition and diminish the need for either punishment or exclusion.

Madness on the Eve of the Republic

Prior to the waning years of the Qing dynasty, the Chinese were aware of mad acts and mad people—but they did not always consider madness a self-contained or discrete condition. Mad behaviors, instead, were largely regarded as symptomatic of some ulterior biological, emotional, supernatural, moral, or social cause, and thereby demanded treatments that corresponded to their perceived origin. Because knowledge of madness was dispersed and hetero-geneous, treatment of the condition oscillated among the physician, the faith healer, and the family itself. Within this etiological web, the question of who should manage madness—and how they should go about doing it—was neither clearly delineated nor epistemologically fixed.

The mad person, meanwhile, also provoked diverse responses. Although families were technically responsible for the domestic confinement of the in-sane, their decision to either incarcerate or liberate the lunatic often depended more on individual prerogative than legal mandate. Confident that madness was only a temporary affliction, and hopeful that their loved ones would soon recover their wits (as well as their ability to contribute to the household economy), families did not consistently abide by the directive to register and confine the insane. Mad people were therefore regularly spotted outside the home: a phenomenon that attracted the indignant attention of the missionary but caused little reaction on the part of the Chinese. Throughout the late Qing, then, the mad person compelled neither the collective intolerance of the com-munity nor the compulsory action of the state.

The epistemic disunity of madness was the very reason that the father of Zhang Shuqin was able to employ such varied methods to treat his son—even going so far as to appeal to the peculiar beliefs of the foreign missionary. But it was also the reason that the state, when confronted with the specter of madness, could not determine precisely what to do with it. If mad people belonged to no jurisdiction in particular, then they became the responsibil-ity of both everybody and nobody. And if madness had not yet become a discrete object, then no specialized profession or institution was required to eliminate it.

The Birth of the Chinese Asylum, 1901–1918

Exactly half a century after the mad boy Zhang Shuqin had been brought to the provincial seat for questioning, a policeman was making his normal rounds in the inner city of Beijing when he came across "a madman [*fengren*] wantonly dancing" near a busy thoroughfare. "He seems to be about thirty years old," the policeman noted in his 1916 report. "I asked his name but he would not speak. When I questioned him later on, he maintained a crazy demeanor [*kuangtai*] as before." The report was filed and passed along to the chief of police, and the unnamed madman was taken to the local poorhouse to be detained indefinitely. Ten days had passed when the man's younger brother suddenly appeared to collect him. The madman's name was Gao Shengwang, his brother told the police, and he had wandered away from his family's home about two weeks earlier. When Gao failed to return, his family had petitioned the police for aid, but it was only after several days that they had learned where he was being held. "Although he is insane," Gao's brother told the police, "he does not have a tendency to make trouble." Satisfied by this assurance, the police released Gao from the poorhouse and sent him back to the supervision of his family at home.[1]

When placed side by side, the case of the madman Gao Shengwang and that of the young boy Zhang Shuqin reveal a critical difference. While the latter had only attracted the attention of the provincial authorities after he had been linked to the burning of a Catholic priest, the former was detained by the municipal police simply for "wantonly dancing" near a crowded city gate. Although both men were ultimately returned to the care and custody of their families, it was only in the case of Gao Shengwang that the local authorities had *preemptively* incarcerated the lunatic in a public house of detention—independent of the fact that he was neither presumed dangerous nor had broken the law. Indeed, by the early Republican period, the Beijing municipality had assumed much of the responsibility for institutionalizing the insane, and it did so both proactively and comprehensively. In public facilities like the poorhouse, workhouse, and asylum, mad people were kept under police custody until they either expired or could be returned to their natal homes. Thus, in contrast to the Qing, when the mandate to confine the insane was considered a primarily familial responsibility and not consistently enforced, Republican authorities increasingly detained mad people regardless of whether they had committed a crime.

This changing approach to the institutionalization of the insane mirrored an overall shift in the relationship between state and society in the late Qing and early Republican periods. As chapter 1 demonstrated, control over madness throughout the Qing dynasty had been largely decentralized to the family and local community—unless, of course, the mad person had run afoul of the law. By the time the Qing was overthrown and a new republic established, however, the policing of madness (alongside the policing of the sick, disabled, and poor) had come to be seen as an integral component of effective governance.[2] Through the erection of a municipal asylum in Beijing, and through an expanded policing apparatus that was tasked with the supervision and restraint of the city's disenfranchised populations, the late Qing and nascent Republican state sought to signal—both to the Western powers and to its own people—that it had grasped the underlying imperatives of modern statecraft. Control over errant bodies, including those of the insane, had become indistinguishable from the practice of effective and self-sustaining governance more generally.[3]

As a result of the Chinese government's changing approach to the management of Beijing's insane, madness itself was imbued with new meanings. While mad behaviors had previously been treated as the symptoms of a dynamic and variable condition—one that did not automatically require recourse to specialized treatment or public institutionalization—the intervention of the state into matters of madness transformed the disorder from a temporary expression of imbalance to a more permanent identity.[4] To the Beijing authorities, people who exhibited mad behaviors necessarily possessed the latent potential for subversion, even if they had not, like Gao Shengwang, acted in an overtly criminal manner. The need for a proactive response to *potential* agitation caused the municipal police to imbue madness with a classificatory power that trumped all other aspects of the individual's identity— and thereby justified the indefinite incarceration of the "madman" under the watchful eye of the local authorities.

Madness and Statecraft

By the turn of the twentieth century, the Qing government had belatedly come to the realization that it would need to undertake significant structural reform. Following their swift defeat by the foreign powers during the Boxer Uprising of 1900, Qing leaders eventually accepted the need to modify their existing institutions if they wished to remain in power. Over the course of the decade, then, Qing functionaries moved to implement the New Policies: a series of sweeping reforms that introduced new institutions and eradicated those considered defunct.[5] Although provision for the insane was not viewed as an immediately urgent issue at the beginning of the decade, growing pressure from Western missionaries, foreign diplomats, and the Chinese intelligentsia eventually convinced the Qing to reevaluate its previously limited role in the management of madness.

Beginning in the late nineteenth century, Western medical missionaries had called attention to what they perceived as the plight of the Chinese insane. The Presbyterian missionary John Kerr (1824–1901), who founded the Kerr Refuge for the Insane in Guangzhou in 1897,[6] bemoaned the "lamentable fact" that "throughout the Chinese empire . . . there has never been any provision for the insane." The madman was instead confined and put in chains, he observed, with his death "hastened by the want of care and ill-treatment."[7] Charles Selden, who assumed the management of the refuge upon Kerr's death in 1901, concurred with his predecessor's assessment. "Knowing nothing of the real nature of the malady," he wrote, "the [Chinese] can have recourse to no other efficient plan of treatment than the use of the chain."[8] Often, Selden continued, all that sufficed for the lunatic's full recovery was his joyous liberation from the fetters of his confinement—even if it meant that he would continue to be detained within the more "civilized" space of the missionary asylum.[9]

Despite vehement denunciations such as these, missionaries were not ignorant to the fact that Western medicine was similarly impotent when it came to the treatment of madness. In annual reports, physicians at the Kerr Refuge readily acknowledged their inability to treat the vast majority of patients who had been brought to their attention—roughly 70 percent, if not more.[10] It was therefore not the efficacy of psychiatric medicine that inspired their charitable work, but rather their fervent belief in the relationships between medical humanitarianism, religious salvation, and national regeneration.[11] The neurologist Andrew Woods, who managed a teaching college in Guangzhou before taking up clinical work in Beijing, was convinced that the spread of Western medicine would ultimately result in the "regeneration of China."[12] John

Kerr similarly linked institutional psychiatric practice to the enhancement of individual, societal, and national well-being. By proselytizing the benefits of the humane asylum, Kerr believed he could diminish "heathen" practices and introduce the Chinese people to the "glory of [W]estern lands."[13] Medical missionaries, in other words, maintained few illusions about the effectiveness of the asylum itself. Their involvement with psychiatric medicine in China, rather, lay in a purely Whiggish concern with social progress, Christian salvation, and the universal convergence toward Western norms.

Over the course of the first decade of the twentieth century, Chinese authorities in Guangzhou progressively came to recognize the utility—if not the efficacy—of the psychopathic institution. By 1908, reports from the Kerr Refuge noted that local officials had begun to send the homeless insane to the hospital for treatment rather than "as formerly, putting the serious cases in prison and setting the harmless ones free in the street."[14] One year later, the provincial government and the Hong Kong police together granted over five thousand silver dollars for the expansion of the facility. With the help of these funds, physicians at the Kerr Refuge agreed to accept every patient that the police brought to their attention.[15] Although local authorities were enthusiastic to expand their work with the refuge, their motivation, arguably, was informed less by the lackluster rates of cure than by the practical and symbolic benefits of cooperation with the West. By placing the troublesome insane under foreign care, the municipality was able to isolate potentially criminal elements while "accommodating the [modernizing] demands of the era," as a later commentator observed.[16]

Pressure to adopt psychiatric institutions stemmed not only from medical missionaries, but also from foreign diplomats who sought to integrate China into the new global order. Throughout the decade, the Qing Office of Foreign Affairs fielded numerous invitations to participate in international conferences on the modern treatment and provision of madness. In 1902, the Qing was invited to send a representative to Belgium, which was convening an international "mad person conference" (*fengren hui*).[17] The gathering, which was known in the West as the "First International Congress for the Care of the Insane," was held in Antwerp in the first week of September and attracted 250 participants from around the world.[18] A few years later, the Office of Foreign Affairs again received word that "each nation would be convening at a conference in Japan on the topic of how to treat mad people and illnesses of the heart-mind [*fengren yu xinbing*]."[19] And in 1910, the Ministry of Civil Administration was invited to the "Ten-Thousand-Nation Conference on the Treatment of Mental Illness" (Wanguo tiaoyang jingshen bing huiyi), which was scheduled to be held in Berlin.[20] The meeting, better known as the "Fourth

International Congress on the Care of the Insane," was concerned not simply with the proper treatment of the mentally ill but also with the prevention of "psychical abnormalities."[21]

At each of these congresses, representatives of the Qing were gradually initiated into global psychiatric discussions. In Antwerp, for instance, Chinese functionaries compiled a fourteen-page document outlining a major debate on the relative merits of institutionalization versus familial care. While some physicians maintained that "the proper place for the lunatic is within an asylum," others pointed out that domestic supervision served to relieve the asylum system of overcrowding and disease. Following a series of heated discussions on the subject, participants were invited to travel to the neighboring town of Geel, a lunatic "colony" where the insane boarded with local families and were free to roam wherever they pleased. Ultimately—and somewhat ironically, given that medical missionaries in China had so recently disapproved of such methods—the congress resolved that the Geel model should be widely implemented and adopted wherever possible.[22]

Regardless of their specific content, international congresses such as these served to awaken the Qing to new ideas and practices concerning the treatment of madness. Through memorials circulated from abroad, government functionaries learned that the "madman" was a discrete object of medical inquiry: one who required specialized treatments and the specifically tailored knowledge of the trained psychiatric professional. No longer the mutable and heterogeneous disorder described in the previous chapter, madness in the twentieth century had become an explicit focus of medical expertise. In addition, and perhaps more urgently for the Qing functionaries who perused them, these memorials also suggested that the management of madness required the attention and proactivity of the paternalist state. The public asylum—free of cost and maintained by the municipality—exemplified, according to one government emissary, the very notion of "a magnanimous act undertaken for the public good [yiju]."[23] Institutionalization was thus not simply a medical initiative but also a political one. If the Qing truly wished to consider itself among the ranks of the civilized nations, then the dynasty would need to become far more involved in the management, health, and policing of its population—including the insane—than it had been in the past.

There was no clearer example of this point than the recent advances that had been made in Meiji Japan. As several scholars have convincingly shown, the Japanese had discovered in the mid-nineteenth century that government attention to, and policing of, the health of its citizenry was an essential component of an effective and powerful state. Invoking the modern concept of "hygiene" (eisei), Japanese physicians, policemen, and government bureaucrats argued that the fitness of the "national body" (*kokutai*) was inherently linked to the fitness of the people who comprised it. The government subsequently inaugurated numerous public health initiatives that were meant to both strengthen the individual constitution and reinforce the sovereignty of the Meiji regime; as the historian Susan Burns has suggested, Japan's efforts to make medical practice a part of state jurisdiction enabled the polity to more easily "exercise control over the body of its citizens."[24]

The Meiji government's sponsorship of new psychiatric institutions was one such way that the state sought to impose itself into matters that had previously been considered a primarily familial concern. As early as 1886, a chairmanship in neuropsychiatry was officially instituted at Tokyo Imperial University, and by the turn of the century, a variety of public and private asylums had been erected throughout the country, eight of which were located in Tokyo alone.[25] In 1900, moreover, the National Diet moved to adopt the "Law for the Care and Custody of the Mentally Ill," which aimed to regulate confinement of the insane and prevent wrongful imprisonment.[26] In practice, as Akihito Suzuki has pointed out, the law basically served to codify existing practices of familial guardianship. But unlike the relative laxity with which these earlier practices had been enforced, the 1900 law regulated confinement through the expansion of local government supervision and intervention.[27]

By the first decade of the twentieth century, the relationship between hygiene and state power had progressively entered the Qing imagination as well. Throughout the decade, Chinese intellectuals and government bureaucrats embarked on investigatory "tours" of Japanese prisons, asylums, and hospitals, and several of these visitors specifically remarked on the heightened role of the state in the management of the mentally ill (*jingshen bingzhe*).[28] As a "model of nonwhite modernity," as Ruth Rogaski once put it, Japan served to mediate between Western ideologies and Chinese norms. Particularly following China's humiliating loss to the Japanese during the First Sino-Japanese War (1894–1895), Qing leaders were effectively awakened to the idea that state control over bodies was categorically linked to the preservation and expansion of political sovereignty and strength.[29]

On the eve of the 1911 revolution, in short, the problem of madness was confronting the Qing from three separate directions: the medical missionaries on its soil, the Western governments that aimed to incorporate China into a new world order, and Meiji Japan, whose effort to extend state power into the bodies of its citizenry was viewed as a benchmark of its modernizing success. Chinese editorialists, recognizing the urgency of the situation, implored the Qing to enact institutional reforms. In England and Germany, they suggested, the erection of asylums had greatly reduced problems like vagrancy and criminality. "Nobody is destitute and homeless," an anonymous editorialist optimistically remarked. "[Isn't it] wonderful!"[30] Closer to home, too, writers entreated the Qing to adopt a more proactive stance on the management of madness. One author, describing a mad woman in Beijing who assaulted a pedestrian, pleaded with local authorities to better control the scores of insane who populated the city. "Only then," he concluded, "can this be considered benevolent governance [*dezheng*]."[31] Due to long-held assumptions about the relationship between successful statecraft and dynastic paternalism, statements such as these were likely intended to strike a chord with the floundering Qing state.[32]

When late Qing authorities finally resolved to open the first public asylum in Beijing, they did so not because they were entirely convinced of its therapeutic efficacy. Rather, having recognized the symbolic and practical value of such an institution, dynastic leaders realized that an asylum would serve to both bolster their own legitimacy and better control their people. The birth of the Chinese asylum, in other words, was motivated by distinctly political forces. Just as colonial asylums in the British and French empires promised to "regulate public order" and evoke "national prestige and power," the Chinese asylum was similarly inspired by the political desire for sovereignty, strength, and social control.[33] Upon its erection in 1908, accordingly, the Beijing Municipal Asylum was utilized as a primarily managerial apparatus, one that was meant to keep troublesome elements off the city streets and away from public view. The "madmen" who were confined within it, likewise, represented an amalgam of dispossessed, vagrant, and otherwise bothersome individuals whose institutionalization reflected as much a custodial impulse as a therapeutic one.[34]

The Beijing Municipal Asylum

"China is the only nation that does not yet have specialists in the study [of psychiatry]," the Qing Office of Foreign Affairs wrote to the Japanese consul in 1907.[35] The sober admission was written in response to an invitation to attend a Japanese conference on the treatment of madness the following month. Although the Qing declined to participate in the affair, foreign pressure to adopt new psychiatric norms eventually compelled the dynasty to reconsider its long-established technologies for managing madness. The following year, the government decided to revoke the legal substatute that required families to register and confine the insane within the home. As the legal scholar Shen Jiaben (1840–1913) acknowledged, this substatute had rarely been upheld in practice, and he consequently recommended abrogating it completely.[36] Yet,

if the family was no longer liable for managing the insane, who would be responsible for policing their behavior? Following the example that had already
been set by the Western nations and Japan, the Qing ultimately concluded
that the management of madness, at least to a certain degree, must belong to
the *state*.

In the years leading up to the revision of the penal code, the Qing had
been experimenting with the adoption of Western disciplinary and charitable
institutions as part of its New Policies effort to demonstrate that it was capable of undertaking substantive reform. The New Policies, according to the
historian William Rowe, were China's first entrée into the world of "big government."[37] Beginning in 1901, the governor general of Zhili province, Yuan
Shikai (1859–1916)—who would later go on to become the first president of the
republic—joined forces with a Japanese military expert named Kawashima
Naniwa (1865–1949) to develop China's first modern police academies. Prior
to this time, order was maintained throughout the empire by a mixture of
community watch groups (*baojia*), neighborhood defense committees, and
(in Beijing specifically) a gendarmerie of ten thousand troops. Yet it was
not until the turn of the century that specialized police forces—composed
of trained, equipped, and salaried recruits—began to spread throughout the
country.[38] The early success of these police academies persuaded Yuan Shikai
to turn his attention to the equally pressing problems of poverty, vagrancy,
and idleness within the burgeoning city of Tianjin. Inspired by Japanese models of criminal reform that emphasized the ameliorative properties of labor
and discipline, Yuan spearheaded the establishment of a criminal workhouse
in 1904 and a vagrant workhouse the following year. The model soon spread
to the capital in Beijing. Convinced by Yuan's reports that "positive results
[could] already be observed," Beijing officials optimistically established the
Capital Workhouse in 1906 and the Inner City Poorhouse in 1908.[39]

In tandem with their efforts to establish institutions for the poor, vagrant,
and criminal, local authorities in Beijing also decided to erect a small public
asylum (*fengren yuan*) for the city's insane in 1908—the first in China's history.[40] In a circular report, the Qing explained its reasons for doing so. "We
have investigated all of the countries in the east and in the west," the report
noted, "and each has established institutions for the elderly, the young, and
the infirm, as well as those who cannot survive on their own." The government in Beijing, the report continued, had decided to "imitate" (*fangzhao*)
this model and establish charitable institutions for the poor and insane, the
latter of which would "only receive those with a mad illness" (*zhuanshou
fengji zhiren*).[41] The Qing's decision to undertake psychiatric reform, in other

words, was motivated by its desire to better conform to the practices of Japan and the modern West.

Despite the dynasty's articulated desire to "imitate" the norms of the international community, the early asylum was almost entirely a product of the Qing's own making. When the facility was first erected, it was not treated as an independent, stand-alone institution but rather as an "attachment" (*fushe*) to the Inner City Poorhouse.[42] It therefore shared not only the same physical space as the latter institution but also the same residents. (It was for this very reason that Gao Shengwang, the madman who began this chapter, was taken to the "poorhouse" rather than the asylum more specifically.) It would not be until 1918, for reasons of overcrowding, that the asylum was physically detached from the poorhouse, moved to a separate courtyard near Anding Gate in northeastern Beijing, and referred to consistently by its newer name, Fengren shouyang suo (literally, a unit for receiving and fostering the insane).[43] Even so, after this separation had taken place, the poor and the insane continued to be shuffled back and forth between the two units. Because the asylum's regulations specified that the facility would only admit those whose madness was "difficult to treat" (*nanyu*), individuals suffering from relatively minor symptoms of madness were often directed to the poorhouse instead.[44]

One of the reasons that the poorhouse and the asylum retained such porous boundaries was simply because both institutions were overseen by the municipal police. According to Sidney Gamble (1890–1968), a sociologist who extensively surveyed Beijing institutions in the 1910s, "The management of the [asylum] is entirely in the hands of the police, who not only appoint the manager, vice-manager, doctors and guards, but also pay all the bills."[45] The only way to have a case admitted was to bring the mad person to the attention of the local police precinct, which would then keep the suspect imprisoned until the chief of police approved her transfer to the asylum. Similarly, a person could not be released from the facility until the police approved the discharge and ensured that she was returned to her relatives or spouse. If the person's family members either could not be located or refused to take responsibility for their charge, the facility's regulations stipulated that she be turned over to the workhouse or poorhouse for an indefinite period.[46] Thus, regardless of whether the individual was insane, poor, criminal, or sick, the police were almost entirely—and singlehandedly—responsible for her welfare.

A short list of regulations guided the management of the facility, but it was not consistently observed. In theory, inmates were supposed to be segregated by sex and by the severity of their disorder, such that the violently insane would reside alone and the more manageable cases would live in rooms

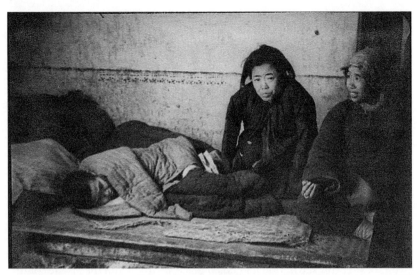

FIGURE 2.1. Women on a *kang* (brick bed) at the Beijing Municipal Asylum (from the collection "Old and New with the Insane in Peiping"; courtesy of Rockefeller Archive Center)

of three to four people. In practice, however, overcrowding prevented the proper adherence to these regulations. Although an effort was made to keep men and women in separate compounds, the seriously insane were not consistently removed from the general population.[47] When Sidney Gamble visited the asylum in 1918, he noted that all of the inmates—violent and peaceful alike—were clustered together in large rooms lined on three sides with brick beds (*kang*); the only difference between them was that the dangerous lunatics had their hands bound with rope.[48] Lax supervision further eroded the preservation of order. At any given time, four guards and a head watchman were expected to maintain a constant patrol over the facility. As police records make clear, though, these wardens not infrequently took bribes or "indulged themselves" while on the job—at one point allowing an inmate to leave his room, scale a wall, and abscond into the suburbs of Beijing.[49]

The asylum itself was a no-frills institution. Allocated a budget of only 2,400 yuan a year, the manager of the facility could not afford to spend frivolously on its upkeep or improvement. Inmates were provided a meager ration of two meals a day, consisting mainly of corn, millet, and pickled vegetables. There was no space for an infirmary, so the sick were treated on the same *kang* where they ate and slept (see figure 2.1). And while a few separate rooms were reserved for those of "wealth and position," most inmates could not have dreamed of such a luxurious expense; as the next chapter will discuss in more detail, most of the facility's charges were so poor that they were entirely reliant on municipal charity for survival. To save money, moreover, the manager of the asylum performed his duties on a completely voluntary basis. Simultaneously employed at a separate municipal institution, he received no remuneration for his work at the asylum whatsoever.[50]

When inmates were received, they were examined and treated by practitioners of Chinese medicine, who did little to incorporate biomedical methodologies into their therapeutic repertoire. Noting that inmates suffered from conditions like "*qi* confusion," "overabundant mucous," and "empty, thin pulses," physicians spoke about madness in a vocabulary that diverged little from that of their Qing-era predecessors.[51] Yet despite the availability of medical treatment, doctors at the asylum played a relatively minor role in comparison to that of the guards and police. Only one medical practitioner was employed at a time, and he was expected to visit the institution a mere four days per week.[52] The task of determining a person's lunacy or sanity, meanwhile, was not considered part of the physician's purview. This responsibility, instead, was entirely the domain of the police, who made their determinations at the local precinct without the counsel of doctors or psychiatric specialists.[53] Appealing to a shared bureaucratic understanding of what it meant to be mad, the police justified their assessments by invoking stock phrases and descriptive tropes, many of which had been used in Qing dynasty legal cases as well.[54] Madmen and madwomen, they wrote, spoke "confused words" that "lacked logic" or "upside-down words" that were "very strange." They were described as "being in a trance" or in a "stupor." They "stared blankly," "hit and cursed and destroyed things," or "jeopardized order and harmed public safety." At no point in the adjudication of madness were physicians consulted or medical experts notified; even the manager of the asylum, Zhang Mengxiong, was simply a career bureaucrat who was given no specialized training prior to accepting the position.[55]

The peripheral role played by physicians at the municipal asylum raises an important question. Considering the centrality of psychiatrists to the treatment of the insane in the Western world, why had the asylum in Beijing been placed under the leadership of a primarily disciplinary profession? Certainly, the lack of Chinese psychiatrists had much to do with it; as chapter 5 will show, it was not until the 1930s that psychiatric instruction even became available in China. But the decision to leave the management of the asylum to the direction of the police—rather than the practitioners of Chinese medicine who periodically worked there—calls for a deeper discussion of the role and responsibilities of the municipal police force itself. To answer this question, then, we must examine the contemporary confluence of sociopolitical change, evolving expectations about the nature of madness, and the expanding functions of the nascent Republican state.

Policing Madness

As the historian Janet Chen previously observed, the workhouse and the poorhouse, much like the asylum, "functioned in the space between punishment and charity." On the one hand, these institutions provided much-needed social services to the poor and dispossessed. On the other hand, they also "created new forms of criminality" by stigmatizing their residents as useless, lazy, deviant, or unproductive.[56] Although poverty, vagrancy, and insanity did not necessarily provoke moral censure throughout the imperial period, these issues progressively came to be reinterpreted as "social problems" by the early twentieth century—problems, in other words, that required the proactive intervention of the civilizing state.[57] Municipal institutions thus played a dual role in the shifting political order. At the same time that they offered charitable relief to a wider swath of the population, they also served to legitimate the extension of the government into previously unpoliced realms of urban life.

The expansion of the Beijing municipal police exemplified the widening, and more intrusive, role that government agents were coming to play in the regulation of everyday activities. After the fall of the Qing dynasty in 1911, the Beijing police not only grew to an unprecedented size but also assumed responsibility for various disciplinary, moral, and administrative tasks that had previously been outsourced to informal social groups, such as families and mutual aid societies.[58] As the eyes and ears of the bureaucratic state, the police were not just viewed as fighters of crime, but as the very people responsible for the preservation of social order, the maintenance of moral authority, the advancement of public hygiene, and the promotion of "civility."[59] Indeed, as David Strand has noted, the power of the Beijing municipal police extended into almost every corner of political, social, and charitable work, causing them to function like "street-level bureaucrats."[60]

Police recruits learned the full scope of their responsibilities while being trained at the Beijing Police Academy. Under the tutelage of constables and military officials, many of whom had been educated in Japan, local cadets were told to do everything in their power to maintain social order and eliminate threats to the general peace. Preemptive arrests were not only legal but also encouraged, at least to some degree; at the police academy, lecturers emphasized the "anticipation and prevention of crime and disorder" and instructed recruits to "nip problems in the bud" before they had gotten out of hand.[61] As Neil Diamant has shown, furthermore, police guidebooks offered only a loose description of what constituted an "infringement" of public order. In daily practice, patrolmen were given "wide discretion" to arrest those they deemed deviant or transgressive, even if these people had not actually broken the law.[62]

To the Beijing municipal police, the problem of madness became interlinked—and often conflated—with many of the other "social problems" facing the young republic. Since patrollers were not given specific instructions on how to identify or manage the insane, they tended to police madness in much the same way as they policed problems like malingering, criminality, and other forms of social deviance. Frequently, men and women were classified as insane simply for having "lingered" in the streets without an obviously identifiable purpose. Tian Feng'er was brought to a local police precinct in 1913 after a patrolman found him aimlessly wandering the Beijing alleys. Upon questioning him, the policeman declared that his words were "confused" and that he was almost certainly mad. (Tian was later released when a neighbor testified that he lived in the city and that he was, in fact, perfectly lucid.)[63] Mrs. Jian (née Xue) was picked up by the police and accused of being insane after she was found meandering the streets at two in the morning. (Her husband soon thereafter came to claim her, stating that they had just arrived in Beijing and had been separated outside of the train station.)[64] And Zhang Baochang was detained under suspicion of lunacy after he was noticed "loitering" (*douliu*) and "lingering" (*panxuan*) near Gongfu Gate in the spring of 1915. (He, too, was later cleared of the charge, but remained under police custody until his death less than a year later.)[65]

The above cases signal a particular trend in the early policing of madness. In the examples of Tian Feng'er, Mrs. Jian, and Zhang Baochang, the police uniformly equated lunacy with displacement or dislocation. These individuals had neither broken the law nor shown an obvious need to be institutionalized.[66] Rather, they had attracted the attention of the police mainly because they did not appear to belong to a particular address or social network—a concern that had long preoccupied government officials throughout the Qing dynasty, as well.[67] To remedy the problem, the police did not necessarily expect their charges to demonstrate that they were "sane," per se, but instead to provide proof of their embeddedness within a recognizable social structure—be it the family, the neighborhood, or the workplace. Thus, Tian Feng'er was released when his neighbor could attest to his fixed address within the city, while Mrs. Jian was released when her husband came to collect her. For both, sanity and social rootedness appeared as two sides of the same coin, though the adjudication of the latter often took precedence over the former.

The reason Zhang Baochang was *not* released—even after the police recognized that he was mentally sound—had less to do with his psychological
state than with the fact that he could not provide the necessary legitimation
of a nearby social network. Zhang, who had traveled from the southwest of
China to Beijing in search of work, offered the police his home address in
the remote province of Yunnan but could name neither relatives nor relations within the capital itself. "He seems like a country bumpkin," the chief
of police matter-of-factly concluded after reviewing Zhang's file. "We must
find a way to put him up so that he doesn't wander around destitute." Zhang
was soon thereafter transferred from the asylum to the poorhouse, and in the
process, his designation in police records was changed from "madman" to
"vagrant" (*youmin*).[68]

The easy slippage between the designations of lunacy and vagrancy ex-
poses the peculiar logic that informed the policing of madness in the early
Republican period. Having internalized the imperative to sustain public order, the police targeted people who appeared to transgress against it—either
due to their unfixed physical residence or to their uncertain social identity
within a city whose human geographies were constantly in flux. The problem
with Zhang, in the eyes of the police, was not necessarily that he appeared to
be insane but, more importantly, that he was both geographically and socially
disenfranchised. By placing him under police control, the municipality was
able to rectify the pressing issue of his dislocation; in so doing, it was also able
to transform him from an anonymous wanderer into a "knowable" disciplinary subject.[69] In the end, it mattered little if Zhang was insane or if he was a
vagrant, since the policing mechanism for both designations—incarceration
within a municipal institution—was almost entirely the same.

The relationship between madness and social displacement is likewise ev-
idenced by the way the police tended to associate mental rehabilitation with
labor and economic viability.[70] Before a lunatic was released from the asylum,
he was often made to promise that he would henceforth engage in productive work. (Women were not expected to make such a claim, though their
return to a domestic setting likely implied a similar outcome.) In 1914, for example, Shang Guoqi was transferred from the poorhouse to the asylum after
he had "contracted a mad illness." After five months, the police reported that
he had made a full recovery and sought to "return him to his home so that he
could seek a livelihood and engage in business [*mousheng yingye*]." The relative who came to collect him likewise assured the police that he would "take
Shang home so that he could earn a living."[71] The case of Liu Bowen, detained
by a patrolling guard in the fall of 1913, was much the same. Liu had been
loitering outside of Tiananmen when an officer spotted him. "His words were

topsy-turvy, like the 'mad illness type' [*leiyou fengji*]," the guard reported. After five months in the municipal asylum, Liu was reportedly cured. "I will immediately return to my hometown and I wouldn't dare linger in the capital," Liu testified prior to his discharge. "Please release me so I can go home and work the land."[72]

Although police functionaries likely manipulated such testimonies in order to appeal to the sensibilities of higher authorities, their inclusion in case files signifies an explicit attitude on the part of the state that linked rehabilitation to economic productivity. Just as the Republican penal system (based on the Japanese model) assumed that convicts could be reformed through physical labor, the municipal agents who policed madness also believed that the *desire* to labor could stand as proof of mental recovery.[73] By emphasizing labor as a precondition of discharge, the police were not simply hoping to achieve the moral reformation of the prisoner or the lofty goal of national economic salvation, however.[74] They were also, and perhaps more urgently, attempting to immobilize and neutralize deviant elements by binding them to a particular geographical and socioeconomic space. This was the reason that a lunatic's testimony was almost always accompanied by an external assurance from a relative, neighbor, or friend: release from the asylum was contingent on the guarantee that the madman would be moved from an overtly *policed* network to a *self-policing* one.

Subversive Speech

It was not just the physical displacement of sojourning individuals that aroused the attention of the municipal police. In the early years of the republic, the police were also highly attuned to any illicit speech or unorthodox writings that could potentially undermine their goal to regulate and monitor the bodies under municipal control. Although late imperial authorities had also arrested—and sometimes even executed—mad people for having written or spoken seditious words,[75] the Republican police were concerned with far broader forms of speech and script than those that directly incited insurrection against the state. To the municipal authorities, words and texts could easily contain the *potential* for subversion even if they were not overtly criminal, and their possession by mad people only served to increase the risk that they might be deployed for incendiary purposes.

Throughout the 1910s, the police sent numerous people to the municipal asylum at least partly because they possessed suspicious written materials. In the spring of 1915, a man named Yin Yuan was found "lingering" outside of a government office holding a letter and a name card; although he insisted that he was merely looking for employment, he was taken to the precinct for questioning and slapped with the label of madness.[76] In 1913, a "mad woman criminal" named Mrs. Wang (née Yang) was detained after the police noticed her carrying "two sheets of yellow paper with characters on them." The paper was sent, along with Mrs. Wang, to the precinct for further investigation.[77] Liu Bowen, described above, was apprehended under the suspicion that he was an "insane criminal" after he was found loitering in front of Tiananmen with a chop and a book of rubbings.[78] And Zhang Baochang—the presumed madman discussed earlier who was found to be perfectly sane—had initially aroused the attention of the police for having been spotted with an inkstone, pen, scroll of red paper, handwritten poem, and the books of John and Daniel.[79]

What was the relationship between literacy and lunacy? In itself, the ability to read and write was not necessarily cause for concern; what the police found problematic, rather, was the potential instability that the written word could incite. To illustrate this point, let us look at the case of Shu Xinglin, who was arrested in 1913 for having "stirred up trouble through rumor-mongering." On November 23, a patroller was making his regular rounds when he spotted Shu referencing a book of the Eight Trigrams in order to tell fortunes. As Shu's performance became more animated, a crowd gathered around him. "He seemed to be the 'madness type,'" the patroller reported before bringing Shu to the precinct for further questioning. When Shu was interrogated, he revealed that he was fifty-two years old and had come to the capital from Shandong province in the hopes of "telling people's fortunes and making a name for himself." Referring to him as a "criminal" (*fan*), the police suggested that his words "lacked logic" and that the fortune-telling books he carried contained "absurd words and phrases." By the time the case had been passed along to the chief of police for further instruction, Shu was no longer being classified as a "criminal" but rather as a "madman." He was sent to the asylum soon thereafter for treatment.[80]

In Shu's case, the liminal space between criminality and madness was bridged through the use of a potentially subversive text. Because the text (and Shu) spoke in a language that was outside the realm of sanctioned speech— and because the ideas contained within this text had managed to incite the formation of a large and disorderly crowd—Shu had attracted the attention of the municipal police, who were unsure of whether to label him a criminal or a lunatic. Although Shu had not technically committed any crimes prior to his arrest, he was nevertheless held under suspicion of criminality simply because his words and writings contained the potential for civic disruption. As Steve Smith has shown in the case of the early People's Republic, the Chinese state was highly wary of "unauthorized speech" because it "reflected a potential threat to social stability."[81] In the Republican period, too, the use of writings to spread illegitimate ideas appeared to be acutely threatening to a state that was still unsure of how to govern the masses under its control.[82]

It was likely due to the destabilizing power of illicit speech—and its subsequent ability to galvanize the masses or subvert political authority—that the municipal police implicitly grouped superstition and evangelization alongside the equally disruptive condition of madness. In the spring of 1918, for instance, a vagrant named Yin Ruxin was spotted sleeping in the woods and was taken to a local police precinct to be interrogated. Although the police accused him of having "unclear speech," the transcript of his oral testimony appears entirely lucid. As Yin told his examiners, he was from Guangping County in Zhili province and had recently come to the capital in search of work. In Beijing, he had found employment at a variety of odd jobs and had lived in several residences, but he had recently spent his days preaching Christian sermons and sleeping in the woods. "He is a Protestant," the chief of police summarized upon reading the case file. "He doesn't have a fixed residence. During the day he preaches, and at night he sleeps outdoors. His mind is muddled and his words approach superstition [yujin mixin]. It is madness. Send him to the asylum." Three weeks after Yin was institutionalized, he was found dead from a fever.[83]

A similar scenario occurred in the case of Yang Chengdian, who was observed at a crowded intersection holding a white flag and burning incense. When brought to the police precinct and questioned, Yang insisted that he was simply "being a good Buddhist." He burned incense three times a day, he related, and carried the flag in order to "disseminate information." Like Yin Ruxin, Yang was born into an exceptionally poor household in neighboring Zhili province and had come to the capital after a spirit (shenren) visited him in a dream and persuaded him to search for his uncle in the city. Unable to locate his relative, however, Yang stayed in an old temple at night and begged and prayed during the day. The chief of police reviewed the case and determined that all of Yang's words were "heretical [zuodao]. He is certainly insane." Yang was sent to the asylum, where he spent the next seven months. When the police finally managed to persuade one of Yang's relatives to come to the capital to collect him, the madman was deemed cured and released from the facility. Upon his discharge, Yang offered the following statement: "[Because] I carried a flag and lingered in the streets, I was taken by the police into the precinct for questioning. Since I was insane, they sent me to the asylum for treatment. Now I'm completely better. . . . It is currently the planting season. Please release me [so I can return home] to work the land."[84]

In the examples of both Yin Ruxin and Yang Chengdian, the chief of police—without having ever met either man in person—directly passed from

a determination of "superstitious" or "heretical" to a classification of "insane."
Although both men may have indeed been physically compromised by their
itinerant lifestyles, the uneasy transition between heresy and lunacy signals that
other calculations had also come into play. In order to better parse these incidents, it is useful to examine a comparable case that unfolded in the United
States in the late nineteenth century, one that explicitly linked ideological nonconformity to madness. In 1864, a woman named Elizabeth Packard (1816–
1897) made national headlines when she claimed to have been wrongfully institutionalized by her husband. Packard, who was sent to an asylum after having
challenged her husband's religious views, was able to secure her freedom only
by taking the case to court. In a treatise she later published, Packard drew a
damning conclusion about the reason for her confinement. "Instead of calling
me by the obsolete title of heretic," she explained, "[my husband] modernize[d]
his phrase by substituting insanity instead of heresy as the crime for which I
[was] sentenced."[85] In this scenario, which Packard suggestively referred to as
a "Modern Inquisition," the asylum had replaced the church as the sanctioned
locus of social control. Insanity, likewise, became the accepted label by which
deviance and female impertinence could be policed.

For Yin and Yang, similarly, it is possible to make the argument that the
chief of police—consciously or otherwise—conflated the overlapping problems of social nonconformity, ideological heterodoxy, and madness. Although
Buddhism and Protestantism were not technically disallowed as forms of religious practice, public acts of proselytization necessarily raised the eyebrows
of the municipal authorities. Not only did "superstitious" behaviors run counter
to the state's articulated desire for scientific modernity, but religious speech
often functioned as a means of expressing political discontent—and hence
acted as a catalyst for mass mobilization.[86] When combined with the fact that
both men actively pursued a rootless lifestyle and were unwilling to labor,
Yin and Yang easily slipped from the margins of deviance into the concrete
realm of the pathological. It makes sense, then, that as a precondition for
his release from police custody, Yang was forced to repeat and renounce the
charge that had originally been lodged against him. In this way, he explicitly
demonstrated his acknowledgment of, and submission to, the vision of order
and stability he had earlier transgressed.

The easy slippage among vagrancy, heresy, and madness signaled that the
Beijing municipal police were aware of the destabilizing potential of nonconformist individuals but were not necessarily concerned with enforcing a
strict delineation between them. Indeed, because the police oversaw all of the
criminal, charitable, disciplinary, and reformative institutions within the city,
there was neither a practical nor legal need to distinguish between the various

categories of social deviance; the police merely desired that the transgressive person be detained *somewhere*. The inattention to explaining precisely what differentiated a madman from a vagrant, a criminal, or even a religious zealot helps explain the permeable borders that formed between the asylum, the poorhouse, and the prison, as the next section will show. Under police supervision, in other words, madness more closely approached other types of "social problems," both in the way that it was identified and in the methods through which it was managed.

This is not to say that madness was only a constructed designation used to retroactively justify an otherwise illegitimate arrest. In many cases, archival documents paint a vivid picture of individuals who had genuinely lost their grip on reality. But other cases were not nearly so cut-and-dried, and they suggest that a more complex bureaucratic mechanism was often at work. It was in these latter cases that the police blurred the boundaries between madness and illicit speech, transgressive activities, and superstitious beliefs, thereby justifying the incarceration of people who had not actually broken the law. In contrast to the Qing, which had called for the preemptive confinement of the insane but had often only enforced the measure after the lunatic committed a crime, the Republican police widely detained the insane even in the absence of overt criminal activity—and without explicit legal justification. This evolving approach to madness signals a distinct paradigmatic shift. In the early republic, the mad person no longer had to *do* anything to provoke police attention; he simply had to *be perceived as* mad in order to attract the intervention of the state.

Penalizing Madness

Were the municipal police placed in charge of the asylum because of the implicit association of madness with social deviance? Or did madness only continue to be conflated with criminality because the police, rather than physicians, were held primarily responsible for managing the city's insane? It is difficult to distinguish the order of cause and effect. What is certain, however, is that the progressive convergence between madness, vagrancy, superstition, and delinquency signaled that the bureaucratic construction of madness under the new republic was not entirely distinct from the bureaucratic construction of deviance and criminality more broadly. Thus, while the Beijing municipality recognized, at least ostensibly, that madness was as much a medical problem as a social one, the fledgling state's primary preoccupation with order and control caused the police to emphasize the latter construction of madness over the former.

The connection between insanity and deviance is exemplified through the vocabulary that policemen employed when handling cases of lunacy. When the insane (and potentially insane) were brought to the municipal asylum, they were not admitted to be "treated" but rather to be "detained" (*jujin* or *kouliu*), "taken into custody" (*kanya*), or "incarcerated" (*jianjin*); upon their release, likewise, they were "set free" (*kaishi* or *shifang*).[87] Within the asylum, too, policemen often accorded more priority to restraint than rehabilitation (or more optimistically, rehabilitation *through* restraint).[88] The American physician J. H. Ingram, who was employed at the nearby Peking Union Medical College, observed that the asylum "is nothing more nor less than a prison where the insane are confined, and put in chains when necessary." At the time of his visit, the facility "was overrun with about one hundred and fifty petty thieves, for whom no other jail accommodations could be found."[89] Sidney Gamble was somewhat more optimistic about the status of the institution but nonetheless pointed out the widespread use of the chain. "Those who are violent are shackled and placed on a rug on the floor," he wrote. All others were kept "confined in large rooms," with "practically no use [being] made of the courtyard for giving the patients any exercise"[90]—a direct violation of the asylum regulations, which stipulated that the insane be let outdoors once or twice per day.[91] Even if the municipality distinguished between the asylum and the prison in theory, in practice the two shared both a common population and a similar disciplinary impulse (see figure 2.2).

One of the reasons that criminals and the insane so easily coexisted within the asylum was likely due to the ambiguous way that madness had been framed in the early Republican penal code. A temporary draft of the code, which was published in 1912, diverged little from its predecessor, the New Qing Penal Code by Imperial Decree (Qinding da Qing xin xinglü), which had been promulgated just a few months before the dynasty was overthrown.[92] Like its forerunner, the Republican penal code also stated that deviant acts committed by the insane should "not be considered a crime" (*buwei zui*) but that the lunatic should nevertheless be "incarcerated and penalized" (*jianjin chufen*) according to the facts of the case.[93] The purposely vague wording of the clause—incarcerated where? penalized how?—perpetuated a certain confusion about how to handle the criminally insane, as well as where to put them.[94]

Throughout the first decade of the asylum's existence, the police puzzled over what to do with criminals who had gone mad or lunatics who had committed crimes.[95] In one case, the Xianghe County Jail asked to transfer two prisoners, Ma Hong'en and Wang Liu, to the municipal asylum. Both men had

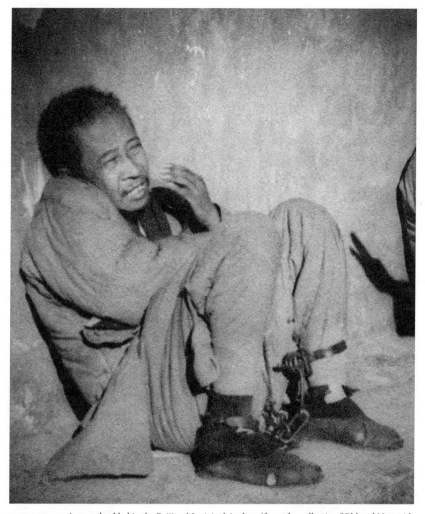

FIGURE 2.2. A man shackled in the Beijing Municipal Asylum (from the collection "Old and New with the Insane in Peiping"; courtesy of Rockefeller Archive Center)

been sentenced to prison for aggravated assault, but the prison soon found that it lacked suitable arrangements for their management. According to the testimony of a prison guard, Ma had begun showing signs of lunacy in the midst of serving his sentence, while Wang had been classified as insane even prior to being sent to jail. "As per article twelve of the penal code, [Wang's behavior] should not be considered a crime," the prison warden wrote to the chief of police. "Should we keep him locked up forever? The prison is over-crowded as it is."[96] Citing an earlier precedent in which the municipality had permitted a transfer from the Number One Capital Prison to the asylum, the warden attempted to shift the burden of madness onto another agency entirely.

Complicating the issue even further, the municipality had not developed a precise mechanism for determining how to adjudicate criminal madness—a conundrum even in today's legal system.[97] From as early as 1906, the Qing had moved to replace its board of punishments with an independent judiciary based on Western and Japanese models; by the time the dynasty was overthrown, 345 courts had been established throughout the country.[98] When individuals who were suspected of being insane committed a serious crime, such as injury or homicide, they were forced to stand trial and undergo sentencing in accordance with the 1912 penal code. In Beijing, the judges who presided over these courts regularly debated the sanity of convicted felons and struggled to retroactively assess lunacy at the time a crime had been committed. In 1916, for example, the Beijing high court tried a criminal case for a man who experienced intermittent insanity. At the time of his trial, the man's mental state had returned to normal (*ruchang*), but the prosecution had no way to know if he had been lucid at the time of the crime itself. Reaching out to the asylum, local hospitals, and Chinese and Western doctors alike, the police attempted to seek answers within the "specialized art" (*xueshu*) of psychiatry. They quickly learned, however, that nobody was "equipped" to provide this type of critical determination.[99]

These legal complications were exacerbated by ongoing debates about the appropriateness of the new penal code. According to Jan Kiely, the early years of the republic were a time when "considerable confusion and ambivalence reigned with respect to new laws," particularly when such laws conflicted with late imperial "notions of justice and social morality."[100] Although Republican legal statutes technically affirmed that the actions of the insane "should not be considered a crime," judges sometimes ignored the letter of the law if they found it antithetical to Confucian ethics.[101] In 1916, the Beijing high court was confronted with the case of Zhang Xitun, who had injured and ultimately killed his paternal grandmother. The court decided that since Zhang was clearly insane, he should not be found guilty of the crime but should instead be "placed under restraint" in the asylum until he recovered his senses. A tribunal reviewing the case "refused to accept this verdict" and sought to overturn the original ruling. Because Zhang's actions "violated proper human relationships" (*nilun*), the tribunal believed that the verdict of "not guilty" was insufficient. Instead, it recommended that Zhang be "imprisoned and punished in full accordance with the law." Although Zhang passed away from illness before a final verdict was returned, his case nevertheless exemplified the legal, moral, and practical difficulties involved in "incarcerating and penalizing" insane criminals.[102]

By relieving the insane of legal culpability while simultaneously requiring their physical confinement, the 1912 penal code solidified the place of the asylum within the administrative order. Since the actions of insane criminals were not considered a "crime," the insane could not be sent to prison; yet, if they could not be sent to prison, how were they supposed to be "incarcerated and penalized" in accordance with the law? The murky space between outright punishment and absolute freedom came to be filled by the municipal asylum. Throughout the early years of the republic, the institution occupied a gray space in Beijing's jurisdictional layout. Populated with the city's delinquents, vagrants, and people who, by their very words and deeds, posed a threat to the stability of the Republican state, the asylum functioned less as a strictly therapeutic institution than one that could control, monitor, and restrain the individuals who refused to abide by the shifting norms of their society. It was, as Sidney Gamble succinctly put it, a primarily "custodial" unit.[103]

Madness and Social Control

Although the waning Qing state belatedly came to recognize the relationship between madness and modern statecraft, it was the early Republican government that fully embraced the evolution from theory to practice. Through the establishment of the municipal asylum-cum-poorhouse, and through the expansion of the nascent police force, the Beijing municipality made the policing of madness a practice that was inextricable from the preservation and augmentation of state power more broadly. The municipal police, as a "semi-paternal" organization, played a central role in this process.[104] Emboldened by the prerogative to eliminate potential problems before they began, local patrollers not only intruded into previously unpoliced realms of urban life but also prosecuted a range of activities that, while technically legal, were increasingly being viewed as politically problematic or socially destabilizing.

While the police sometimes struggled to differentiate madness from other "social problems," their desire for taxonomic specificity was ultimately far less important than their desire for social control. Thus, it did not necessarily matter whether incarcerated individuals were mad, homeless, superstitious, criminal, or some combination thereof. What mattered, instead, was that they be taken off the streets and removed from public view. The blurred line that distinguished mad acts from deviant ones allowed the police to pass seamlessly from one categorization to the other, thereby legitimizing the porous boundaries among the asylum, poorhouse, and prison. And in the pursuit of social order, the police occasioned a casual convergence of madness, uprootedness, vagrancy, and illicit speech. Even when mad people were found to be sane, therefore, they were forced to remain under police custody until they could be returned to the informal supervisory networks of their family, community, or native place.

The increasingly intrusive role played by the Beijing authorities caused the policing of madness to undergo a paradigmatic shift. Rather than prosecuting mad people only after they had committed a crime, municipal agents began to preemptively institutionalize the insane (and potentially insane) even if they had not technically broken the law. While the Qing penal code had allowed—and indeed mandated—that such measures be taken, prevailing public notions about the ephemerality and harmlessness of the disorder had previously served as a check against the indiscriminate confinement of the insane. It was only once the Republican state had thoroughly embraced the relationship between authority, legitimacy, and social control that mad people were systematically arrested, confined, and erased from the urban landscape. In the process, madness gradually evolved from the intermittent expression of psychosomatic distress to a regulatory *identity*—one that could be upheld as justification for incarceration even in the absence of criminal activity.

This particular construction of madness did not exist prior to the reconfiguration of the bureaucratic state at the turn of the twentieth century. It was, instead, an act of political invention that came into being as a result of the historically contingent demands facing the doomed Qing dynasty and early Republican government. Yet, while the municipal police played a significant role in the evolving imagination of Chinese madness, their actions constitute only one part of the story. In order to understand how this vision of madness came to be popularly institutionalized—and thus reproducible outside the supervisory realm of the police—we must turn our attention to the broader society.

3

The Institutionalization of Madness, 1910s–1920s

When the American social scientist Sidney Gamble paid a visit to the Beijing Municipal Asylum in 1918, he marveled at the low rate of insanity within the capital city. "The phlegmatic temperament of the Chinese and the lack of strain in their life," he reasoned, "save many who under other conditions might be insane."[1] Gamble's sanguine observation was widely shared among foreigners in China, who attributed the health of the native psyche to the relative primitiveness of Chinese civilization. While the incidence of madness appeared to be on the rise in Western Europe and the United States, the Chinese presented themselves as happily exempt from its depredations; as one commenter noted, "no saner body of men exists anywhere" in the world.[2] Madness, it was widely believed, was directly proportional to the degree of civilization that a nation had achieved. It was therefore no wonder that a simple country like China had emerged from the incubus of insanity relatively unscathed.[3]

In Gamble's mind, the low incidence of insanity in the city helped explain why so few inmates were being held at the municipal asylum at the time of his visit. Although accommodation had been made for up to eighty people, Gamble noted that only thirty-two inmates—twenty-three men and nine women—were currently in residence. Yet, as he passed through the rooms of the recently erected facility, he could not help but wonder *why* more lunatics were not being held there. Gamble himself had seen "imbeciles and low-grade morons" wandering the streets of Beijing, and he had even heard rumors about families who made use of violent tactics to keep their insane relatives restrained within the home. Given such poor alternatives to institutional care, he wondered, why had families not availed themselves of municipal resources? "The people are slow to make use of [the asylum]," Gamble concluded after having finished his tour. "There is a feeling throughout the city that a family ought to do almost anything rather than send a person [there]."[4]

While it is unclear how Gamble came to these conclusions, historical records show that his assertions were almost entirely incorrect. First, it was certainly not the case that the Chinese were immune to madness. In 1920, the American neurologist Andrew Woods estimated that there were at least ten thousand visibly insane men and women in and around Beijing and that there were "constant . . . local demands in connection with the insane."[5] Some put the numbers even higher, at one in four hundred persons, or approximately one and a quarter million insane throughout the entirety of the country.[6] And others, still, were forced to admit that insanity among the Chinese was "as common as, if not more common than, it is in the West."[7] By the first decade of the republic, the long-standing myth that insanity did not affect the Chinese was progressively, though not entirely, being put to rest.

Second, Gamble's claim that the Chinese refused to pursue institutionalization was also largely inaccurate. Although it was true that most well-to-do families typically kept their insane relatives at home,[8] large numbers of the urban poor gradually came to recognize the economic and practical utility of public institutionalization. Particularly for those of the lowest socioeconomic classes, madness could easily drain the household's limited financial resources and place insupportable logistical and emotional demands on the family and community. Over time, and as word continued to spread about the existence of the municipal asylum, families actively pursued institutionalization for their relatives and neighbors—at times outpacing the ability of the municipality to provide accommodation for their requests. Indeed, if only a few inmates were being held at the asylum when Gamble recorded his observations, it was mainly due to the timing of his visit. The asylum, which had been separated from the poorhouse and reopened to the public in January 1918, had only been in operation for a few months prior to Gamble's survey of the city.[9] By the early 1920s, however, the facility was constantly filled to the point of overcrowding.

The very possibility of institutionalization transformed not just how local families dealt with the insane but also how they conceptualized insanity itself. As this chapter will show, the availability of municipal aid enabled families to invoke the charge of madness not only for those who were severely and demonstrably mad but also for those who simply disrupted the normal patterns of life. Women who challenged patriarchal norms, men who stirred up trouble, and elderly parents who were becoming an unwanted financial burden all came to fall under the expanded rubric of the "mad person." The prospect of municipal intervention, in other words, allowed families to demonstrate a decreased tolerance for behaviors that, in other circumstances, might have been deemed little more than bothersome, inconvenient, or typical challenges of everyday existence.[10] In the process, they also pushed the boundaries of what types of people could legitimately be considered pathological.

The changing ways that madness was both handled and conceptualized throughout the 1910s and '20s were thus not simply the consequence of an expanded municipal apparatus, as chapter 2 has shown. Equally important, these changes were also the result of ordinary people deploying the charge of madness as a means of obtaining municipal aid. In the daily fight for survival, families actively utilized madness as a strategic means through which they could procure scarce resources and take advantage of government social services. In contrast to what Gamble theorized—that families would do anything in their power to avoid contact with the municipal asylum—the reality of the situation was often exactly the reverse. In the context of the early republic, the label of madness was not just a tool of control wielded by an apprehensive state. It was also a strategy employed by ordinary people to gain a modicum of power over their uncertain existence.

A Police Matter

The presidency of Yuan Shikai, the first leader of the Chinese Republic, was embarrassingly short-lived. In 1915, moved by his own monarchical aspirations and convinced that the Chinese nation needed to be ruled with an authoritative hand, Yuan decided to revive the imperial system and declared himself emperor of the new Hongxian dynasty. His political machinations, which few supported, caused tumult to erupt throughout the empire. Intellectuals and commoners alike rebelled against the news of the revived monarchy, and Yuan was forced to capitulate to public pressure by shelving his imperial ambitions. Even so, the pressures and humiliations of leadership had been too much for him to bear. Sick with uremia and weakened by the embarrassment of his political defeat, Yuan died only a few months after the imperial government had been restored.

In the aftermath of Yuan's death, the country was plunged into a political vacuum. Several provinces had responded to the restoration of monarchical rule by declaring independence from the central government, and Yuan's Beiyang Army quickly disintegrated into competing cliques known as warlords. Control over Beijing passed from one military power to the next, and roving armies roamed the countryside in the fight to establish dominance over their rivals.[11] Despite the fluctuations in national- and municipal-level

politics, however, Beijing institutions like the asylum and poorhouse continued their operations as usual. Since the municipal police board and Beijing
Municipal Council—the governmental body responsible for public works
projects—were managed separately from the central government, the day-to-
day functioning of the municipal asylum remained relatively stable regardless
of political change.[12] Records from the institution proceeded apace, with little
hint that the country was immersed in a state of chaos and turmoil; indeed,
throughout these political changeovers, municipal services not only persisted
but may have actually expanded.[13]

The police, too, remained ubiquitous. Particularly following the advent
of warlord factionalism throughout northeast China, policemen appeared
more and more like "the government of the street,"[14] to borrow David Strand's
terminology. As policemen proliferated, the popular media documented their
expanding role in the maintenance of municipal order. Pictorial artists depicted the local authorities as upright, courageous citizens who boldly confronted the troublesome insane. In images such as those shown in figures 3.1
and 3.2, the ragged, patchwork clothing of the lunatic and the implied un-
predictability of his movements stand in stark contrast to the police, whose
deliberate advances and authoritative uniforms serve to assuage the anxiety
of the reader. With headlines like "Madmen Are Frightening" and "Madmen
Should Be Controlled," pictorials both thrust the lunatic into the realm of
the threatening "other" and effectively demonstrated how the mad person's
management belonged to the jurisdiction of the police. Cut off from his familial context, and portrayed as alone and disenfranchised, the madman all
but demanded the salutary intervention of the state.[15]

As the historian Barbara Mittler has shown, the literate and semiliterate
audiences of late Qing and early Republican China frequently turned to the
news media for guidance and insight into recent trends.[16] Newspapers therefore played a key role in conveying the idea that, in the new political order,
the police had become at least partially responsible for the management of
the city's insane. In periodicals and tabloids, the positive contributions of the
police featured prominently. The highbrow newspaper *Shishi gongbao* (Current affairs), for example, detailed how the police had expertly handled the
case of a "madwoman" found walking barefoot in the rain in the spring of
1913: first by taking her into the local precinct to be housed and later by dispatching an officer to locate her husband.[17] The Japanese-managed newspaper *Shengjing shibao* (Shengjing times) similarly praised the police on several
occasions, such as when they apprehended a madman named Mr. Li, who
had grabbed a young boy returning home from school, and when they had
succeeded in tying up a madwoman named Mrs. Li (née Lei), who had been

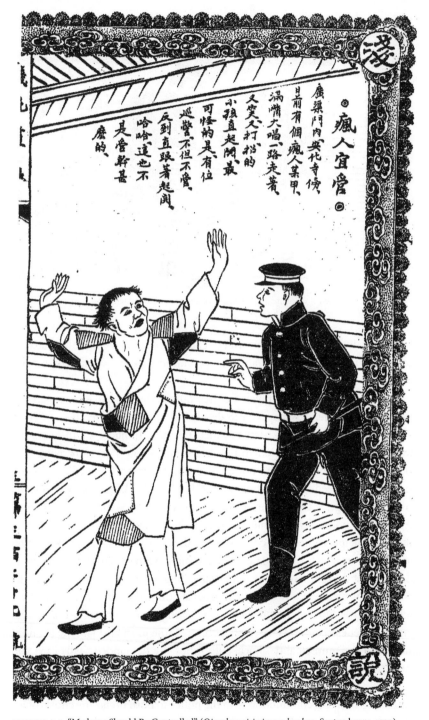

FIGURE 3.1. "Madmen Should Be Controlled" (*Qianshuo riri xinwen huabao*, September 21, 1909)

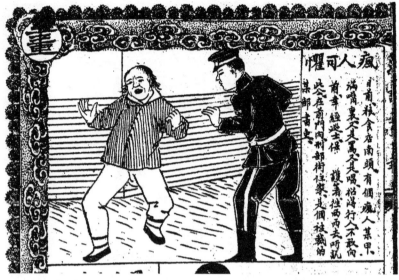

FIGURE 3.2. "Madmen Are Frightening" (*Wushen quannian huabao*, September 5, 1909)

"making a loud ruckus" in the street. The police let her go, the newspaper satisfactorily concluded, only after she promised that she would "correct her errors and make a fresh start."[18]

While commending the police for their quick thinking and expert management of the insane, newspapers also derided local officers when they failed to perform with the gravity expected of their position. In figure 3.1, the assumed professionalism of the policeman is belied by the image's accompanying text. "The policeman not only did not control [the madman]," the editorialist laments, "but caused a commotion alongside him. Ha! What the hell does he think he's doing?!"[19] Other journalists, foreign and Chinese alike, similarly condemned the police for not doing enough to keep madmen off the streets and under municipal control. An editorialist for the *North China Herald*, describing an incident in which a madman struck a foreign woman across the face, complained that the Chinese police were doing "little or nothing" to eliminate the "menace" of madness.[20] A Chinese journalist adopted a similar tone in an article titled "Madmen Should Be Detained." Citing the example of a lunatic who cursed at pedestrians and chased after children, the journalist laid the blame at the feet of the municipality. "Local authorities," he demanded, "why can't you more rigorously crack down on [the insane]?"[21]

Such condemnations, however, were few and far between. In most cases, the press worked in conjunction with the police to both praise the efforts of local authorities and publicize the whereabouts of unidentified lunatics. When a migrant named Jian Luowang appeared at the municipal asylum to claim his wife in the spring of 1914, for instance, he had been led there with the aid of a vernacular tabloid. The incredulous man could not contain his emotion when he was finally reunited with his wife, Mrs. Jian, whom he feared had been lost to the chaos of the city. As Jian told the police, the two had come to the capital from their small village in search of a relative. After disembarking at the train station, they had gone as far as Xuanwumen Avenue when they were suddenly separated. "I blinked and she was gone," he maintained. Less than a week later, Jian happened to be perusing an edition of the *Aiguo baihua bao* (Patriotic vernacular news) when he spotted an announcement about a woman whom the police had assumed was insane. "It was only then that I realized she had been sent here [to the asylum]," he told the police. Mrs. Jian was ultimately released to her husband's care, but only after Jian testified that he would look after her under all circumstances.[22]

Even if the Beijing public somehow managed to avoid such images and expositions in the local news, the increasingly visible relationship between policing and madness was ultimately inescapable. As the police became more involved in the arrest and detention of the vagrant insane, they announced their broadening responsibilities through the dissemination of missing persons notices in markets, stores, and local police precincts. We have already seen in chapter 2 how the police had publicized the location of Gao Sheng-wang to such success that his brother was able to identify and claim him at the poorhouse only one week after he had gone missing. Throughout the 1910s and '20s, descriptions of other unclaimed lunatics also began to populate the city's streets. "His face is yellow, he has no pockmarks, and he wears a queue," the police wrote about the "madman" Wang Tiancai, who was captured by a patrolling officer in 1915. "He has been sent from the police station to the Inner City Poorhouse for temporary accommodation."[23] The prostitute Mrs. Song (née Duan), who was found wandering the streets in a mad daze and taken to the asylum, was made known to the public in a similar way.[24] And for the many insane men and women who had died under municipal custody, the police urgently publicized their names so that their bodies could be returned to their families for burial. Announcements for these individuals frequently graced the city walls, sometimes accompanied by an image of the face and torso.[25]

As the bodies of lunatics were plucked off the streets and redirected to the asylum or poorhouse, the proliferation of street-corner announcements and pictorial images ironically caused madness to become more visible (and more ubiquitous) than it had ever been before.[26] As such announcements expanded in scale and scope, moreover, local families not only learned about the existence of the asylum but progressively came to recognize its potential utility. By availing themselves of municipal resources, they realized, they could achieve multiple objectives at once: poverty relief, medical attention, and a temporary reprieve from the emotional and practical demands of madness at absolutely no cost. Beginning in the 1910s, families actively and aggressively sought municipal aid in connection with the insane. In so doing, however, they also (though perhaps unintentionally) sanctioned the augmented role of the municipality in the regulation of everyday life.

Desperate Measures

For many Beijing dwellers, life was lived on the precipice of utter destitution. In fictional stories, hardship and desperation were omnipresent and unremitting. Lao She's famous novel *Camel Xiangzi*, whose main character aspired to pull himself out of poverty only to be consistently frustrated by forces beyond his control, highlighted the precarious existence of the urban poor and the oppressive nature of industrial capitalism.[27] Lu Xun's fictional subjects also showcased the ubiquity of poverty, the growing disparity between rich and poor, and the insensitivity to the plight of the dispossessed. In his short story "An Incident," an unnamed narrator feels nothing but resentment for an old woman, clothed in a tattered jacket and rags, who is struck by his rickshaw and delays his commute across the capital city.[28] Yet poverty was more than mere fiction. As warlordism exacerbated famine-like conditions in the countryside, refugees left their natal homes en masse and resorted to begging in the city.[29] By the early 1920s, lagging economic conditions, rising inflation, and a lack of steady employment had forced many urban residents to the brink of economic collapse. Census data from 1926 show that close to three-fourths of the city's inhabitants were considered either part of the "lower class" or the "poor and extremely poor," while many lived on less than thirty yuan a month.[30]

Throughout the 1920s, newspapers detailed the atrocities of urban life. Journalists, capitalizing on the fetishistic horror of dead bodies, routinely calculated how many corpses they had seen in the city streets; one noted in 1923 that over 467 people had died from cold and hunger just in the span of one winter alone.[31] "Yesterday I saw three dead bodies," one reporter casually noted, including the locations that their corpses could be found.[32] But while the winter months posed their own hazards, the summer months contained hidden dangers, too. Bodies froze in winter but rotted in summer, and municipal authorities were often slow to respond to the pressing hazards of decomposition and disease.[33] As the poor-relief services offered by the municipality failed to keep pace with the sheer scope of urban need, the poor themselves often took to the media to seek aid from willing philanthropists.[34] Yet even as philanthropy expanded to fill gaps that the municipality had left behind, the power of wealthy donors also proved limited. As one editorialist somberly concluded, when political and economic instability touched the lives of every urban resident, "the upper class becomes the middle class, the middle class becomes the lower class, and the lower class all become beggars."[35]

The families on the furthest edges of destitution were often the ones to most actively seek the assistance of the municipality when it came to matters of madness. Lacking the means and the resources to care for the insane at home, they had little choice but to implore the police for aid. As survey data from Republican Beijing have shown, households with lower median incomes typically had fewer average members.[36] While wealthy families could afford to produce more offspring and hire live-in servants, poorer families could accommodate no such expenses. As a result, when sickness or madness struck, the lower classes were left with little recourse to meet its challenges. They could neither entrust the care of the compromised person to a servant or relative nor offset the loss of labor by hiring domestic help. When the urban poor could barely make ends meet under normal circumstances, the unwelcome presence of lunacy was sufficient to push the household to the edge of financial ruin.[37]

Police records confirm the extent of this destitution. Although the asylum did not maintain detailed records on the socioeconomic background of its residents, evidence of their poverty can nevertheless be deduced in alternative ways. In 1921, for instance, the asylum cataloged the possessions that had been left behind by the deceased insane. A ragged piece of cloth, a copper key, a pair of worn shoes, and a single coin—these were the only worldly belongings that the insane had brought with them to the facility.[38] Most did not even have this much. Only fifteen inmates out of a total of sixty-two were listed as having entered the asylum with any property; the majority were simply registered as having owned nothing whatsoever.[39] Indeed, when the asylum published its first set of statistical materials in 1927, it was noted that close to 70 percent of inmates were either "poor" or "extremely poor."[40]

Given the magnitude of their privation, many of the insane succumbed to illness during the period of their detention. Charles Selden and J. Allen Hofmann (1878–1933), superintendents of the John Kerr Refuge in Guangzhou, remarked that their facility experienced "a large number of deaths" due to the fact that many of their patients had arrived "in a state of physical exhaustion." Ironically, the facility also experienced a disproportionately large number of recoveries for the very same reason.[41] The psychiatrist Richard

Lyman (1891–1959) noted a similar phenomenon at the Peking Union Medical College many years later. Families of "comfortable circumstances" rarely admitted their relatives to the facility, he observed. Instead, most patients hailed from situations of abject poverty in which their families had found "no way to keep them." These types of patients, Lyman lamented, generally displayed a high incidence of "purely physical or symptomatic psychoses" due to obvious factors like "nutritional defects and infections."[42] Although the rate of mortality was not documented at the municipal asylum, medical records show that death from illness was common; when an inmate passed away and his or her family could not be located, the police prepared a simple coffin and buried the body outside of Desheng Gate.[43]

In a way, then, it was the very conditions of Beijing life that caused the symptoms of insanity to arise in the first place. Intellectuals and the urban poor alike certainly perceived this to be the case, and they frequently highlighted the reciprocal relationship between poverty and madness as a way to both appeal to the sympathies of the local police and obliquely impugn the municipality for failing to take care of its people. In popular publications like *Dongfang zazhi* (Eastern miscellany), writers often ascribed madness to the socioeconomic instability that had accompanied the rise of warlord regimes.[44] "Because unemployment is so high, the people are poverty-stricken," one editorialist lamented. "Suffering from this economic pressure . . . they either commit suicide or go mad."[45] Insanity, according to these writers, was nothing more than a response to the anxieties and pressures of contemporary society, and it was no surprise that so many of the urban poor fell victim to its grasp.

Families of the insane articulated their plight in a similar language. "Because we were in financial straits and my son could not find a job, he became very anxious and eventually went crazy," Wang Fu told the police in his oral testimony.[46] The same excuse was given for Mrs. Meng (née De), who was sent to the asylum by her younger brother. "Because our household circumstances are extremely bad, my sister became anxious and contracted a mad illness," he rationalized.[47] And Zhao Jingxi blamed his wife's madness on the near-starvation conditions in which his family lived. "Her poor diet caused her thoughts to be muddled and her words to become confused," he reported in 1926.[48] Such testimonies generally concluded with a formulaic, though heartfelt, plea: "Our household is very poor and we have no means by which to provide treatment. We beg you [the police] to institutionalize this patient."[49]

So deeply had this rationale been internalized that even the insane, when lucid, tended to attribute their illness to the stress of urban poverty. The Manchurian Guan Yanchang, for instance, arrived at a local police precinct hoping to gain admission to the asylum in the winter of 1918. Guan was thirty years old and had previously worked as a secretary for the Bureau of Transportation. After three years of gainful employment, however, he had lost his job and had been unable to find any work since. "Because I am poor and unemployed, the stress has caused me to go mad," he told the police. "I am destitute and have no work. This is why I came into the precinct to beg to be housed and treated [anzhi yizhi]."[50] A similar situation occurred with Fang Yujing in the spring of 1925. Fang, who was forty-three, had recently come to the capital from Zhili province in search of the wife of his deceased older brother, whom he hoped could lend him money. Finding himself "in economic straits," he "contracted symptoms of mad confusion" (de fengmi zhizheng) soon after arriving in Beijing and presented himself to the police hoping to undergo treatment at the asylum. Both men were admitted to the facility, where they were fed, treated, and released after a few short months.[51]

The stories of Guan and Fang reveal that, though poor, the lower classes were not entirely helpless. Appealing to long-held notions of state paternalism, they emphatically invoked the extreme nature of their economic plight as a way to receive municipal favor—particularly at a time when city resources were already stretched dangerously thin. In most cases, the police recognized the precariousness of their situation and agreed to feed, house, and treat them at absolutely no cost. At other times, the police went one step further to provide the most desperate families with a modicum of financial support. In 1919, a man petitioned the municipal police to send his wife to the asylum after an illness had left her insane and physically disabled. He made only five yuan a month, he told the police, and could not afford to care for a family of four—an old woman, a four-year-old daughter, and a terminally ill wife—on such a meager salary. The police, upon inspecting the living conditions of the family, determined that they were "exceptionally poor" and not only granted the man permission to send his wife to the asylum but also approved the allocation of one yuan to the family "as a means of showing empathy."[52] While such people were undeniably constrained by the severity of their economic hardships, they nevertheless fought to obtain sparse government resources and the limited attention of the overburdened police.

From the perspective of the urban poor, gaining admission to the asylum may have meant the difference between life and death. This outlook contrasted greatly with that of the Western physicians and foreign-educated Chinese who denounced the facility as nothing more than a primitive, abusive prison—a place that appeared more like punishment than reprieve, more like condemnation than salvation. "Even speaking about it made me want to die of humiliation," the Japanese-trained physician Tang Erhe (1878–1940) wrote of the asylum in 1924,[53] while the German-trained Weng Zhilong (1896–1963) compared the facility to a penitentiary where the insane were "completely deprived of their right to freedom." The repressive conditions within the asylum, Weng concluded, helped to explain why poor and wealthy alike would not dare enter it of their own accord: funds were never sufficient, food was sparse, and facilities were simple and crude.[54] Indeed, sentiments like these help to explain why the sociologist Sidney Gamble automatically assumed that the Beijing people would do everything in their power to avoid the institution, even if it meant resorting to the confinement of the insane within the home.

Despite such scathing condemnations as the ones above, however, the Chinese elite could not always sympathize with the patterns of life that the urban poor experienced on a daily basis. Certainly, conditions within the asylum were far from ideal: hygienic standards were lax, inmates were offered only two bowls of porridge and pickled vegetables a day, and criminals were sometimes kept there alongside patients. But from the perspective of impoverished Beijing families, the asylum promised at least a temporary reprieve from the pain and deprivation of urban life—guaranteed food, the warmth of a brick *kang*, and the therapeutic attention of doctors and staff—without so much as asking for a single dollar in return. Although the idea of willingly sending relatives there may have seemed counterintuitive to the sensibilities of the elite, the asylum was sometimes all that separated men like Guan and Fang from the hundreds of urban poor who each year were found dead in the city streets. With aid only forthcoming once the insane had encountered the institutions of the state, is it truly so shocking that such individuals fought to be allowed in?

Working the System

Once the Beijing people had discovered the asylum, it was only reasonable that they would try to take advantage of its services. By the 1930s, it was estimated that close to two-thirds of all asylum inmates had been brought there by their families rather than by the police.[55] Armed with the knowledge that the municipal authorities responded earnestly to accusations of madness, families frequently invoked the affliction in order to obtain police intervention and government aid. Over time, the scope of what could be considered a mad behavior—and who could be considered a mad person—progressively began to expand. In addition to claims that linked madness to poverty, local families also started to use the vocabulary of madness as a way to describe bothersome behaviors and inconvenient people. By claiming that an individual was pathological, rather than merely disruptive, families and members of the community were able to couch their concerns in a language that was intelligible to the state—and thus able to warrant police involvement.

The ability of local families to turn municipal policy into personal benefit exemplifies what Eric Hobsbawm has referred to as "working the system . . . to [one's] minimum disadvantage."[56] Rather than resisting the intrusion of the state into matters that might have otherwise been considered private, the Beijing people welcomed the intervention of the police—when it could be used to suit their own ends. With few other resources at their disposal to call for substantive sociopolitical or economic reform, ordinary people found that they could most easily promote their own interests not by resisting the state, but by manipulating it to their own benefit.[57] Invoking the label of madness thus became a tool that individuals wielded in order to convince the police to intervene in problematic (though not necessarily criminal) matters. In so doing, however, members of the lower and middle classes legitimated new municipal norms that linked madness to civic disruption—and hence sanctioned the broadening role that the police were coming to play in familial, personal, and community affairs.

We can see how this process unfolded in the summer of 1921, when a patrolling officer received a complaint from Mrs. Li (née Shi), the proprietress of a Beijing guesthouse called the Hongshun Inn. The complaint concerned a certain resident of the guesthouse, Dong Wenlong, who had been staying at the compound for a few days. "His words lack logic and he seems to be insane," Mrs. Li told the police when they arrived at the inn to investigate. When the police pressed her to explain the accusation further, she regaled them with tales of Dong's bothersome activities. In his room, he loudly recited the scriptures and kowtowed in the four directions; he tried to tell people's fortunes by using the Eight Trigrams; he stirred up trouble when he insisted that the inn was haunted; and he used his magical powers to eliminate the "evil" that resided there. "When he speaks of ghosts and spirits, his words depart from reality," Mrs. Li continued. "I'm afraid he'll cause a dangerous situation." Although the proprietress had tried to persuade Dong to move to a different guesthouse, he would only agree to leave once he had succeeded in "making the inn clean" from the spirits that inhabited it.

When the police investigated Dong's room, they found several questionable materials: a medicine pouch, a glass jar containing medicinal powders, a copybook with prescriptions, a book of the Eight Trigrams, a small drum, and four yellowed pieces of paper. Such items necessarily raised their suspicions. But after questioning Dong and finding his words lucid, the police were

unable to determine whether the man was truly mad or if he was simply
overtaken by his religious beliefs. When the case was forwarded to the chief
of police, the latter made his final verdict in bright red ink: "Dong's superstition is extreme. He studies Buddhism and Daoism, sees ghosts, and wants
to rid people of evil. He isn't mentally ill. He's just too superstitious [*mixin
taishen*]." In the assessment of the chief of police, in other words, Dong was
psychologically stable—just a bit idiosyncratic. Despite this determination,
Dong was nevertheless removed from the inn and taken to the police precinct, where he was held in custody for five days and made to promise that
he would "not dare be superstitious" or "linger in the capital" from that point
forward.[58] The case was thus satisfactorily concluded from the perspective of
everyone involved—except, perhaps, Dong Wenlong.

The confrontation between Mrs. Li and her lodger reveals a surprising twist
in the adjudication of madness. As we have seen in chapter 2, the municipal
police frequently fused madness with superstition in their effort to justify the
incarceration of deviant individuals. Yet, in this particular instance, it was *not*
the state that had made such a claim—it was the proprietress of the Hongshun
Inn. Had Mrs. Li sincerely believed that her lodger was insane? Was she truly
convinced that his religious practices signaled a deeper pathology? It is impos-
sible to know for certain. But regardless of what she may have thought, the
significance of this story lies less in her beliefs than in her actions. By invoking the charge of madness, Mrs. Li was able to secure police intervention into
an entirely harmless—albeit bothersome—affair. In short, it did not matter if
Dong Wenlong was truly disordered, or even if Mrs. Li believed him to be.
What mattered, instead, was that municipal norms and individual needs had
coalesced around the pivot of madness in order to achieve a common goal: the
expulsion of a troublesome person from the Hongshun Inn and, ultimately,
from Beijing altogether.

With its overwhelming ability to delegitimize the reality of the implicated individual, an accusation of madness functioned as an effective way to
gain power over inconvenient people. Because the municipal police had no
greater insight into the authenticity of madness than anyone else, and since
the police were more often compelled by the reinstatement of order than by
the adjudication of "truth"—if it is even possible to speak of such a thing in
this scenario—families and neighbors increasingly alleged lunacy as a way
to achieve municipal intervention. The case of the supposedly mad Mrs. Gu
(née Li), which unfolded in the summer of 1916, attests to the ways in which
an accusation of madness could unite state and society in their mutual desire
to silence problematic people. In July of that year, a woman named Mrs. Wang
(née Gao) called the police to her courtyard complex with the complaint that

her neighbor, Mrs. Gu, was insane. "Day and night Mrs. Gu curses at people," Mrs. Wang alleged, "and on the twenty-fifth of the month, she attacked me relentlessly with a slur of obscenities." On the day that Mrs. Wang had sent for the police, Mrs. Gu had apparently brandished a knife and threatened to assault her with it. "Mrs. Gu ripped my clothes, so I grabbed her pants and I ripped them too," Mrs. Wang reported to the police. "She is certainly insane."

The police were not automatically convinced by Mrs. Wang's story, but they became even more perplexed upon hearing the testimony of Mrs. Gu. The fifty-two-year-old widow, who lived alone and supported herself by sewing and washing clothes, described herself as the lone upright citizen in her courtyard complex. As she told the police, her neighbors would often invite "unemployed wanderers, prostitutes, and strangers into their homes to gamble together." While the women "cuckolded their men," the men "brought loose women to spend the night with." Because Mrs. Gu disapproved of their behaviors, she made her position known. "I'm a pain in the ass," she willingly admitted to the police. "But because I give them a hard time, they'll get into fights with me and say that I'm crazy. Ever since moving into this courtyard, I keep getting my money stolen. In the past two days alone, I've lost six copper coins." Mrs. Gu told the police that she had never intended to harm her neighbor, but when tensions had escalated, she found herself wielding a cleaver against Mrs. Wang in self-defense. "I might be sick with other illnesses," she definitively concluded, "but I am certainly not insane."

The main difficulty with this case, according to the police who were called to adjudicate it, was that both women had managed to tap into a vocabulary that resonated with the concerns of the municipality. While Mrs. Wang had accused her neighbor of being insane, Mrs. Gu had claimed that her courtyard complex was populated with deviant, promiscuous thieves. A scribbled note in the margin of the case file revealed the crux of the issue: "Did Mrs. Wang typically behave improperly, or was Mrs. Gu actually insane?" Lacking alternative means to verify one woman's claim over the other, the police had no choice but to question the remaining neighbors in the compound—people who, as Mrs. Gu had already stated, were already allied with Mrs. Wang in their mutual distaste for her. Although at least one other resident corroborated Mrs. Gu's interpretation of events, the general consensus was that Mrs. Gu "spoke crazy words, cursed, and yelled." This evidence was compelling enough. The police declared Mrs. Gu insane and brought her to the asylum that very evening, where she would remain for a mere three weeks before being deemed "fully cured." Since she lacked family in the city, however, the police decided not to release her but rather to transfer her to the poorhouse. It was only after Mrs. Gu contracted tuberculosis that the police discharged her to the care of a distant relative.[59]

Similar to the case of the lodger Dong Wenlong, the accusation of madness against Mrs. Gu had achieved its purpose: to shift the burden of responsibility for a problematic person away from an informal supervisory network (the inn or courtyard complex) and toward the formalized surveillance of the municipality.[60] Mrs. Wang, much like the proprietress Mrs. Li, had therefore been able to "work the system" to her minimal benefit. Invoking madness as a way to obtain municipal intervention, she succeeded in washing her hands of her bothersome neighbor once and for all. In both examples, then, the charge of madness functioned as a tool by which inconvenient people could be silenced and expelled. Particularly when coupled with other suspicious factors, such as superstitious activity (in the case of Dong Wenlong) or social alienation (in the case of the widow Mrs. Gu), an accusation of insanity propelled the bothersome individual from the realm of eccentricity into the realm of the pathological, thereby justifying the involvement of the police.[61]

By linking disruptive behavior to madness—and madness to the municipal police—the women who lodged these accusations not only legitimized the intrusion of the state into their everyday lives but also subtly expanded the scope of what could be considered "insane." Just as the municipal police conflated madness with vagrancy, superstition, and failure to conform to certain social norms, ordinary people like Mrs. Li and Mrs. Wang progressively came to view inconvenience as a type of pathology. When the police responded positively to their demands for incarceration, the relationship between insanity, problematic people, and troublesome behaviors became further institutionalized in the minds of the Beijing public. The broadening scope of madness was therefore not simply the result of an expanding state apparatus, but also the result of a decreased tolerance on the part of the community for inconvenient individuals; while the former may have introduced the possibility for municipal intervention, the latter was all too willing to push the boundaries of police cooperation in the pursuit of their own minimal interests.

And Being Worked by the System

This is not to say that the police automatically accepted any case of madness that appeared on their doorstep. By the early 1920s, the municipal asylum had become so overcrowded that the police were often far more interested in taking people *out* of it than putting them back *in*. In 1921, frantic reports from the manager of the asylum noted that the "people were overcrowded" in rooms that were "too narrow" to hold them.[62] In 1922, the asylum began turning away requests for inmates to be transferred there from surrounding counties.[63] And in 1924, the manager bemoaned that there were over 120 inmates at the facility—forty more than could be safely accommodated. "Everyone is crowded together and rubbing up against one another," he reported to the chief of police.[64] Fearing an outbreak of disease, the municipality sought desperately to ease the influx of the insane but could find no satisfactory solution to the unremitting problem.

Given the trend toward overcrowding within the asylum, the municipality was sometimes forced to deny admission to the facility when incarceration within the home remained a possibility. Although the police continued to institutionalize insane men and women who were simultaneously homeless, socially disenfranchised, violent, or poor, they were far less willing to incarcerate people whose families were able to look after them on their own. In 1920, the Beijing government produced a new set of interim legal statutes that once again upheld the centrality of the family in the management of madness. If a lunatic committed an offense or disturbed the peace, the code stated, the police were required to notify the mad person's father, elder brother, or caretaker, who would then be responsible for appropriately detaining his charge outside the purview of the state. If the lunatic's family members failed to do so, they would be punished on the mad person's behalf. According to article thirty-two, "Those who negligently allow lunatics, rabid dogs, or other dangerous animals to roam the streets or enter other peoples' houses" could be detained for up to fifteen days and fined up to fifteen yuan.[65] As the code made clear, the lunatic, like an animal, was a matter of familial responsibility first and state responsibility second; although the municipality would willingly detain the mad person if her family could not be located, her regular custody remained in the home.[66] Ironically, then, while local families were beginning to more proactively seek municipal services in connection with the insane, the municipality itself was attempting to curb these requests by resurrecting earlier laws that mandated domestic confinement.

In addition to new municipal legislation, the asylum also developed informal protocols that intended to both stymie the influx of new inmates and more efficiently process their releases. In 1921, the manager of the asylum, Wang Baohua, wrote a memorial to the chief of police with a series of suggestions for how to limit overcrowding. "From this point forward," he wrote, "anyone who seeks to send a mad person to the asylum for care and treatment must petition to do so with his or her police precinct." The precinct would then investigate the severity of the disorder and the extent of the family's need before making a final determination. Once these individuals had been cured, moreover, the asylum reserved the right to return them to their families "at any time and in an expedient manner."[67] A later manager of the facility, Wang Chengxun, further proposed in 1924 that lunatics who had shown any sign of improvement whatsoever be removed from the asylum and housed in an independent institution, such as the poorhouse. "There are not enough rooms to accommodate everyone," he wrote to the chief of police, "and so everyone is jostled together and crowded beyond measure."[68] Although it is difficult to assess if these suggestions ultimately came to fruition, they nevertheless signaled the facility's growing desperation at the unrelenting rise of the incarcerated insane.

Throughout the 1920s, the police frequently denied requests for institutionalization when the family did not display obvious signs of need and the individual in question was neither violent nor seriously deranged. The municipality's continued emphasis on domestic management had two important consequences. On the one hand, by refusing to formalize legislation that enabled the widespread and systematic internment of the insane—as France had done in 1838, England had done in 1845, and Japan had done in 1919[69]—the Beijing police unintentionally defended against the mass incarceration of inconvenient people that Michel Foucault so famously documented in *Madness and Civilization*.[70] Although Republican Beijing shared certain similarities with the so-called Great Confinement that Foucault claims took place in eighteenth-century France—in particular, the indiscrete lumping of idle, vagrant, and mad individuals into houses of institutionalization—the Chinese experience was nevertheless tempered by the continued primacy that was placed on familial care.[71]

On the other hand, the prioritization of domestic management served to frustrate families—and jeopardize the health and safety of insane people—who were denied municipal aid. Two examples will illustrate this point. In the summer of 1925, a patrolling officer came across an eighteen-year-old woman, Mrs. Zhang (née Xiao), who was yelling and cursing at her mother-in-law in the street. Because the young woman refused to be pacified, the officer brought her (along with her mother, husband, and mother-in-law) to the nearest police precinct for questioning. According to Mrs. Zhang Xiao's oral statement, she had been engaged to her husband from the time she was nine years old and had moved into her mother-in-law's house when she was sixteen. From that time on, her mother-in-law had constantly tyrannized her. She mocked and beat her, bit her, and kicked her in the ribs. One month earlier, the abuse had reached its climax when Mrs. Zhang Xiao's sister-in-law took a belt and wrapped it around her neck. The ill treatment triggered headaches and shortness of breath and caused her to neglect her household duties. "Because I didn't take care of the cooking, they refused to feed me," she told the policeman. "This is why I was angrily accusing my mother-in-law, and why I am supplicating the police to find accommodation for me [*qingqiu anzhi*]."

Mrs. Zhang Xiao's mother, distraught over the affair, confirmed her daughter's statement. But when Mrs. Zhang (née Bai)—the young woman's mother-in-law—presented her side of the story, the two tales did not match. "My daughter-in-law is insane," Mrs. Zhang Bai told the police. "Last July, she misplaced a silk undergarment [doudu]. Fearing that I would hold her responsible [for the loss], she became anxious and suddenly contracted a mad illness [hude you fengbing]. I treated her and she recovered, but in the last few days, she felt sick to her stomach and the madness returned. She frequently wanders off by herself and has broken glass and furniture at home. She is crazy, and I most certainly did not abuse her." The son of Mrs. Zhang Bai (and husband of Mrs. Zhang Xiao) confirmed his mother's account. "Last July my wife contracted a mad illness. Currently, her confusion makes her think that people are hitting and cursing at her." Mother and son finished their testimonies with a final plea. "We beg you to take Mrs. Zhang Xiao in [to the asylum] to be treated."[72]

Aside from these testimonies, the case file provides few clues about how the police eventually mediated between the two parties. What we do know, however, is that by the end of the day, Mrs. Zhang Xiao had decided to revoke her accusation of abuse and return home with her husband and mother-in-law. Although the latter continued to insist that Mrs. Zhang Xiao was indeed insane and required treatment—and despite the fact that Mrs. Zhang Xiao *herself* had also implored the police to intervene on her behalf, albeit for different reasons—the police determined that the woman's recuperation could just as easily be achieved within the home as in the asylum. Upon the conclusion of the affair, the mother of Mrs. Zhang Xiao gave a succinct (albeit unsettling) summary of the day's events. "My daughter was abused by her mother-in-law and accused her [of ill treatment]," she stated matter-of-factly. "Her mother-in-law denies the charge. My daughter will return home with them." (The chief of police, reviewing the file, crossed out the last sentence and replaced it with a subtle, but all too important, change. "My daughter *is willing* to return home with them," he corrected.) All four individuals were then released from the precinct and the case was considered closed.[73]

Let us compare this case with a similar incident that occurred a few years later. The incident began when a man named Zhang Fuzeng wrote a letter to the municipal police with the complaint that his fifty-two-year-old mother, Mrs. Zhang (née Wang), had suddenly gone insane. "She curses at people, cries and laughs irregularly, and displays world-weary thoughts," he informed the police. In Fuzeng's letter, he tried his best to depict himself as the typically doting son. "I secretly weep to myself [about my mother's problem]," Fuzeng admitted to the police, "but I still try my best to be filial and loving to her, and

I spare no effort to tend to her in a way that fulfills my filial responsibility."[74] Frightened that his mother might cause trouble or hurt herself, however, he pleaded with the police to have her detained in the asylum.

When the police sent an agent to Zhang's house to question him and his mother, the woman denied her son's allegations. Arguing instead that Fuzeng was only attempting to incarcerate her so that he could gain access to a family-owned parcel of land, Mrs. Zhang maintained that she was of sane mind. "My son accuses me of being insane and plots with his wife's family to have me institutionalized," she claimed. "When my husband was alive, we owned two parcels of land. . . . Ever since my husband died, though, my son began living apart from me, and rented out sixty *mu* of land from the second parcel.[75] I never received any money from it, which made me extremely angry, but I am certainly not insane." After recording the confessions of both parties and sending them to the chief of police for further instructions, the municipality eventually decided that Mrs. Zhang's madness was not severe enough to require institutionalization; instead, they demanded that Fuzeng bring his mother home and attend to her there.[76]

The examples of the abused Mrs. Zhang Xiao and the world-weary Mrs. Zhang Wang reveal several points about the adjudication of madness, the pride of place given to the familial home, and the role of gender in the negotiation between public and private forms of management. In both cases, the police were arguably less concerned about the welfare of either woman than the need to reach an expedient resolution—which they did by returning both families to their status quo ante. To the police, it did not necessarily matter if Mrs. Zhang Xiao and Mrs. Zhang Wang were legitimately insane or if they were the victims of mistreatment and neglect; what mattered, instead, was that they could be reintegrated into their families, kept within the home, and removed from the purview of the already overburdened state. Through an insistence on the primacy of domestic management—particularly for cases involving women[77]—the police relieved themselves of responsibility for the problematic person in question. At the same time, though, they also achieved their goal to preserve social stability by returning the woman to her rightful place within the home. It was for this very reason, as later survey data suggest, that the municipal police were "more conservative in their arrest of [insane] women" than men, preferring to leave the former under the supervision of their husbands and parents.[78]

Although this approach certainly served the interests of the state, it also functioned as a check against the indiscriminate confinement of what Michel Foucault has termed "an abusive amalgam of heterogeneous elements"—in other words, the incarceration of those who might not have been insane but who simply "disturbed their families' peace or who squandered their goods."[79] Indeed, it was not purely coincidental that the aforementioned allegations were both aimed at women. Given the woman's traditionally marginalized role vis-à-vis her husband, son, and parents-in-law, it was not surprising that wives and mothers could become easy targets of disavowal and abuse.[80] Just as a claim of hysteria in the West functioned to undermine the woman's subjectivity and justify her institutionalization, accusations of madness in Republican China could easily achieve a similar end.[81] In Shanghai, for instance, the tabloid press capitalized on a scandalous affair in which a man had accused his wife of being insane and locked her away in a private asylum; he had done so, the press revealed, because his wife had stood in the way of his ongoing dalliance with a younger woman.[82]

The reason these sorts of scandals were not more prevalent in Republican Beijing, however, was simply because the municipality had neither an economic incentive nor ideological interest in incarcerating such cases. Since the public asylum did not charge for its services, the police could not profit from the insane in the same way that British "mad doctors" had done;[83] and unlike the governments of France, England, and Japan, the warlord government in Beijing had never attempted to expand its control over the insane beyond the initial measure of funding the asylum.[84] As Francis Hsü (Xu Langguang, 1909–1999), a social worker at the nearby Peking Union Medical College observed, the police were more than happy to "loosen [their] control of any mental patient" so long as his or her family was able to "bear the responsibility."[85] Hsü provided two examples to bolster his point: first, a deranged lunatic who had hacked ten people to death with a cleaver but who was returned to his family because his wife wished to keep him at home; and second, a young woman who went mad in a public square but who was denied entrance to the asylum even after her mother had petitioned for aid. It was only once the woman became considerably more violent that the police eventually acceded to taking her in.

Because the municipality neither wanted nor could afford to assume a broader role in the supervision of the insane, a disjuncture arose between the demands of the society and the priorities of the state. Although the existence of the local asylum had awakened families to the possibility for external care, limited financial resources and insufficient space had forced the police to turn down requests for institutionalization in all but the most desperate cases. Thus, while the municipality's approach to handling madness might have been bureaucratically necessary, it was also entirely insufficient. *What if* the families of Mrs. Zhang Xiao and Mrs. Zhang Wang had been sincere in their requests for police intervention—not just because they wished to relieve themselves of an inconvenient person, but because their relatives sincerely needed attention beyond that which the family could provide? The failure of the police to offer alternative arrangements for such families left a conspicuous gap on the continuum between state incarceration and domestic management. This lacuna, which caused families and sick individuals alike to be left vulnerable to the long-term burdens of madness, necessitated the development of new possibilities for psychiatric care.

New Solutions for Old Problems

In 1924, the tabloid *Shehui ribao* (Social daily news) described the case of Yan Zhongyou, who "had gone crazy due to everyday hardships." Business at his store had been in a slump, he was ridden with debt, and his life had become exceptionally difficult. Due to the stress of his financial burdens, Yan eventually "became sick and went mad." On the night of June 13, he grabbed a kitchen knife and burst into his wife's room while she slept. There, he stabbed his wife until her "fresh blood gushed" and then proceeded to the kitchen where he boiled his young son alive. There was no doubt that Yan's actions were exceptionally heinous. But even so, the author of the report did not hold the man morally accountable for his crime. Instead, the tabloid laid the blame for Yan's mad actions on the unrelenting pressures of urban life.[86]

In popular imaginings throughout the warlord period, madness remained inextricably linked to poverty, displacement, and the anxiety associated with political instability and financial distress. As migrants flocked to the city to escape famine and war in the countryside, and as established residents of Beijing were forced to combat an economic slump following the end of World War I, beggary, homelessness, destitution, and death became common landmarks on the urban terrain. Although the municipality attempted to combat the privation of its people through charitable services, the city was ultimately unable to provide enough relief to meet the growing demand for food, shelter, and steady employment. Moved by a sense of hopelessness, people began to break down. And while the story of Yan Zhongyou was certainly an extreme case on which the popular press sought to capitalize, the theme of misfortune and madness was a common enough refrain that readers would not have questioned the inherent relationship between them.

Even if the poorest classes had few resources at their disposal to escape the devastating challenges of their time, this chapter has shown that they were not entirely helpless. As migrants and city residents became more familiar with municipal services and institutions, they increasingly used this knowledge for their own ends. Some appealed to police aid when relatives or neighbors displayed strange or bothersome behaviors, while others pursued treatment for conditions that had originated from deprivation, exposure, and stress. Although accessibility to charitable services was unevenly spread across gender and class, and although some individuals—like the lodger Dong Wenlong and the widow Mrs. Gu—had little recourse to unwanted police intervention, archival records nevertheless reveal that large numbers of the urban poor took advantage of limited state resources in order to achieve temporary relief from their routine hardships. In so doing, however, they also sanctioned and perpetuated the expanding role of the police in the governance of everyday life.

Throughout this process, unforeseen consequences occurred. First, the possibility of municipal involvement served to decrease familial and community tolerance for actions that would not have been thought to require external intervention in the late imperial period. By extension, moreover, decreased tolerance for deviant behaviors also broadened the scope of what types of people could legitimately be considered mad. It was no longer just the severely deranged or the criminally insane who were thought to require the attention of state functionaries. Rather, those with subtler tendencies became fair game for police involvement, as well: individuals who were bothersome, who drained familial resources, or who refused to submit to their proper place in the patriarchal household. By calling such people "mad," the Beijing public sanctioned a discursive shift whereby troublesome and pathological behaviors became intrinsically linked.

Second, and in direct contrast to the above, the expansion in appeals for police aid taxed municipal resources and forced the police to develop alternative solutions for both short- and long-term institutionalization. Recognizing that overcrowding in the municipal asylum was becoming a habitual problem, the police continued to emphasize the primacy of the familial home in the management of the insane. Particularly when accusations of madness proved convoluted or suspect, the police demonstrated that they were less concerned about the welfare of the individual than the preservation of social order. Families with enough means to support themselves were therefore told to resolve the situation internally, even if it meant that the well-being of the person in question might continue to be compromised by abuse or inattention.

A strange juxtaposition thus arose. While families were beginning to recognize the possibility of pushing the insane out of the house, the municipality was trying to put them back into it. The disjuncture between familial demand for institutional services and municipal norms of domestic control eventually culminated in a third avenue for rehabilitation and care: the psychiatric entrepreneur. It is to this transition that we now turn.

The Psychiatric Entrepreneur, 1920s–1930s

If provision for the insane had begun to change by the early 1910s, treatment for the disorder largely had not. At the Beijing Municipal Asylum, physicians continued to employ therapeutic regimens that remained firmly embedded within traditional medical paradigms. They did not speak of brains and nerves but of mucous, fire, and *qi*; they diagnosed patients not with schizophrenia or paralysis of the insane but with spleen vacuity, abundant mucous, and excessive wetness.[1] Outside the asylum, too, options for the rehabilitation of madness were little different than they had been before the fall of the Qing. Although a small number of biomedical hospitals, erected under the auspices of Westerners and the Japanese, had begun to appear on the urban landscape, few Chinese families made use of them for the specific treatment of mad disorders. As the neurologist Andrew Woods caustically observed, "There are extremely few [Chinese] physicians . . . who could recognize a disease of the nervous system as such, and none who would think of referring the patient to a hospital for care." Citing the example of a well-to-do Beijing family who refrained from bringing their father, a "paretic dement," to a hospital despite living only a few blocks away from it, Woods noted that the family simply "didn't think of that."[2]

When someone fell ill with madness, Beijing families instead did what they had always done. Those who could afford private treatment hired practitioners of Chinese medicine, who prescribed an assortment of drugs involving roots, tubers, and ground-up animal bones. Diagnosing their patients by feeling the pulses and looking at the color of the tongue, physicians located the roots of madness in the gall bladder and spleen, in the chest and in the diaphragm.[3] When the luxury of a private physician was unavailable, Beijing families pursued alternative avenues. In local temples, individuals enjoined priests to pray on their behalf or made direct offerings to Daoist gods. A foreign visitor to Beijing observed that the Daoists, in their quest to "rout the demons causing *malaise*," kept up an "incessant din" of chanting, punctuated by an intermittent clash of drums and cymbals, over the course of three days and nights.[4] Those with a few extra coins to spare hired exorcists and shamans to visit the patient directly; reciting prayers and spells, they sought to purge the sufferer of the evil spirits that plagued him.[5] And if such religious methods proved ineffectual, the temple market provided pills and potions for every ailment known to man. Displaying a dizzying array of concoctions from powdered silkworms to pickled sea horses, medicine men inveigled buyers into offering their limited dollars to the "oriental Aesculapius."[6]

Although these trends persisted throughout the Republican period, they would eventually be forced to confront—and adapt to—the evolving socioeconomic context of 1920s Beijing. Throughout the first three decades of the twentieth century, the progressive marketization of the urban economy transformed patterns of consumption and created new possibilities for the provision of medical care. Private clinics and mass-produced medications competed with Chinese medicine practitioners for the dollars of desperate invalids. Meanwhile, the continued expansion of Chinese print culture facilitated the commercialization of medical services to a degree that had not been possible even a few decades earlier.[7] In local and national newspapers, medical advertisements offered new solutions to long-standing problems, thereby challenging the cultural power of preexistent networks and therapeutic strategies. But while most of these advertisements only targeted ailments like coughs and constipation, provision for madness remained noticeably absent in the burgeoning medical marketplace.

This would change by the mid-1920s with the rise of a new type of health purveyor, someone I shall refer to as the psychiatric entrepreneur.[8] Similar to other "agents of consumer culture," to borrow Sherman Cochran's words, psychiatric entrepreneurs both responded to and perpetuated popular demands, desires, and fears pertaining to sickness and health.[9] Through the power of the print media, they sought to capitalize on the distresses associated with madness by offering new and affordable solutions to a problem that had never been adequately resolved—either by medical practitioners or by the municipality. Extending the possibility for private hospitalization of the insane, and promising an immediate cure for madness through the ingestion of proprietary medicines, psychiatric entrepreneurs readily filled the void between domestic management and public institutionalization.

Yet, the rise of the psychiatric entrepreneur did not simply *reflect* a growing demand for alternative solutions to madness. As part of their goal to turn psychiatric services into a profitable commodity, psychiatric entrepreneurs also worked to *create* this demand. They did so primarily by rebranding madness in a way that appealed to the sensibilities of the moneyed elite, the intelligentsia, and the petty urbanites (*xiao shimin*, moderately educated and marginally well-to-do people like students, clerks, and teachers).[10] By depicting madness as a singularly biological affliction that mainly affected those who labored with their minds, advertisements aimed to divorce the disorder from its connection to poverty and deviance. Moreover, in their efforts to appeal to a wealthy clientele, advertisers also introduced their readers to foreign "nervous illnesses" like neurasthenia, illnesses that appeared wholly removed from the madnesses of the urban poor.[11] In so doing, psychiatric entrepreneurs legitimized the anxiety and malaise of the moneyed classes while making it acceptable—and perhaps even fashionable—for them to pursue specialized remedies for their psychic distress.

Advertising thus functioned as a way of "making known" new psychiatric concepts, etiologies, and therapeutic possibilities to the Beijing public.[12] In a way that complemented—and in many ways anticipated—the increasing intellectual interest in neuropsychiatry that would take root in the 1930s, psychiatric entrepreneurship helped shape the contours of new forms of mental distress while simultaneously creating new demographics of psychiatric sufferers. This chapter therefore treats commercialism as a persuasive and influential form of knowledge production, and shows how an emerging capitalist impulse helped to commodify the very experience of mental illness itself. At the same time that advertisers were marketing new products and services, they were also selling new ideas about the nature of madness—as well as new ontological possibilities about what it meant to be "mad."

Selling Madness

Illness, though a bane to those who experienced it, proved a boon to those who could profit from it. Chinese medicine men knew this principle all too well. The temple fair, where urbanites and rural dwellers alike perused the latest knickknacks and novelties, had long been a central location for the peddling of health. In bustling outdoor markets, hired actors complained of unseen pains and unspeakable discomforts, only to be magically healed by panacean potions; and bombastic quacks, gesturing emphatically toward their prized herbs, roots, and animal bones, inveigled their audiences into buying medicinal mixtures of questionable content and efficacy. Throughout the late imperial period, the temple fair had been a vital location for the spread of medical knowledge, the exchange of information, and the purchase of necessary remedies.[13]

Although temple fairs and markets persisted throughout the Republican era, their form was irrevocably altered by the exigencies of the time. As Madeleine Yue Dong has documented, the shift from a lunar to a Western calendar forced buyers to adapt to new consumerist rhythms that mapped onto a seven-day week. Meanwhile, the Republican state's opposition to certain forms of religious practice caused some temple fairs to shut down entirely. As permanent commercial centers gradually came to replace itinerant markets, many fairs were displaced to the outskirts of the city or forced to relocate to impoverished neighborhoods. Consequently, while the petty urbanites and wealthy elite began to patronize department stores and indoor markets, temple fairs remained the bastion of the urban poor—people who, as Dong writes, were "excluded from the emerging world of new-style consumption."[14] By the 1920s and 1930s, the geography of consumerism had undergone a visible shift, and the demographics of marketgoers reflected a socioeconomic stratification that had not been nearly as salient during the late Qing.[15]

Evolving modes of consumerism were reflected not only in the rise of new commercial spaces but also in the advent of mass advertising in the popular press. As early as the late Qing, Chinese newspapers had been inundated with advertisements for various goods and services, many of which featured foreign businesses hoping to make their fortune in an untapped Asian market. By the end of the First World War, however, Chinese entrepreneurs had also joined the consumerist frenzy by urging customers to purchase only "national goods."[16] The advertisements they published, though ostensibly marketing new and necessary products, also subtly communicated changing consumerist norms. Enjoining buyers to pursue a cosmopolitan, scientific, and patriotic lifestyle through the purchase of domestically manufactured items, advertisers skillfully intertwined the act of consumption into broader concerns over national viability and economic growth.[17] In this way, advertising functioned in both a commercial and a didactic capacity. By suggesting that consumption was a political act, advertisers sought to convince their middle- and upper-class audiences that the types of products they purchased—as well as who they purchased them from—both reflected and advanced their identity as modern consumers and national subjects.

Yet, even as Chinese manufacturers encouraged consumers to purchase national brands, they could not ignore the unmistakable allure of foreign items. In order to better compete with the credibility and cultural cachet of imported products, Chinese manufacturers sometimes mimicked the form and content of foreign advertisements to (ironically) make their products seem more Western.[18] In the case of medical advertisements, Chinese pharmaceutical companies gradually adopted Western techniques for depicting the contours of the material body, both visually and textually. As Eugenia Lean has insightfully demonstrated, Chinese medical advertisements in the late Qing could be characterized by an *absence* of physiology; the body, when depicted, lacked discrete anatomical units, and health was implied through reference to Daoist immortals rather than flesh-bound men and women. By the 1910s, however, many advertisements had begun to mimic the mechanistic shape of the body as it was imagined in Western biomedicine. Illustrations delineated disembodied parts (heads, lungs, abdomens), while the accompanying texts described specific disease *entities*, such as headaches and heartburn, rather than underlying disease patterns.[19]

From as early as the mid-1920s, medical advertisements had begun to frame madness as a stand-alone disorder—one that necessitated a specific type of medical intervention. The decision to do so represented a sharp contrast with earlier configurations of the "mad illness." As chapter 1 has shown, Chinese medicine tended to frame mad behaviors less as a discrete pathology than as a manifestation of an underlying imbalance or malfunction. Consequently, when Chinese physicians and old-style apothecaries prescribed medications for the symptoms of madness, they often targeted the perceived *source* of the somatic disorder rather than the "madness" itself. In a manual produced by the Beijing pharmacy Hongren Tang, for instance, a medication called "White Dragon Powder" claimed that it could cure "excess heat in the heart and stomach, agitation and fidgeting, indigestion and dull pain in the five organs, constipation, fever, and going crazy [*fakuang*]."[20] Listed alongside a host of associated problems, madness merely appeared as a symptom of an ulterior pathology; it was not, however, described as the isolated target of the medication in question.

In contrast to the above, Beijing-based tabloids, dailies, and handbills progressively began to market madness as a discrete problem that required a specialized solution. Given the rising demand for alternative forms and sites of medical treatment—a demand that was both evinced and amplified by the ubiquity of advertisements for pills, potions, and hospitals in local newspapers—psychiatric entrepreneurs wagered on the possibility that the urban public desired, and would actively pursue, radically new solutions to the hitherto-unsolved problem of madness. Starting in the 1920s and continuing with increasing frequency into the 1930s, these solutions typically took one of two forms: private hospitals and proprietary medicines.

THE PRIVATE HOSPITAL

Just as the asylum represented a new feature on the urban terrain, so too did the hospital. Although medical clinics for the poor had periodically been established throughout Chinese history, their responsibilities often blurred with the broader charitable functions undertaken by local philanthropists: housing the homeless, feeding the hungry, and confining the diseased.[21] For the most part, when people fell ill, gave birth, or required any sort of medical attention, these transactions took place within the confines of the home.

It was not until the arrival of medical missionaries in the mid-nineteenth century that the hospital was introduced as a viable alternative to domestic care. While Western medicine at the time was hardly more advanced than its Chinese counterparts, missionaries endeavored to prove the superiority of their practices by emphasizing the orderliness and cleanliness of their facilities: places, they believed, that stood in stark contrast to the dirty and poorly ventilated space of the native domicile.[22] Yet despite this hygienic vision (or perhaps because of it), the Chinese people were slow to make use of foreign-managed clinics. Not only did Western physicians speak in an unintelligible biomedical vocabulary, but the hospital, as a new type of therapeutic space, contrasted uncomfortably with traditional family-centered regimens.[23] Similar to the nineteenth-century United States, where hospitals were publicly regarded as "institutions for the desperate" and "unsuitable places for ordinary people to patronize," those who could avoid institutional treatment in China far preferred to receive medical attention within the more welcoming space of their own bed.[24]

By the early Republican period, however, Chinese opinions on the hospital had started to change. The urban poor, when given the opportunity for free or low-cost treatment within Western clinics, gradually came to recognize biomedicine's efficacy in performing routine operations such as setting broken bones and removing cataracts—often to the financial detriment of the hospital itself, which was forced to foot the bill.[25] The middle and upper classes, meanwhile, were persuaded to pursue treatment in an institutional setting for altogether different reasons. Moved by contemporary discourses that linked Western medicine to national health and civic progress, urban elites tried to distance themselves from traditional medical practices that they increasingly viewed as backward or superstitious.[26] When the esteemed statesman Sun Yat-sen (1866–1925) sought treatment for cancer at the American-managed Peking Union Medical College, this decision only further cemented the compelling symbolic relationship among Western medicine, the hospital, and the evolutionary advance of Chinese nationhood.[27] Indeed, as de jure president Li Yuanhong (1864–1928) stated in a 1923 speech in Beijing, "Nothing has done so much to modernize China as modern medicine."[28]

Psychiatric entrepreneurs, though perhaps less moved by an overtly nationalistic impulse than a commercial one, attempted to capitalize on the recent attention being paid to the Western hospital. In the mid-1920s, private institutions for the treatment of the insane began to emerge in the wealthier enclaves of Beijing. Although advertisements for these clinics did not outwardly implicate a specific clientele, it is easy to deduce that the middle and upper classes were the likely targets of such services. Located in the western part of Beijing's inner city, these hospitals were strategically established in areas of relative prosperity alongside Western medical institutions.[29] Furthermore, although fees for their services were advertised to be relatively inexpensive—one hospital noted that an exploratory appointment cost only forty cents[30]—inpatient expenditures and the associated costs of prescription medications would have been unaffordable for the vast majority of the urban poor.[31]

By adopting the institutional format of the modern psychopathic hospital, Chinese-managed clinics strove to achieve the same legitimacy as their Western counterparts. Yet, regardless of their similarity in form, Chinese clinics often phrased their treatments in a vocabulary that had little to do with neuropsychiatric ideas or concepts. For example, the Natural Healing Hospital (Ziran zhiliao yiyuan), which was established in the relatively prosperous neighborhood of Xidan in 1924, described the symptoms of madness in a language that would have been largely unintelligible to a contemporary biomedical physician. The owner of the hospital, Li Xingxin, claimed to cure madness (*fengkuang*), along with its affiliated conditions of stagnant mucous and pathogenic *qi*, simply by harnessing the natural principles of the universe. Eschewing potentially harmful medicines, Li's therapies depended on nothing but the skillful manipulation of "*qi*, blood, spirit, and the meridians" in order to "reconcile body and mind" (*shenxin*).[32]

While facilities like the Natural Healing Hospital employed a primarily traditional vocabulary, other hospitals interwove psychiatric neologisms into their advertisements in an effort to bolster their therapeutic legitimacy. In the same year that Li Xingxin boasted of his ability to treat madness through natural means, a physician named Shi Sunzhi began publishing a series of similar advertisements in the Beijing newspaper *Chen bao* (Morning post). The facility over which he presided, which was also located in Xidan, promised to treat all of the illnesses that "could not be cured with medicine," including mental illnesses (*jingshen bing*), nervous disorders (*shenjing bing*), brain illnesses, and all manner of "unnamed evil sicknesses and strange and bizarre ailments." Without resorting to pills and nostrums, Shi promised to achieve "the health of mind and body" (*xinshen jiankang*) in five minutes or less.[33]

Although Shi's advertisements do not reveal how, exactly, he planned to cure these inscrutable disorders in such a short period of time, later advertisements provide clues about his particular approach. By 1928, Shi had begun to advertise separately for a teaching institute that would instruct students in his "new science" (*xin xueshu*) of mentalism. Participants in his training courses would not only learn the "fast and effective" techniques of hypnotism, meditation, and breathing therapy but would also be instructed in the arts of mind reading and X-ray vision.[34] Tapping into the widespread contemporary interest in statuvolism (self-hypnosis)—a "science" that had attracted the fascination of Chinese and Western audiences alike since the turn of the century—Shi sought to profit from the fact that stubborn disorders of mind had consistently eluded even the most skilled of native physicians.[35]

Over the course of the next decade, advertisements for private psychopathic hospitals became even more explicit about the content of their services. The bluntly named Madness Hospital (Fengdian yiyuan) offered "specialized" treatments for insanity, epilepsy and palpitations, paralysis and numbness, and women's *zangzao* (a condition that was often compared to hysteria).[36] The Baikui Hospital, located on Xuanwumen Avenue in the western part of Beijing, not only specialized in the treatment of madness but also produced its own "particularly effective" medicine for sufferers of mad disorders, simply called "N.O.P."[37] And Xu Fu'an, a self-proclaimed "specialist in madness medicine" (*fengke zhuanjia*), boasted that he had become an expert in the treatment of madness after having studied the disorder for a number of years. Under promise of a full refund, Xu guaranteed that his "special new discoveries" would allow him to cure "all types of insanity."[38]

Given the brevity of these advertisements, it is difficult to say for certain how such institutions cared for their patients. Fortunately, the records produced by one facility, the Wei Hongsheng Psychopathic Hospital (Wei Hongsheng jingshen bingyuan), provide a more detailed look at the background and therapeutic approaches of contemporary psychiatric entrepreneurs. Wei Hongsheng, a self-taught intellectual, founded his eponymous hospital in Beijing in 1934 after two decades of study. According to his writings, Wei had not originally intended to become a physician. Instead, he had devoted his early years to the study of classical Chinese texts, and he had only developed an interest in human physiology out of a desire to obtain a more complete understanding of the universe.[39] In his pursuit of medical knowledge, Wei had left Beijing in the 1920s and joined a research society in Shanghai that had been founded by a hypnotist named Bao Fangzhou.[40] The main premise of Bao's teachings was that madness was not an illness of body but rather one of mind (*xin*); accordingly, the disorder could not be cured through material procedures alone.[41] In place of treatments like medication and acupuncture, Bao developed an alternative regimen that he claimed could cure over 70 percent of mad patients.[42] His methods eventually became so popular that Bao later boasted of having trained "all the psychiatrists in the country"— including one of his more esteemed graduates, Wei Hongsheng.[43]

Upon completing his training, Wei returned to Beijing, where he continued to pursue the study of Confucian, Buddhist, and Daoist texts. Eventually, he integrated his philosophical and medical knowledge into a specialized regimen that could cure even the most intractable illnesses, madness among them. Wei's curative philosophy owed much to his mentor, Bao Fangzhou. Like Bao, Wei believed that "material medications" were insufficient to cure mad illnesses. Because man's soul (*lingxing*) and consciousness (*juexing*) were both immaterial, he argued, madness could be counteracted only through formless (*wuxing*) means.[44] At his psychopathic hospital, he renounced all types of medicine, acupuncture, and surgery and instead employed several techniques that aimed to "facilitate the flow of blood and *qi*, straighten out the meridians, restore the spirit, relieve mucous fire, clear the heart cavity, and return the patient to normalcy." These techniques, which included hypnotism, talk therapy, and a specialized regimen involving meditation and guided breathing, were effective even for patients with such severe forms of madness that they "talked to themselves and spoke nonsensical words."[45]

Wei's patients were encouraged to document their experiences at the hospital for publication in his institutional records. One of his charges, a former soldier named Ma Muzhao, claimed to have developed schizophrenia (*xinli fenlie*) and nervousness (*shenjing jinzhang*) after having "taxed his mind" (*laoxin*) at work. Although he had visited both Chinese and Western doctors, none could treat his illness, and he continued to languish in his pathological state until he happened to see an advertisement for Wei's hospital in a local newspaper. At the hospital, Wei met with Ma personally to teach him the methods of his therapeutic practice. Ma began his treatment by sitting quietly in a meditative stance with his hands hanging loosely on his knees, his mind rejecting earthly desires, his body closed tight against external pathogenic influences,[46] and his attention focused on the *qi* flowing throughout his body. After one week of this regimen, Ma observed that a strong *qi* had begun to ascend from his lower abdomen, causing his body to drip with sweat and his limbs to go limp. Ten more days passed, and his body felt drunk with the *qi* circulating throughout him. Slowly, he began to regain his health. By the time his treatment was over, Ma estimated that his condition had improved by 70 to 80 percent.[47]

Wei Hongsheng's therapies, which represented a mongrelized version of Chinese and Western medical theory, were likely not far removed from those of his competitors. Like other psychiatric entrepreneurs, Wei adopted the institutional format of the psychopathic hospital and frequently invoked psychiatric neologisms; at the same time, he also distanced himself from the actual practice of Western medicine. Claiming that biomedicine and Chinese medicine were both fundamentally unable to treat madness, Wei and others like him attempted to capitalize on a lacuna in the contemporary therapeutic landscape. Integrating pseudoscientific approaches (such as hypnotism) into long-standing, albeit repurposed, curative and philosophical regimens (such as meditation), Wei offered an appealing alternative to existent medical models. In so doing, he also redefined the etiology of the mad condition. By framing madness as a formless disorder of "mind," Wei inched closer to a Cartesian model of mind-body dualism—yet he did so by following a logic that was far more rooted in traditional medical principles than neuropsychiatric ones.

PROPRIETARY MEDICINES

Not all psychiatric entrepreneurs possessed sufficient capital, resources, or training to provide this level of personalized care. For those who still wished to participate in the growing "trade in lunacy" but did not have the means or desire to open a private psychopathic hospital, an alternative route was also available: the proprietary medicine industry. Proprietary (or patent) medicines, as one nineteenth-century observer defined them, were "drugs compounded of unknown ingredients" that were "intended for the relief or cure of the various ills that flesh is heir to."[48] Many were harmless but also ineffective; others, consisting of analgesics like heroin, cocaine, opium, and alcohol, might have temporarily relieved headaches and coughs but produced "insidious developments" that could lead to addiction and sometimes even death.[49] Their continuing popularity, therefore, was not always related to their efficacy. Rather, as James Harvey Young has argued, proprietary medicines emerged at a particular historical juncture in which physicians were still powerless to cure disease, the medical industry was largely unregulated, and urban populations had begun to demand inexpensive and expedient solutions to the innumerable ailments from which they suffered.[50] Although Young was referring to the situation in nineteenth-century America, this description was equally applicable to Republican China.

Proprietary medicines were vigorously introduced into the Chinese market just prior to the fall of the Qing dynasty.[51] The first Western pharmaceutical companies infiltrated Asia in the last quarter of the nineteenth century and, through "judicious and persistent advertising," gradually gained a foothold in China by the 1910s.[52] Chinese entrepreneurs, inspired by both nationalist sentiment and the pursuit of profit, soon followed suit. By the 1920s, advertisements for a wide array of "nourishing" tonics and "bolstering" elixirs had become ubiquitous in newspapers and pictorials. They were so widespread, in fact, that some scholars have estimated that as much as one-third of non-news-related content in major urban newspapers consisted solely of medical advertisements.[53] As Hugh Shapiro has concisely summarized, "The scale of the Republican medical industry, and the interdependence of pharmaceutical houses, hospitals, practitioners, and newspapers was unprecedented," as dailies "pandered to advertisers . . . [and] inveigled readers into swallowing medicine."[54]

Proprietary medicines claiming to specifically target madness first appeared in the Beijing press in the early 1920s. Throughout 1922, the newspaper *Chen bao* ran an advertisement for a "miraculous drug" that could eradicate the problem of madness at its root. At only thirty cents per pill, the drug cost approximately the same amount as a one-day stay in a lower-class ward of a municipal hospital.[55] The "Madness Suppressing Pill," which cost forty cents per capsule, claimed to ease the symptoms of "hysterical madness and *qi* confusion" by opening up the heart cavity and dredging the stagnant mucous that had accumulated there.[56] And the "World's Number One 'Mucous Confusion and Madness' Pill" proved to be a particularly long-standing mainstay in the Beijing newspaper world; across four years and at least three different newspapers, the advertisement confidently asserted that its "miraculous secret prescription" could treat all types of madness, including cases where the sufferer "speaks illogical words," "sees ghosts and spirits," and "laughs and curses, while the mouth flows with sputum." For only one and a half yuan per bottle, the patient could finally "escape from the bitter sea of suffering."[57]

Much like advertisements for private psychopathic hospitals, proprietary medicines adopted a modern form—the mass-produced capsule—but spoke to their consumers in a relatively traditional vocabulary. Madness remained etiologically linked to pathogenic *qi* and an accretion of mucous in the heart cavity, and the symptoms that accompanied the disorder—such as "laughing and cursing" or "seeing ghosts and spirits"—were no different from the four-character stock phrases that had typically been used to describe mad people throughout the imperial period. As Sherman Cochran has observed in the case of the Chinese pharmaceutical magnate Huang Chujiu (1872–1931), medical entrepreneurs often used familiar terminologies so as to make their products "seem intelligible and unthreatening."[58] Thus, despite the newness of their form, they did not overtly challenge preexistent conceptions about the nature and cause of madness. Functionally, too, proprietary medicines acted on the body in much the same way as their traditional counterparts. While some served as purgatives and emetics, others merely functioned as temporary sedatives.[59]

Although these new-style products may not have introduced new etiologies of madness, they did contribute to evolving psychiatric discourses in other ways. More specifically, many of these advertisements subtly attempted to undermine the negative connotations that were associated with madness and mad people. As discussed in the previous two chapters, the municipal police and the Beijing public tended to conflate madness with social deviance and transgressive behaviors. Widespread discomfort with the insane—if not outright fear and hostility—was further compounded by the unsavory ways in which the disorder was typically depicted in the popular press. Throughout the early republic, the print media often presented madness as violent, salacious, and obscene. In tabloids, mad people yelled and cursed, disemboweled themselves and slit their own throats, disrobed in the streets and caused public commotions. They were, at best, objects of public fascination and, at worst, targets of public disgust.[60]

In order to combat these connotations, advertisements for proprietary medicines presented the disorder as banal and routine. One of the ways that they did so was by employing first-person testimonials. The tactic of using testimonials to sell proprietary medicines had originated with the American pharmaceutical industry, which frequently included pictures of "rehabilitated" customers alongside personalized statements of gratitude.[61] Foreign businesses continued this strategy in China, changing little from their original templates save the names and images of their satisfied clientele.[62] In the case of madness, Chinese proprietary medicine companies adopted a similar strategy by showcasing testimonials such as the following:

> I previously worked at the post office. Every day, work was busy. As a result, my brain sometimes felt confused, and I would get worried and depressed at home. Last winter, I suddenly contracted the symptoms of a mad illness [*hude diankuang zhi zheng*]. My movements were abnormal, and whenever I regained consciousness I became enraged. I would rave and hallucinate. I didn't know if I was starving or full. I reluctantly received treatment and took medicine, but nothing worked. Then in March of this year, I saw an ad in the paper for the "Number One Madness Pill." I bought three bottles and took them all, and I got a little better. So I bought some more and my illness was

completely eradicated at the root. I would like to offer my gratitude to this miraculous medicine, as well as to this newspaper for printing [the advertisement]. To those who are sick, don't just wait around; quickly buy this medicine and escape your suffering![63]

My younger brother had been sick with madness for three years. He visited many doctors to no avail. He took the "Spirit Quieting Powder" a few times and it completely eliminated the root [of the illness]. . . . I want to express my thanks to this miraculous medicine. Signed, Wang Fumin, statistician for the city government.[64]

Though couched in a vernacular and otherwise unremarkable vocabulary, testimonials such as these aimed to "rebrand" madness. In contrast to the scandalous ways that madness was often depicted in the popular press, advertisements for proprietary medicines presented the disorder as morally neutral. It affected hardworking, middle-class individuals and their families—even the siblings of public officials—and could be "contracted" and "eradicated" as easily as the common cold. In the advertising imaginary, madness was etiologically understandable, readily curable, and ultimately a quotidian disorder that was democratic in its epidemiology.

This particular portrayal of madness represented a strategic business decision, of course. By altering the public discourse associated with madness, proprietary medicines sought to reduce the stigma of the disorder and thereby appeal to the needs and desires of the petty urbanites.[65] But even if psychiatric entrepreneurs were motivated more by profit than a genuine concern for the insane, they nonetheless introduced new paradigms by which madness could be evaluated and treated. As a routine disorder that affected ordinary people, madness was progressively dissociated from the homeless, the deviant, and the poor, and as an illness that could be cured merely by swallowing a pill, madness no longer required the arcane knowledge of the literati physician. In this sense, advertising served to generate new forms of psychiatric knowledge by reframing both the moral and biological content of the condition.

Elite Madness

Psychiatric entrepreneurs did not just imbue existent mad disorders with new meanings. In certain cases, they also introduced new forms of insanity altogether. One of the most widespread—and persistent—disorders that was unveiled to the Chinese people in the early republic was the nervous condition known as neurasthenia (*shenjing shuairuo*).[66] Discovered by the American physician George Beard (1839–1883) in 1869, neurasthenia (also known as nervous exhaustion) was originally considered a prototypically American malady. The illness was taxonomically linked to madness and shared some of its symptoms, but it differed from other types of insanity in the sense that it primarily affected intellectuals, bureaucrats, and those who labored with their minds. Characterized by headaches, insomnia, depression, and a host of other physical and emotional symptoms, neurasthenia was to the nervous system (a deficiency of "nervous force") what anemia was to the vascular system (a "want of blood").[67] The reason for its development, Beard surmised, had much to do with the conditions of contemporary American life. "Civilization," he explained, "is the one constant factor without which there can be little or no nervousness, and under which in its modern form nervousness in its many varieties must arise inevitably."[68] Neurasthenia, in other words, was a disease of the refined, civilized, and eminently modern man.

After its discovery in the mid-nineteenth century, neurasthenia soon became an epidemic of unimaginable proportions. Men and women who had succumbed to the malaise and intensities of modern life suddenly had a name to give to their sufferings, and they invoked the term with the same pride that one does with a wound sustained in the course of battle.[69] Over time, the disease spread across the Atlantic to England, France, Germany, and the Netherlands, where native practitioners endeavored, albeit unsuccessfully, to find an effective cure. "Neurasthenia has swept over the whole civilized world," one observer frantically reported in 1915,[70] while others, with more moderate tone, noted that the ailment had undoubtedly become "a condition of everyday occurrence, and therefore one of considerable importance."[71] Although some physicians bemoaned the classification as uselessly vague, others rejoiced at the fact that neurasthenia had isolated a common somatic root—the nerves—for a host of mysterious disorders that defied organic explanation. Thus, while there was no known cure for the affliction, a diagnosis of neurasthenia could nevertheless "validat[e] both the doctor's ministrations and the patient's suffering."[72]

The explanatory power of neurasthenia was so potent that it quickly spread to emerging parts of the civilized world. Beginning in the last decade of the nineteenth century, discussions of neurasthenia gained considerable traction in Japan. Appropriating Beard's argument that the illness derived from modern civilization, Japanese intellectuals invoked the term to explain a range of otherwise inexplicable symptoms, from indigestion and heart palpitations to sudden fits and depression.[73] Some intellectuals spoke publicly about their frustrations with the disorder. Ishikawa Hanzan (1872–1925), a well-known newspaper editor, published an account of his lengthy recovery from neurasthenia in 1907, in which he described the illness as the "twentieth-century disease of civilization."[74] The writer Natsume Sōseki (1867–1916) similarly suffered from neurasthenia, and characterized it as an affliction that had been "contracted by many modern people."[75] As Yu-chuan Wu points out, the Japanese had no prior conception of the nervous system, but the theory behind neurasthenia was both sufficiently convincing and culturally desirable that the affliction readily penetrated Japanese life.[76]

Scholarly interest in neurasthenia was somewhat slower to take root in China. Although a handful of Chinese intellectuals had contracted the ailment while studying abroad in Japan—the revolutionary Song Jiaoren (1882–1913), for example, had to be institutionalized at a neurological hospital in Tokyo after becoming sick with neurasthenia in 1906[77]—the disorder would not become a widespread subject of intellectual discourse until close to two decades later. Indeed, the first Chinese-language books on the subject did not appear until the late 1910s and early 1920s, though even these were translations of Japanese or English works that were written in a stodgy, classical language.[78] And despite the fact that medical missionaries had been extant in China from the mid-nineteenth century, most did not prioritize the treatment or prevention of nervous ailments. Focusing the brunt of their energies on problems related to public health, foreign-run facilities were far more preoccupied with degenerative conditions like neurosyphilis than functional disorders like nervous exhaustion.[79]

When knowledge about neurasthenia initially penetrated China, it did so primarily via commercial means rather than purely discursive ones. More specifically, the Japanese patent medicine industry played a critical role in introducing the concept of neurasthenia to Chinese consumers. In Japan, the proprietary medicine trade had already been in existence for several decades by the time the fervor had reached China; the industry was so profitable, in fact, that the Meiji government had begun regulating and taxing it from as early as 1877. In order to maximize profits from the trade, however, the Japanese Diet had passed an additional bill in 1905 that exempted medical exports from taxation. As a result, pills, powders, and pastes began making their way from Japan to its colonial outposts in Korea and China in the first decade of the twentieth century.[80] These products, much like their British and American counterparts, flagrantly claimed to cure all types of ailments that were resistant to modern medicine. One such product, named after the eminent seventeenth-century Japanese physician Bandai Jokan, even went so far as to claim that it could "bring the dead back to life." As one British observer reported in 1908, "Most people probably regard America as the chosen land of the patent medicine vendor, but Japan would seem to be able to 'give points' to the great Republic in this respect."[81]

The Japanese patent medicine industry quickly flourished in China. Thomas Sammons, the United States consul general in Shanghai, noted in 1917 that the sale of Japanese proprietary medicines in China was "nearly equal to those of all the other foreign firms combined." Although Sammons partially attributed this success to "similarity of language [and] racial characteristics," he also acknowledged that Japan's business acumen was unrivaled by any of its foreign competitors. Through advertising and publicity campaigns, the Japanese pharmaceutical industry managed to "exploit thoroughly and systematically the whole of China," even bringing its offerings to remote outposts that no Western firm cared to penetrate.[82] With over three thousand licensed manufacturers exporting their goods directly to at least eight different ports, Japanese products had effectively flooded the Chinese market by the early years of the Republican period.[83]

Due to the sudden ubiquity that neurasthenia had gained in Japan, Japanese proprietary medicine manufacturers began to vigorously promote antineurasthenic pharmaceuticals to both domestic and Chinese consumers. The "Brain-Strengthening Pill" (Japanese: *kennōgan*; Chinese: *jiannao wan*), which was produced by the Tampei Manufacturing Company, first emerged on the Japanese market in 1896.[84] It was then exported overseas, where it appeared in newspaper advertisements throughout northeast China and Shanghai beginning in the first decade of the twentieth century. "Brain-Strengthening Pills" were specifically targeted at consumers who "frequently overexerted their brains." Developed by a Japanese physician, the product claimed to heal neurasthenia; strengthen the memory; and cure headaches, insomnia, and nervous exhaustion. It could be found at "all pharmacies and wherever medicine is sold" in prices ranging from twenty cents to five yuan, depending on the quantity being purchased.[85]

Similar Japanese products, following the same template as the "Brain-Strengthening Pill," also claimed to target the nervous weaknesses of the petty urbanites and intellectual elite. The "Efficacious Pill" for brain and nerve disorders (Japanese: *rēben*; Chinese: *lingpian*), which was developed by ten Japanese medical specialists in conjunction with several prominent Beijing physicians, combated such illnesses as neurasthenia, dizziness, and headaches. Consumers who were skeptical of its efficacy were encouraged to "try a tablet" at a local pharmacy; once they experienced its "particularly effective" curative abilities, they could then purchase as many as seven hundred tablets at a time.[86] The "Efficacious Brain Bolstering Potion" likewise asserted that it had been developed in the "Great Japanese Empire" by a physician who specialized in neurological disorders. The medicine's "secret formula" could cure all diseases of the brain and nervous system, including depression (*xinshen yumen*), insomnia, neurasthenia, and mental confusion (*jingshen huanghu*). Like its competitors, the "Efficacious Brain Bolstering Potion" also targeted an elite clientele who "used their minds but did not labor." Students, teachers, gentry, merchants, lawyers, bankers, and even Buddhist monks and Daoist priests were enjoined to purchase the medication, which would quickly cause "the hundred illnesses to disappear."[87]

As tensions between Japan and China escalated throughout the late 1910s, the cachet of Japanese goods progressively diminished. Although these products continued to advertise in Chinese newspapers well into the 1930s (excising, however, all references to their Japanese origins), Chinese manufacturers capitalized on the increasing demand for domestic commodities by developing their own anti-neurasthenic goods and services. The "Wonderful Medicine for Neurasthenia," which began advertising nationally in 1925, boasted that "everyone who works their minds cannot afford to *not* take it."[88] The Baikui Pharmaceutical Company in Beijing produced an assortment of medications that were "particularly effective" at treating neurasthenia, revitalizing the brain, combating memory loss, and strengthening the mental faculties.[89] And numerous tonics and potions, including the "Brain-Bolstering and Nerve-Strengthening Pill," targeted those who were "overworked" and who resultantly suffered from symptoms such as depression, mental confusion, headache and blurry vision, and seminal emission.[90] Even the famous Ailuo Brain Tonic, which first appeared in Chinese newspapers in 1905, began to include specific references to neurasthenia by the 1920s.[91]

Physicians who claimed to "specialize" in the treatment of nervous disorders also advertised in Beijing newspapers, often in the form of signed testimonials from rehabilitated patients. In 1924, for instance, a local resident named Li Yunfei thanked the Harada Hospital for having cured his neurasthenia. A self-proclaimed "member of the journalism world," Li had ostensibly developed the illness "due to constant overwork":

> I brought my illness to the attention of many doctors, but to no avail. Recently, I again fell ill and could not get out of bed. I reported the details of my sickness to the doctors at the Harada Hospital. Mr. Harada himself examined my serious illness and was able to cure it. I decided to publish this special announcement to thank him, and to publicize his name so that other patients will know whom to ask for. Signed, Li Yunfei.[92]

Li, though perhaps more vocal about his condition than other sufferers, was certainly not alone. Just like in Japan, petty urbanites and intellectuals alike proved extremely receptive to both the concept of neurasthenia and the salutary promises of medical advertisements. Even well-respected writers like Lu Xun and Xu Zhimo (1897–1931) left evidence that they consumed "brain-bolstering" proprietary medicines, such as the imported Western brand Sanatogen.[93] By the 1930s, neurasthenia had reached such epidemic proportions in China that the Beijing municipality was moved to approve the erection of a specialized facility for the treatment of nervous disorders in 1936. Managed by a neurologist named Wang Jiaxiang (d. 1937), the "Mental Convalescence Clinic" (Jingshen xiuyang yuan) ministered specifically to the wealthiest classes and charged a cash deposit of up to one hundred yuan for first-class patients.[94]

Advertisements for anti-neurasthenic products and services, the earliest of which predated Chinese-language tracts on the subject by a full decade, functioned as an initial means by which psychiatric and neurological discourses penetrated Chinese society. Much like advertisements for other madness-combating proprietary medicines, those for anti-neurasthenic products acted as a compelling didactic force. By targeting members of the intellectual elite, such advertisements introduced new information about the populations at risk for nervous disorders. Moreover, by emphasizing the brain and nerves (rather than the heart) as the locus of "mental" distress, proprietary medicines also subverted how human physiology had traditionally been conceptualized in the Chinese medical canon.[95] These advertisements thus did not solely promote modern medical commodities, though that was certainly their primary intent. Equally important, they served as a vehicle through which new ideas about the etiology and epidemiology of "mental" and "nervous" illnesses could be popularized.

Claiming a Neurasthenic Identity

Epistemic contributions aside, what strikes me as equally significant about these advertisements was their ability to create—and to sell—a particular social identity. By explicitly reinforcing the link between neurasthenia and mental overwork, such advertisements underscored the elite nature of the consumers to whom their products were being sold. The allure of the medication was therefore not simply its utility, but also its ability to confirm the consumer's identity as a member of the intellectual upper class. The historian Stuart Ewen has referred to this tactic as a "self-conscious change in the psychic economy."[96] In order to induce consumers to purchase certain goods, he suggests, advertisers emphasize not just the efficacy of the product itself but also an experience, identity, or form of cultural capital that the product can help its consumers to achieve. In other words, by forging a definitive relationship between neurasthenia and the elite classes, Republican-era advertisers were striving to "define customers as an integral part of the social meaning of goods."[97]

In China, intellectuals proved extremely amenable to claiming the title and identity of the neurasthenic sufferer. Just as in Japan, where members of the intelligentsia spoke publicly about their experiences with the disorder, self-proclaimed neurasthenics in China also composed their own public and private illness narratives as a way to come to terms with the chronic condition.[98] Zhou Zuoren (1885–1967), the younger brother of the well-known writer Lu Xun and a prominent essayist in his own right, detailed a prolonged experience with neurasthenia in his diary and in letters to close friends. In the summer of 1921, Zhou fell seriously ill with pleurisy and moved outside of Beijing to the neighboring Fragrant Hills (Xiangshan) to convalesce. Although he eventually recovered from his sickness, he noted in a letter that his "neurasthenia was easily excited" and that it had become "much worse" in the ensuing months:

> During the daytime there is always a period when I feel depressed [*yinyu*]. That period is in the afternoon, after the postman delivers the newspaper. Even trivial matters cause me to feel agitated [*fanzao*], and it's almost like I've developed a fever. Because of this, I generally try to avoid [reading the paper] altogether. Every day's paper is chock-full of unhappy news. Upon seeing it, I can't help but feel vexed [*fannao*]. In other words, since [the news] is always like this, how could it be anything but beneficial to avoid it? But then again, I can't *not* look. It's like there's an injury on my body, and while I realize that touching it will cause pain, I can't help but reach out and feel it with my hands.[99]

Even after having shut himself off from the outside world, Zhou found that he could not escape its unhealthy stimuli entirely. His "bad nerves" continued to plague him throughout the warlord period, and his neurasthenia caused his thoughts to become "helter-skelter" (*fenluan*).[100] Zhou's authorial output suffered as a result. As he lamented in a letter to a friend, "I haven't written in a very long time, nor have I finished any poetry. Admittedly, my poetic inspiration just isn't there."[101]

The relentless pressures and demands of urban life were sometimes all that was necessary for the symptoms of neurasthenia to arise. The renowned historian Gu Jiegang (1893–1980) was still a student at Peking University when he contracted neurasthenia in the late 1910s—a disorder that would continue to plague him for the next thirty years. As a result of overwork and the various stimuli of his urban existence—including, as he noted in his diary, the poor air and loud music at the Peking opera performances he regularly attended—Gu developed symptoms including insomnia and chronic constipation. His health continued to worsen following the death of his first wife in 1917 and paternal grandmother in 1922. Although Gu struggled tirelessly with the condition, trying vitamin supplements as well as Western and Chinese proprietary medicines, it was not until the early 1950s that he finally recovered from the disorder. Reflecting on his battle with the disease, Gu remarked in his diary that neurasthenia had turned his young adult life into nothing more than "a state of restless anxiety, hesitation, chaos, and pain."[102]

Sufferers of neurasthenia did not just document their travails in private letters and diaries. Throughout the Republican period, several self-help platforms enabled neurasthenics to share their experiences with a sympathetic public, as well. The *Huabei yibao* (North China medical journal) regularly featured question-and-answer forums on the subject of neurasthenia, while the widely read *Dongfang zazhi* (Eastern miscellany) published over 350 letters about neurasthenia over the course of the 1930s alone.[103] Some sufferers, having recovered from the disorder, wrote lengthier articles about their experiences to aid fellow patients in their search for a cure. In 1931, a chronic neurasthenic named Liao Qichong penned an article in *Dazhong yikan* (Medicine of the masses) explaining how he had freed himself from the affliction after having contracted it three years earlier. Practitioners of Chinese medicine were useless and absurd, he exclaimed; insisting that the disorder was related to his liver or kidney, they repeatedly "threw decoctions at [him] that had absolutely no effect." Western-trained doctors were not necessarily any better. Although the physician Liao had visited was able to give his suffering a name—neurasthenia—he had nonetheless conceded that no known medication could help. Liao only found relief when he began to lead a "regulated lifestyle." By going to sleep early, exercising regularly, consuming food sparingly, and refraining from taxing his brain, Liao was finally able to feel livelier, stronger, and more at ease.[104]

While writers like Liao Qichong offered practical advice for fellow neurasthenics, other intellectuals simply sought existential commiseration. In poems and short stories, they documented their struggles to an anonymous, though supportive, readership. Some called attention to their feelings of alienation. ("I call out to the setting sun, but the setting sun doesn't answer me back. The cold wind of dusk picks up, with a 'sou sou' and a 'sah sah.'")[105] Others highlighted their intense frustration with an affliction that was both omnipresent and unrelenting. ("The chronic illness hovers over me, causing me to become anxious and depressed. Sometimes I even go so far as to think about escaping from this vexing world.")[106] By the mid-1920s, Chinese literature had become saturated with terms associated with nervous disorders. Neo-Sensationist writers like Mu Shiying (1912–1940) and Liu Na'ou (1905–1940) described the vibrancy and decadence of modern life alongside its psychological dangers. Some of these authors, as Peng Hsiao-yen has argued, likely interwove their own experiences with neurasthenia into the fictional narratives they created.[107]

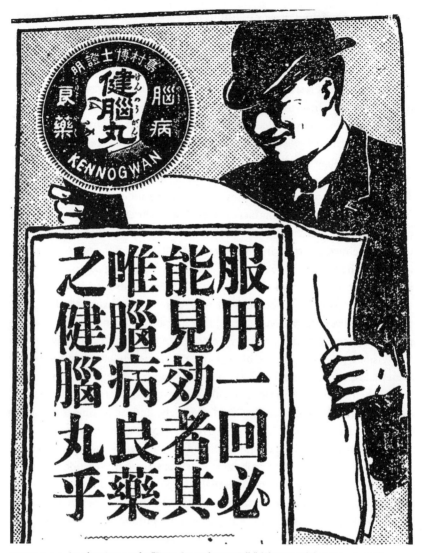

FIGURE 4.1. An advertisement for "Brain-Strengthening Pills" (*Shengjing shibao*, June 22, 1918)

What was it about neurasthenia that attracted both the attention and the financial investment of the intellectual elite? Why were so many writers willing to brand themselves neurasthenics when other forms of psychic suffering did not gain nearly the same level of existential or commercial appeal?[108] The answer to this question, I believe, must be traced to how neurasthenia had been marketed to consumers in the first place. At a time when the traditional roles of the gentry elite were being disrupted by revolution, warlordism, and

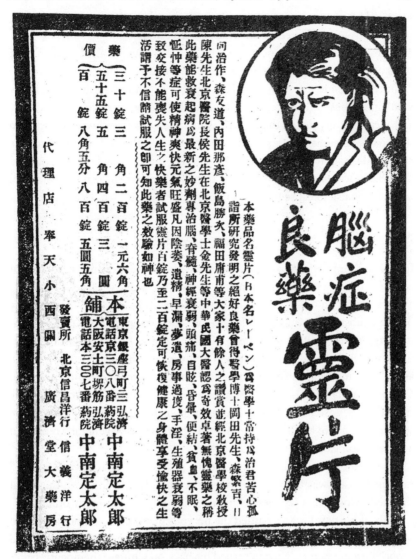

FIGURE 4.2. An advertisement for a brain-bolstering medication (*Shengjing shibao*, February 1, 1921)

imperialism, advertisements for anti-neurasthenic medications responded to anxieties about the unstable and precarious nature of elite identity. By consistently invoking the connection between mental labor and neurasthenia, and by portraying the typical neurasthenic sufferer as a modern man in a Western suit (see figures 4.1 and 4.2), proprietary medicines introduced a new way to define elitism outside of the traditional scope of gentry activity. To be elite, they suggested, one did not have to perform a specific function or social role; one simply had to participate in the adoption of a shared modern subjectivity—one defined by malaise, anxiety, and nervous weakness.

The popularity of the neurasthenic label can thus be attributed, at least partly, to the fact that advertisements for anti-neurasthenic products sold an identity alongside a commodity. Through the act of purchasing proprietary medicines, these advertisements implied that individuals could concretely and meaningfully define themselves as members of an exclusive group.[109] In this sense, capitalism intersected with current social trends to reinforce the cultural desirability of a neurasthenic identity. If consumers readily accepted the label, it was not simply because it resonated with their own psychological needs—but also because it had been purposely sold to them to do so.

The Disunity of Madness

In Lu Xun's famous 1918 parable, "Diary of a Madman," the lunatic protagonist is confined within the family home, "coop[ed] up" as if "a chicken or a duck," and treated by an old-style physician who feels his pulses but can ultimately offer no substantive advice.[110] The parable, though typically read as a scathing critique of traditional Chinese culture, can also be viewed as a lens for understanding the ordinary treatment of the insane in the early republic. Just as Lu Xun's madman is kept within the home and visited by a practitioner of Chinese medicine, so too were countless other insane men and women. Aside from those whose families were too poor to keep them—and who therefore solicited the aid of the Beijing municipality—mad people generally remained a private, domestic affair.

And yet, only a handful of years before publishing "Diary of a Madman," Lu Xun himself was treated for "symptoms [that] indicated neurasthenia" at the Ikeda Hospital, a Japanese clinic in Beijing.[111] Like so many other intellectuals of his day, Lu Xun battled the nervous disorder throughout much of his adult life, even going so far as to treat it by consuming Western-imported proprietary medicines. Having turned his back on Chinese therapeutics after witnessing his father die at the hands of an old-style practitioner, Lu Xun had briefly trained to become a biomedical physician in Japan before turning his attention to the psychologically curative power of literature instead. Regardless of his choice of profession, though, Lu Xun's passionate support of biomedicine—and his equally passionate distaste for Chinese medicine—continued to inform his medical decisions throughout the rest of his life. Persuaded by the superiority of Western forms of healing practice, Lu Xun believed that an ideological commitment to biomedicine was no less important than a commitment to Chinese revolution itself.[112]

The disparity between Lu Xun and his "madman" can be extrapolated outward onto Beijing society at large. While the urban poor continued to pursue therapeutic regimens that were little different from the ones they had employed throughout the late imperial period, petty urbanites, the wealthy elite, and the Western-oriented intelligentsia gradually became attuned to alternative discourses pertaining to "mental" illnesses and "nervous" disorders. Due to changing consumerist practices and the expanded role of the print media, new possibilities for psychiatric care had emerged by the 1920s. The physicians and businessmen whom I have referred to as "psychiatric entrepreneurs" both responded to and helped perpetuate the demand for these novel forms of treatment. Through the promotion of private hospitals and proprietary medicines, psychiatric entrepreneurs swiftly introduced new ideas about the etiology and incidence of mad disorders to an eager, and often desperate, public.

Commercialism thus played a critical role in the production and circulation of modern psychiatric knowledge. In the commercial imaginary, madness was transformed from a mere symptom of an underlying malfunction to a discrete category of disease—one that required specialized forms of medical intervention. In the process of marketing psychiatric products and services, madness itself progressively adopted new forms (the nervous illness), involved new parts of the body (the brain and nerves), and implicated new sufferers (the hardworking petty urbanites and the mentally overtaxed intelligentsia). In this way, psychiatric entrepreneurship predated the formal institutionalization of neuropsychiatry in Beijing, which would not occur until the mid-1930s.

There was one significant way in which psychiatric entrepreneurship diverged from the contemporary theory and practice of biomedical neuropsychiatry, however. While neuropsychiatry conceptualized neurasthenia and other forms of madness as taxonomically related, psychiatric entrepreneurs had dissociated the two from any common medical root. Just as Lu Xun and his "madman" represented two different approaches to managing madness, medical advertisements perpetuated an etiological and demographic divide between high-class nervous disorders and more routine forms of insanity. While the latter remained linked to pathogenic *qi* and mucous accumulation, the former became a disorder of the brain and nerves. And while ordinary types of madness could technically affect any part of the population, nervous ailments were depicted as exclusive to the intellectual elite. In the interests of appealing to the different needs and demographics of urban consumers, psychiatric entrepreneurs had cleaved elite and common madnesses into two separate conceptual categories.

It would not be until the 1930s that these two forms of madness would eventually coalesce. Through the support of the Nationalist government, neuropsychiatry was officially institutionalized at municipal facilities like the local asylum, and Chinese medicine was forced to take a back seat to the ascendant influence of biomedicine. Under the gaze of Western-trained practitioners, the various types of madness that had plagued both the upper and lower classes were ultimately unified into a single neuropsychiatric pathology. Through the authoritative power of medical science, madness would become mental illness.

From Madness to Mental Illness, 1928–1935

If little has been said about neuropsychiatry thus far, it is simply because the Western discipline has played little role in our narrative up until this point. Unlike in Japan, where psychiatric study had become fashionable from as early as the last quarter of the nineteenth century, neuropsychiatric medicine had been slow to take hold among the Chinese. Psychiatric and neurological services did exist in the country, but their scope was extraordinarily limited and resources were few.[1] And though sporadic texts on nervousness and abnormal psychology had appeared in China toward the beginning of the 1920s, most were either direct translations or loose syntheses of Japanese or English works.[2] Neuropsychiatry hence represented a lacuna in the slow but steady expansion of Western biomedicine. As the American physician Richard Lyman correctly remarked, psychiatry was "the Western [medical] specialty last to be recognized in China."[3]

The reason for the limited traction of neuropsychiatry can be traced to both cultural and practical factors. On the one hand, as Lyman observed, mad disorders had traditionally been "absorbed by other agencies," such as the family, the temple, the Chinese medicine practitioner, or (more recently) the police. As a result, "the bulk of the population" did not see the need to incorporate neuropsychiatric regimens into preexistent managerial or therapeutic strategies—particularly at a time when neuropsychiatry had not yet proved its curative worth.[4] On the other hand, and more pragmatically, only a handful of hospitals in the country offered neuropsychiatric services. In a national survey conducted in 1933, it was determined that out of 116 foreign-run hospitals in China, only six provided full care of neuropsychiatric patients, and the rest either did not admit such cases or admitted them on a strictly observational basis.[5] Opportunities for graduate training in neuropsychiatry were also exceptionally limited. A Rockefeller Foundation report from 1931 found that "facilities in China for teaching psychiatry are practically nil."[6] Of the few medical schools that did offer instruction in the discipline, moreover, they necessarily had to do so in English. Due to the paucity of Chinese terms for psychiatric concepts, students with an interest in the field were required to be at least functionally bilingual.[7]

But perhaps most importantly, the influence of neuropsychiatry had remained limited simply because the Beijing warlord government had done little to promote its expansion. In contrast to Japan, where the national government's early sponsorship of psychiatry had served to both legitimize the discipline and create national work for its practitioners, the Beijing municipality never actively pursued the institutionalization of neuropsychiatry at local facilities. Throughout the 1920s, Chinese medicine retained a monopoly at the municipal asylum. Although the country's preeminent Western medical school, the nearby Peking Union Medical College (PUMC), occasionally brought its neuropsychiatric residents to the facility for teaching demonstrations, the municipality remained hesitant about allowing foreigners to expand their role in the management and treatment of the city's insane.[8] Consequently, the PUMC's clinical visits were limited to only twice per week, while patient interviews were restricted to fifteen minutes or less.[9] Throughout the warlord period, in other words, cultural, practical, and political considerations had coalesced to stifle the advance of neuropsychiatric theory and practice.

It would not be until the early years of Guomindang (Nationalist) rule—after Beijing had been merged back into the control of a single, centralized government—that neuropsychiatry was formally incorporated into the municipal apparatus. In 1933, local functionaries of the Guomindang entered into talks with the PUMC to convert the municipal asylum into a state-of-the-art psychopathic hospital. Under the terms of their collaborative venture, the old-style Chinese physicians who had previously worked there were uniformly dismissed and replaced with biomedically trained neurologists and psychiatrists. Madness, these latter physicians insisted, was actually "mental illness," and the various manifestations of the disorder—from schizophrenia and dementia to depression and neurasthenia—all belonged to the unique jurisdiction of the neuropsychiatric specialist. As a result of the collaboration between the municipality and the PUMC, old ideas about the onset and treatment of the "mad illness" were gradually discredited and replaced with biomedical ones. From this point forward, the etiological divide that had emerged between the madnesses of the masses and the nervous disorders of the elite was fundamentally eliminated; in its stead, the PUMC considered all types of "mental illness" to be taxonomically related.

This series of events raises an important question. If neuropsychiatry had remained an overlooked and undervalued practice throughout the entirety of the warlord period, why did it finally gain legitimacy at the time that it did? The reason had nothing to do with the effectiveness or explanatory power of the discipline itself. Rather, this chapter will argue that neuropsychiatry gained authority in Beijing only when the Guomindang—acting in its own financial and political interests—decided to give it institutional support. Prior to the municipality's collaboration with the PUMC, Guomindang functionaries had paid little attention to the cause of modern psychiatry; their concern, like that of their warlord predecessors, lay strictly in routine bureaucratic matters related to the quotidian management and financing of the municipal asylum. The PUMC, conversely, had been attempting to spread neuropsychiatric ideologies to the Chinese public for the past decade and a half but had been consistently frustrated in its attempts to do so. It was only when the Guomindang recognized the expedience of working with the PUMC—and thereby decided to lend its support to the expansion of neuropsychiatry—that the discipline finally achieved epistemic authority within the capital city.[10]

This chapter highlights the critical role of state power in the advancement of new medical paradigms, and suggests that the institutionalization of neuropsychiatry in Beijing was able to occur only as a result of a vested interest on the part of the state. Recognizing the economic and political advantages of working with the PUMC, the municipality supported the development of neuropsychiatry at the Beijing asylum and its legitimation within the city at large. The ultimate triumph of neuropsychiatry, at least on an official level, thus had little to do with its ideological, explanatory, or clinical superiority. Instead, neuropsychiatry was only able to attain power because the Guomindang gave it political support.

The Nanjing Decade

In 1926, Chiang Kai-shek (1887–1975) and his Nationalist Party set off on the Northern Expedition, a military venture that aimed to eliminate warlord factionalism and unite the country under the leadership of a single political party. The movement succeeded far faster than most had anticipated. A mere two years after the expedition had decamped from the southern province of Guangdong, Nationalist troops had already reached Beijing. When they did, they were highly dissatisfied with what they saw. Despite the fact that the city had technically been the capital of the Chinese Republic for the last decade and a half, party bureaucrats perceived Beijing as mired in tradition and obeisant to its imperial roots. "Beijing is the premier region of the country, but facilities and institutions of civilization have not been developed," the Shuntian prefect lamented just prior to the Guomindang takeover. "I feel deeply sorry when I think of it." After the swift capture of the city, Chiang's soldiers began an effort to "wipe out everything"—from clothes and hairstyles to buildings and monuments—in an effort to dislocate Beijing from its imperial heritage.[11] The disorientation that occurred with these municipal renovations was exacerbated by Chiang Kai-shek's decision to move the Chinese capital south to Nanjing, thus beginning the "Nanjing Decade" (1927–1937). On June 28, 1928, the name of Beijing ("northern capital") was changed to Beiping ("northern peace"); from this point on, the city would be forced to adopt a new identity in keeping with its demoted position in national affairs.[12]

In order to solidify their grasp over Beijing, the Nationalists ousted bureaucrats whom they perceived as disloyal to the regime, replaced these vacant positions with direct appointments, and restructured multiple government organs to achieve a higher degree of centralization. The municipal asylum was one of many such institutions to undergo a bureaucratic restructuring. Prior to 1928, the asylum had been directly administered as a branch of the city's police department. Beginning in July of that year, control of the facility was transferred to a new bureaucratic body called the Social Affairs Bureau (Shehui ju), which was responsible for tasks as diverse as population surveys, cultural education, and overseeing the Public Security Bureau (Gong'an ju). While the police would still remain responsible for the quotidian management of the facility, they would henceforth need approval for all major administrative decisions, including the incarceration and discharge of inmates, from the Social Affairs Bureau rather than the chief of police.[13]

Despite this bureaucratic handover, the daily operation of the facility remained little changed from the warlord era. The functionary who had managed the asylum during the latter half of the 1920s, Lin Chuanshu, continued to hold this position after the Guomindang's arrival, and was even reappointed general manager of the facility in July 1929. When he retired a few months later, the Social Affairs Bureau replaced him with an office clerk named Zhao Jiyuan. Similar to the functionaries who had occupied the position before him, Zhao received neither specialized training for the appointment nor additional compensation for his new responsibilities. While acting as interim manager of the asylum, Zhao was simultaneously expected to fulfill the duties of his concurrent clerkship appointment and was only paid a salary commensurate with the latter position. Although the Social Affairs Bureau recognized that the situation was not optimal, it could determine no better solution to the immediate problem; instead, it simply left Zhao with the succinct instruction to expend his efforts on rectifying the facility to the best of his ability.[14]

It is perhaps unsurprising that this thorough rectification did not come to fruition under Zhao's supervision. Concerned more with daily managerial duties than long-term strategies, Zhao was only able to focus his attention on the most pressing matters at hand. Throughout the early years of Guomindang rule, and particularly as China entered an economic depression in the early 1930s, funds remained insufficient and the grain ration inadequate to care for the asylum's consistently growing population.[15] Furthermore, the minimal budget that had been allocated to the facility meant that Zhao could afford to hire only two staff members to assist him with his overwhelming bureaucratic responsibilities—a situation that "made it difficult for them to carry out their work."[16] As Zhao told a foreign visitor in 1932, the asylum was granted only $700 per month for upkeep, a sum that was used to pay not only the rent but also the salaries of physicians, attendants, and staff. After these funds were disbursed, approximately six cents per day remained to feed and care for each inmate. Consequently, no money was left to finance anything beyond the bare necessities of food and warmth, and most of the staff—eking out a living on such meager funds—took their room and board within the facility itself.[17]

Although the Social Affairs Bureau eventually conceded that Zhao Jiyuan should be relieved of his concurrent clerkship responsibilities and paid the salary of a general manager, there was only so much Zhao could do on his own to resolve the administrative issues he had inherited. Throughout his four-year tenure as manager of the asylum, the municipality's general approach to the problem of madness diverged little from that of its warlord predecessors. In fact, upon taking over the facility in 1928, the Guomindang specifically noted that there was "no fundamental need to restructure" the institution; so long as the manager "improved its organization and straightened out its affairs, this would be sufficient [yizu]."[18] The asylum therefore remained a primarily custodial facility that catered to the needs of the urban poor, and the police continued to treat the institution as the most expeditious place in which to detain the city's troublesome, disoriented, and dispossessed populations.[19] As the Austrian journalist Egon Erwin Kisch (1885–1948) tersely summarized upon visiting the asylum, the facility was simply "a police institution, a gaol for the dangerously insane, in design no different from the Peking police prison."[20]

Just as the municipality did little to alter the quotidian management of the asylum, the Guomindang also did not significantly reevaluate earlier attitudes about government responsibility for the criminally insane. The first national penal code, which was promulgated on March 10, 1928, and enacted on September 1, reworked the language of the earlier 1912 code but retained its underlying thrust. According to section four, article thirty-one, "Those who have lost their minds [*xinshen sangshi*] should not be [legally] punished [*bufa*]," but should still be "incarcerated and penalized [*jianjin chufen*] in accordance with the details of the crime."[21] In the same way as the 1912 code, the ambiguous language pertaining to the "incarceration" and "penalization" of the insane reinforced the idea that mad people were more akin to convicts than patients. But because the code again failed to specify *which* institution was responsible for the lunatic's custody, the insane continued to be shuffled among the prison, the asylum, and the familial home.[22] In the spring of 1929, for instance, an insane murderer named Xing Kun—whom the courts determined had "certainly lost his mind"—was brought to the asylum by the local police.[23] Claiming "lack of space," however, the asylum turned him away. The public prosecutor's office suggested returning Xing to his family, but it soon became clear that none of his relatives were able (or willing) to take him in. Although the case does not specify its resolution, it is likely that Xing was returned to the city jail regardless of his unstable mental condition.[24]

Given the municipality's tendency to view madness as a primarily social (rather than medical) problem, it was not coincidental that the Guomindang had decided to place the asylum under the jurisdiction of the Social Affairs Bureau rather than the Ministry of Health (Weisheng bu).[25] This was not just a local phenomenon. Outside of Beijing, too, the problem of madness continued to be treated as a chiefly sociopolitical concern. When the Social Affairs Bureau began drafting plans for the erection of an asylum in Nanjing in 1930, it attributed the urgency of the endeavor to the belief that mad people "not only leave a poor impression, but also affect public order."[26] In a similar government memorandum published a year later, the bureau further underscored the asylum's function as a symbol of engagement with the Western world. "All Western nations boast a flourishing and affluent capital, and each of these capitals has an asylum," the 1931 notice stated. "Since Nanjing is the capital of this country, and since it, too, boasts prosperous businesses and a growing population, it has become imperative that an asylum be established there."[27] Similar to the previous warlord governments, whose dual concern for social stability and political legitimacy informed their support of the Beijing asylum, the Guomindang also justified its decisions on the basis of largely sociopolitical considerations.

Yet, despite its recognition that the asylum constituted a symbolic element of Western modernity, the Guomindang nevertheless failed to acknowledge the pivotal role that *psychiatry* had come to play in the management of madness in the West. At the municipal asylum in Beijing, no attempt was made to introduce neuropsychiatric theories or treatments, and the people who staffed the facility remained skeptical of even the most basic biomedical principles. In a discussion with Egon Kisch, manager Zhao Jiyuan bluntly stated that madness is "never associated with the brain," attributing it instead to mucous and internal fire.[28] Physicians at the facility likewise continued to frame madness in terms of depletion, wetness, and exogenous pathogenic influences and treated the illness with acupuncture needles and various ointments and salves.[29] Although asylum attendants were aware that such treatments were not consistently effective, they were hardly persuaded by the efficacy of neuropsychiatry, either. When Kisch questioned Zhao about his rates of cure, the latter smiled knowingly at his Western visitor: "With us there are just as few results as with you."[30]

In short, throughout the first half decade of Guomindang rule, the municipal asylum retained the same organizational structure and therapeutic regimen that had been in place since the waning years of the Qing dynasty. It would not be until 1933, five years after the Guomindang had taken control of Beijing, that the municipality began to reconsider its approach to managing the city's insane. In that year, the American-run PUMC extended an offer to the Social Affairs Bureau to help transform the asylum into a biomedical psychopathic hospital. In so doing, it also agreed to assume the facility's daily managerial duties and half of its operational expenses. Although Chinese sources are silent on the city's motivation to collaborate with the PUMC, it is likely that the municipality recognized the immediate economic and practical benefits of working with the foreign institution—particularly at a time when the government's finances were being undercut due to the Great Depression.[31] Indeed, while the Social Affairs Bureau had done nothing to sponsor neuropsychiatry in the half decade since the asylum had been placed under its jurisdiction, it was only when the PUMC offered to assume the bulk of the financial and organizational burden that the municipality finally agreed to pursue an alternative course of action.

A Necessary Compromise

While the Beijing municipality had much to gain from the agreement to overhaul the local asylum, the PUMC stood to benefit from the collaboration as well. From the time the PUMC had been erected under the auspices of the Rockefeller Foundation in 1915,[32] the facility's physicians and board of trustees frequently debated how to handle the city's insane. Although both, at least in theory, recognized the need to educate the Chinese people on the "scientific" nature of psychopathology, a variety of deterrents—both financial and logistical—had repeatedly stymied these efforts. Consequently, by the early 1930s, PUMC physicians had made little headway in their goal to disseminate neuropsychiatric ideologies to the local population. When the PUMC eventually extended the offer of cooperation to the municipality in 1933, its decision to do so represented the culmination of close to two decades of frustration in handling the unrelenting problem of Chinese madness.

The Rockefeller Foundation's interest in the cause of mental illness can be traced to the early 1910s, just a few years before the PUMC had been established in Beijing. At the time, and as the next chapter will discuss in more depth, medical and philanthropic organizations had begun to address the long-standing issue of psychiatric mistreatment within the United States. American mental asylums, though managed by medical practitioners rather than the police, had been exposed as mired in scandal and abuse, and the stigma associated with the mentally ill served to perpetuate the neglect that they suffered at the hands of families and physicians alike.[33] By the middle of the decade, the Rockefeller Foundation had emerged as a vocal champion for the humane treatment of the insane. Compelled by the belief that the disorder was "to a large extent both preventable and curable," the trustees of the foundation aspired to promote more "rational" ideas on the care and custody of the mentally ill.[34]

Over time, the Rockefeller Foundation began to turn its attention from a strictly domestic context to an international one. Recognizing the dearth of psychiatric training facilities in China, and disparaging local treatments for the insane as "absurd,"[35] the foundation recommended that Western psychiatric concepts be transported to China alongside biomedical ones more broadly.[36] In 1919, the foundation inaugurated psychiatric and neurological teaching at the PUMC through the hire of Andrew Woods, a University of Pennsylvania–trained neurologist who had earlier served as one of the directors of the Canton Christian College.[37] Woods, like other Western physicians who had come before him, was inspired by both a missionary and a medical zeal. On the one hand, he wished to promote Christian evangelism to the godless and "heathen" Chinese.[38] On the other, he was also deeply moved by what he saw as the barbaric treatment of the mentally ill. "The sufferings of the insane," he noted solemnly at the end of his first year of service, "[are] greatly increased by the cruelties inflicted on them . . . by their own people and officers of the law." Condemning the Beijing asylum as "nothing more than a prison for insane criminals," Woods echoed the Rockefeller Foundation's call to provide both bodily and spiritual comfort to the wretched masses of the Chinese infirm.[39]

To Woods, the numerous problems associated with mental illness could not necessarily be solved through mere treatment but, more importantly, through the training of Chinese psychiatrists. Guided by the assumption that "many insane persons are curable," he believed that the Chinese themselves should assume a more proactive role in the biomedical provision of madness.[40] For this reason, Woods suggested that inpatient treatment of the insane was less pressing than the immediate formation of an undergraduate program in neuropsychiatry. By preparing Chinese "alienists" to serve in their local communities, he surmised that "public opinion in China will be educated[;] proper laws for preventing insanity and protecting the insane will be made and supported; and leaders among the Chinese medical men will be given to the country, who being supported by intelligent public opinion will be able to deal adequately with the problem."[41] With this optimistic vision in mind, Woods established the first department of neurology and psychiatry at the PUMC in 1921 and began to instruct undergraduate students soon thereafter.

Under Woods's leadership, and with support from the board of the medical college, the two disciplines of neurology and psychiatry were institutionalized at the hospital as a unified field of study.[42] The decision to do so was very much in keeping with contemporary trends in German and American medical practice. Beginning in the late nineteenth century, neurology and psychiatry had progressively been merged through an underlying belief that cerebral pathology—either in the form of diseased brains or aberrant brain functioning—was the primary cause of mental disorder. In other words, German and American medical epistemology interpreted both "mental" and "neurological" illnesses as originating from a primarily materialist basis and consequently saw no reason to distinguish organic (i.e., somatic) neuroses from functional (i.e., psychic) ones.[43] While some questioned the reductionism of this model, many of the most influential centers of medical education upheld a predominantly biological vision of both neurological and psychiatric distress—including the PUMC.[44] Indeed, by the close of the 1920s, annual reports from the hospital no longer distinguished between "diseases of the mind" and "diseases of the nervous system." Instead, intake records consolidated all such disorders—from depression and dementia to idiocy and epilepsy—under the shared anatomical classification of "nervous system."[45] Through a common emphasis on the brain and nerves as the locus of neuropsychiatric impairment, the PUMC sought to eliminate the conceptual disparities that differentiated nervous and neurological illnesses from purely "mental" ones.

Yet, despite the PUMC's desire to bridge the gap between neurological and psychiatric disorders in *theory*, the hospital continued to distinguish between the two in practice. Throughout the 1920s, physicians were instructed to refuse admittance to patients who exhibited no organic basis for their mental distress. As Roger Greene (1881–1947), acting director of the PUMC, explained in a series of correspondence, "The establishment of an in-patient service [for the insane] would be attended by some serious embarrassments." On the one hand, he was afraid that placing restraint on violent cases would arouse local resentment against foreign physicians. On the other, he suspected that the ward would quickly be filled with chronic patients who would drain the PUMC's resources and occupy their available beds. Greene accordingly suggested that Woods focus his energies strictly on neurological work; in the case that he required psychiatric patients for pedagogical or research purposes, he would have to make do with periodic visits to the municipal asylum.[46]

The plan for psychiatric treatment and instruction was thus discarded—but not forgotten. Upon Woods's retirement from the PUMC in the spring of 1928, several physicians continued to advocate for the necessary and immediate expansion of psychiatric services. Ernst DeVries (1883–1953), who helmed neurological affairs at the PUMC after Woods's departure, openly expressed his dissatisfaction at the lack of attention given to psychiatric teaching.[47] Francis Dieuaide (1892–1977), a professor of medicine, submitted a resolution that instruction in psychiatry be reintegrated into the teaching hours allotted to neurology. And Ludwik Rajchman (1881–1965), a microbiologist and medical director for the League of Nations Health Organization, complained that the hospital "lack[ed] entirely provision for psychiatry," both in regard to its staff and its clinical facilities.[48] Even Roger Greene, who had sidelined inpatient services for the mentally ill just a few years earlier, eventually admitted in 1931 that the undergraduate curriculum was "fairly complete, with the single exception of the important field of psychiatry."[49]

It is difficult to say why, exactly, the general consensus on the importance of psychiatric instruction had reached such a fever pitch immediately following Woods's retirement, but the timing of his exit might have had something to do with it. As Mary Brown Bullock notes, the consolidation of Guomindang power over Beijing in the summer of 1928 persuaded many in the PUMC chain-of-command that their "social visions might become a reality." With the cessation of warlord fighting, and with the promise that the new government might be more amenable to supporting the aims of the PUMC, reports from 1928 suggest that the governing body of the hospital looked forward to the "crystallization of a new social order in China."[50] It was, perhaps, this renewed faith in the stabilizing power of Guomindang rule that finally convinced the PUMC to move forward with its original plan for psychiatric teaching and treatment. In April 1932, the hospital's board of directors extended an offer of professorship to the psychiatrist Richard Lyman, who had trained at Johns Hopkins and developed clinical experience in Shanghai.[51] With Lyman committed to the project of psychiatric development, Roger Greene agreed to submit a budget proposal to the Rockefeller Foundation's China Medical Board for the establishment of a mental unit of twenty-five beds.[52]

Through no fault of his own, Greene's proposal was rejected almost as soon as it reached New York. This time, though, the problem had less to do with the practical considerations of psychiatric treatment in Beijing than with the unfavorable financial situation in the United States. The Rockefeller Foundation, still reeling from the stock market crash that had plunged the global economy into a financial depression, forced the China Medical Board to postpone the endowment of new funds to the PUMC.[53] Upon receiving word that his proposal had been scrapped, Greene fumed. It was not possible, he gruffly responded, for the PUMC to advance the cause of modern medicine in China given the relatively modest basis on which the college was being supported.[54] But regardless of Greene's complaints, the board remained unmoved. "What are the reasons for which the PUMC should grow," Rockefeller officer Alan Gregg (1890–1957) responded caustically to Greene's frustrated demands, "when every institution in the United States [is] experiencing cuts?"[55]

By 1933, then, both the PUMC and the Guomindang's Social Affairs Bureau had become thoroughly frustrated on the matter of insanity. While the latter had expressed its desire to rectify affairs at the municipal asylum from as early as 1929, this directive had remained easier said than done. Overcrowding and disease were continual problems, functionaries were overworked and undercompensated, and the Social Affairs Bureau had determined no better method for the rehabilitation and release of inmates than its warlord-era predecessors.[56] The PUMC, for its part, was struggling with a different sort of problem. Although physicians at the hospital had developed a feasible plan for the development of a psychiatric clinic, they were alternately straitjacketed by a lack of support and a lack of capital. In light of the problematic financial situation at the Rockefeller Foundation, the board of the hospital recognized that it would take a minimum of two years "under the best circumstances" for their proposal to even be reconsidered.[57] Thus, while the Beijing Municipal Asylum possessed the necessary space for a psychiatric unit, it had neither the finances nor a long-term vision for how the ward should be run; and while the PUMC had developed a strategy for psychiatric instruction and therapy, it lacked both the funds and the accommodations to put this plan into action.

When the PUMC proposed to collaborate with the Social Affairs Bureau on the management of the municipal asylum, it therefore did so as a matter of necessary compromise. Under ordinary circumstances, the PUMC would have had no desire to be hampered by "the quantitative problem" of handling the city's insane.[58] As the situation stood, however, the PUMC recognized that if it was to proceed with its original plans for psychiatric instruction, it would not be able to do so on its own. In May 1933, the PUMC Board of Trustees submitted a proposal to the Social Affairs Bureau suggesting that the two entities work together on the renovation and management of the Beijing asylum. Under the terms of the collaboration, the municipality and the PUMC agreed to share the expenses associated with the upkeep and expansion of the facility, thereby reducing the city's current budgetary contribution. Although the municipality would retain supervisory control over the resulting institution, the PUMC negotiated the right to guide its quotidian management, including the appointment of new physicians and staff.[59] When the agreement was signed in October of that year, it appeared to represent an expedient solution to both parties' problems.

The municipality's ultimate decision to institutionalize neuropsychiatry at the Beijing asylum can hence be considered the coincidental—and largely unforeseen—convergence between the needs of the state, the exigencies of the PUMC, and the timely intervention of an unstable world economy. Neuropsychiatry itself had very little to do with it. Yet, despite the shared sense of desperation that had brought the two together, the municipality and the PUMC gradually came to recognize the mutual benefits of their union. While the city looked forward to the PUMC demonstrating "a considerable showing of improvement" at the asylum, the PUMC also acknowledged the utility of its new position.[60] Through close contact with government functionaries, as well as daily interactions with the families of the mentally ill, physicians and social workers at the hospital recognized the pivotal role that the asylum could play in their goal to "promot[e] modern psychiatry" to both the Beijing municipality and the broader Chinese public.[61]

From Asylum to Hospital

For those even slightly familiar with the history of psychiatry in the early twentieth century, it might perhaps seem strange that the PUMC was so intent on promoting a medical discipline that was almost entirely ineffective at treating the very object of its study. Although neurologists working in Germany and the United States had made certain discoveries about the morphology of the cerebral cortex, these discoveries meant little for the rehabilitation of mental and neurological disorders. Prior to the clinical usage of the lobotomy in 1935, electroshock therapy in 1938, and psychotropic drugs in the 1950s, psychiatrists and neurologists were all but powerless to "treat" (and I use this word generously) the patients over whom they claimed professional jurisdiction.[62] Consequently, at the same time the PUMC was attempting to convert the municipal asylum into a "modern" psychopathic hospital, American psychiatric wards were combating a similarly notorious reputation for their frequent use of restraint and abuse.[63]

Yet, regardless of the empirical limitations of neuropsychiatry, the PUMC still did everything in its power to discredit the Beijing asylum and the medical practitioners who worked there. When Richard Lyman first visited the facility in late 1933, he was compelled to document its obvious hygienic and organizational deficiencies—as well as the structural improvements that it had undergone as a result of the Western intervention. In somber black-and-white, Lyman's camera captured the dirt-encrusted fingernails of the impoverished insane along with their unkempt and matted hair. In one scene, an inspector blew air onto a *kang* and smirked at the ensuing cloud of dust that emerged; in another, a group of three policemen was seen harassing an inmate before chaining his hands together and tying his torso to a pole. "In the summer of 1933, more than one hundred persons were kept in these two courtyards," a caption succinctly noted in order to explain the crowded wards and unsightly inmates. To the intended audiences of this film—the Beijing city government and the Rockefeller Foundation—the footage necessarily conveyed the inherent backwardness of the asylum and its need for immediate rectification.

When Lyman returned with his camera eight months later, the facility had been completely transformed. No longer the asylum of days past, the institution was now referred to as the Beijing Psychopathic Hospital (Beiping jingshen bing liaoyang yuan), and the "lunatics" (*fengren*) under its control had henceforth been rebranded "mental patients" (*jingshen bingren*).[64] The management of the facility, meanwhile, had been turned over to a thirty-five-year-old neurologist named Wei Yulin (1900–1968), who had received his training at both the PUMC and the University of Pennsylvania.[65] Under Wei's leadership, the newly christened patients were given baths and haircuts, and their soiled robes were exchanged for uniform cotton garments. The facility was deloused and the brick *kangs* eliminated; in brightly lit rooms with freshly polished floors, individual beds with grass mattresses appeared to take their place. Doctors perused the wards with white coats and clipboards, assuming a professional demeanor that contrasted with the style of the earlier police

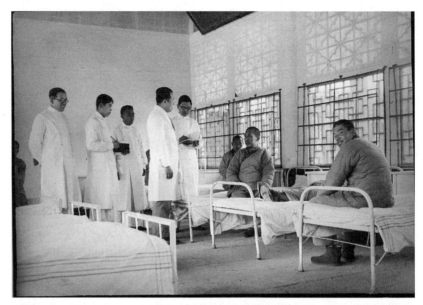

FIGURE 5.1. The newly renovated Beijing Psychopathic Hospital (from the collection "Old and New with the Insane in Peiping"; courtesy of Rockefeller Archive Center)

stewardship (see figure 5.1). And the overcrowded courtyards were expanded into an adjacent residence—five times the size of the earlier facility—that had previously been inhabited by a former Manchu prince.[66]

Moving from room to room with his camera, Lyman revealed the structural changes that had been made in the few short months since the PUMC had assumed partial command. No longer were inmates forced to eat, sleep, and receive medical treatment in the same cramped and unlit rooms where they had previously been cloistered. Following the expansion of the facility, there now existed separate spaces for nursing and administrative offices, classrooms, showers, laundry rooms, and occupational therapy, as well as separate wards, divided by sex, for "excited," "quiet," and "deteriorated" patients. Most residents took their meals in a communal canteen, where they were fed a standard diet of noodles, steamed buns, and boiled vegetables, and during the day, patients who exhibited a modicum of lucidity were encouraged to cultivate themselves through painting, calisthenics, and moderate labor. The silent film, which Lyman titled *An Eight-Month Experiment*, pithily revealed how the everyday bodily realities of the insane changed in tandem with the restructuring of their environment.[67] (See figures 5.2 and 5.3.)

In addition to implementing new hygienic standards, the PUMC also consolidated its jurisdiction over the hospital by attempting to monopolize

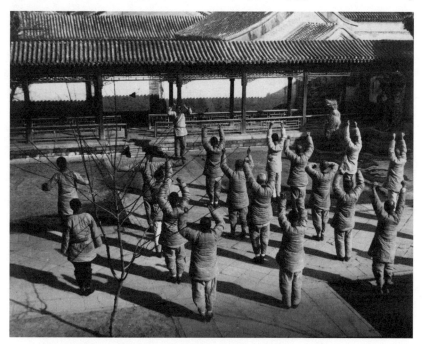

FIGURE 5.2. Patients at the Beijing Psychopathic Hospital performing calisthenics (from the collection "Old and New with the Insane in Peiping"; courtesy of Rockefeller Archive Center)

psychiatric knowledge. The new regulations for the facility, promulgated in the summer of 1934, stated that any prospective admittances to the hospital had to first be examined and confirmed insane by one of the PUMC's own physicians.[68] In contrast to the earlier asylum, which processed admittances solely on the basis of informal police assessments, the new psychopathic hospital reaffirmed the specialized and exclusive nature of biomedical expertise. This professional exclusivity was further bolstered by the complete erasure of Chinese medicine. As soon as the PUMC had taken control of the asylum, Wei Yulin dismissed its Chinese medicine practitioners and replaced their services with a coterie of biomedical physicians, pharmacists, nurses, caretakers, social workers, and occupational therapists, many of whom had been trained at the PUMC itself.[69] When families visited their relatives during strictly regulated hours, moreover, they were prohibited from bringing outside foods and medications—a statute that contrasted uncomfortably with popular modes of expressing care, but that nonetheless reinforced the exclusionism of the psychiatric specialist.[70]

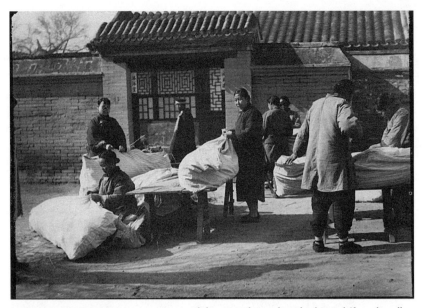

FIGURE 5.3. Patients engaging in occupational therapy at the psychopathic hospital (from the collection "Old and New with the Insane in Peiping"; courtesy of Rockefeller Archive Center)

In seeking to strengthen the epistemic power of neuropsychiatry within Beijing, PUMC physicians relied to a large extent on their privileged ability to categorize and name the various manifestations of mental illness. Unlike the police, who segregated inmates based solely on the severity of their disorder, the psychopathic hospital indicated its precise knowledge (and hence control) over the mentally ill by classifying patients according to their specific symptoms. The once monolithic category of "madness" was thus expanded to include everything from general paresis and idiocy to dementia and manic depression, while patients were no longer classed as mere "madmen" but rather as "hysterics," "paranoiacs," and "schizoids."[71] The symbolic power of psychiatric nosology not only legitimated the exclusive authority of the biomedical specialist but also allowed for greater patient diversity, both medical and socioeconomic. In the interests of attracting a moneyed clientele—who, unlike the general population, would be expected to pay for their psychiatric services—the PUMC installed first-, second-, and third-class wards.[72] By 1937, social workers at the hospital had made note of the increased economic and educational diversity of the individuals under their care; out of three hundred cases surveyed, forty-nine were students, twelve were teachers (including one college professor), and forty-eight had careers in public service (either as civil or military officers, policemen, or office clerks).[73]

But perhaps the most significant, and most obvious, changes that the PUMC implemented involved new forms of psychiatric treatment. Despite its inability to cure most forms of mental distress, the PUMC aimed, at the very least, to temporarily manage patients' symptoms in a way that exemplified the materialist orientation of contemporary neuropsychiatric practice. To that end, physicians like Wei Yulin and Richard Lyman predominantly employed whatever medicinal therapies were available at the time.[74] Barbiturates, for instance, had been clinically manufactured from as early as 1904 and served a range of functions at the psychopathic hospital: from sedating manic individuals and inducing sleep in insomniacs to relieving convulsions in epileptic patients.[75] Protracted narcosis was employed for a variety of conditions, but was most often used on people suffering withdrawal from drug addiction.[76] And fever therapy, the most promising medical breakthrough in the early treatment of neuropsychiatric disease, was believed (though never clinically proven) to be effective at killing the neurosyphilitic spirochete that caused general paresis.[77]

For most types of mental illness, however, medicinal and surgical treatments were not yet existent. Psychiatrists at the PUMC were thus forced to employ provisional, and largely managerial, remedies, whose efficacy they nonetheless sought to justify through the invocation of biological language. Hydrotherapy was one such method; consisting of baths, steams, and warm water wraps, it was believed to work by eliminating toxic impurities from the brain and spinal cord.[78] For patients whose illnesses appeared to derive from social causes, physicians occasionally employed a form of psychotherapy that was meant to bolster other somatic treatments.[79] And patients who were afflicted with a relatively mild form of mental illness were also persuaded to participate in occupational (work) therapy. At the psychopathic hospital, women washed clothes and sewed linens, while men constructed matchboxes and ground soybeans into paste.[80] Although occupational therapy had been used to varying extents in Western asylums throughout the nineteenth century, it had not gained biomedical credence until 1929 when the German psychiatrist Hermann Simon (1867–1947) attempted to explain its efficacy using scientific language. Claiming that the focused use of motor skills had a beneficial impact on the brain, Simon asserted that labor could play a critical role in maintaining "cerebral hygiene."[81]

Regardless of the seemingly objective language in which these therapies were embedded, they were generally unable to achieve a permanent cure. In the summer of 1935, the city government compiled statistics on the number of patients who had been admitted, discharged, and cured from the psychopathic hospital over a six-month period. The results were woefully underwhelming. Out of a total of 292 patients, approximately two-thirds remained in residence at the end of the investigation period. Of those who had been released, moreover, most had either died at the facility or been discharged for reasons that did not relate to their health; only forty patients during this time were said to have been "cured."[82] These statistics, however, do not account for the patients who were later readmitted to the facility upon suffering a psychiatric relapse. According to sociological data compiled at the hospital, approximately 12 percent of cases were admitted either two or three times over the one-year period from October 1934 to October 1935.[83] Low turnover rates caused available beds to quickly become occupied by chronic, recidivist, and incurable cases; as a municipal communiqué succinctly observed, "Those who enter are many, while those who are released are few."[84] The problem of overcrowding was so urgent, in fact, that Richard Lyman later admitted that the facility was "dangerously near [to] becoming just a custodial institution."[85]

Setting aside the rhetoric and trappings of scientific modernity for a moment, it becomes apparent that the PUMC's approach to managing mental illness was perhaps not as distinct from the earlier police approach as it might have seemed on the surface. While the two certainly differed in certain regards—particularly in terms of how they framed the underlying source of mental distress—in many other ways the PUMC merely legitimized former strategies by couching them in the rhetoric of scientific rationalism. Both the PUMC and the municipal police believed that the best recourse to mental illness was confinement within an institutional setting. Both employed methods of restraint, and freely admitted to the use of ropes and chains.[86] Both treated the mad condition primarily through therapies that acted on the material body. And both underscored the close relationship between mental convalescence and an ability or desire to labor. What neither could achieve, however, was a surefire remedy, and so both the psychopathic hospital and the previous asylum accumulated chronic patients while being critiqued as mere "custodial" institutions.

Despite its low rate of cure, the PUMC-managed facility nevertheless gained the vocal and wholehearted support of the Beijing city government. The reason it did so was not because the municipality was convinced of the functional superiority of neuropsychiatry; indeed, as one government memorandum bluntly acknowledged, biomedicine contained "no medicinal cures for mental illness" but could only "calm [the patient], and that was all" (*zhenjing eryi*).[87] Rather, local bureaucrats threw their support behind the PUMC for altogether different reasons: specifically, because they recognized that the psychopathic hospital could be invoked as a symbolic marker of *difference*. In other words, by maligning the previous asylum and praising the new facility, the Guomindang strove to distinguish itself from the earlier warlord governments. As a 1934 report suggested, the police-managed asylum "just took people in but did not treat them," and therefore "those who entered it rarely came out alive [*xian shenghuan*]."[88] The new psychopathic hospital, by contrast, had "renovated everything." By emphasizing hygiene, rehabilitation, and personalized care, the facility strove to offer "curative opportunities to mentally ill people at all levels of society."[89] Conveniently overlooking the fact that these changes had been made only half a decade into Guomindang rule—and that the municipality, just a few years earlier, had seen "no need to fundamentally reorganize" the warlord asylum—the report aimed to drive a wedge between the benevolence of the new government and the cruelty of the preceding regime.

For the Guomindang, the pursuit of neuropsychiatry was intimately linked to the cause of government legitimacy—and relatedly, to the consolidation of its political power. It therefore made little difference that neuropsychiatry was no better at curing madness than Chinese medicine had been before it. What mattered instead was that the new facility embodied the intensely modernist characteristics of hygiene, bureaucratic rationalism, and scientific expertise—characteristics that could easily signal the Guomindang's distance from its warlord forerunners, and hence provide justification for its political mandate to rule. This position was concisely articulated in the preface to a lengthy municipal report. The previous government, the report noted, had "produced no noticeable progress or results" when it came to the health of its citizens. In contrast, it was only after the Guomindang had ascended to power that these past failings were "wiped clean and corrected" to directly "benefit the people."[90]

Spreading Scientific Psychiatry beyond the Hospital

Having gained the support of the Guomindang, the PUMC endeavored to further extend its influence by integrating psychiatric principles into law, policing, and general domestic care. While this had long been a goal for physicians like Andrew Woods and Richard Lyman, the PUMC was able to make headway only once it had obtained the backing of the municipal government. Prior to that time, practitioners at the PUMC had generally believed that the diffusion of psychiatric knowledge would mainly occur through the training of Chinese doctors. When the Guomindang agreed to collaborate with the PUMC on the renovation of the psychopathic hospital, however, the latter's unique position as head of psychiatric work for the city enabled its physicians to rethink their earlier position. By working closely with the municipal

government, they realized, the PUMC would be able to pursue more immediate action toward the large-scale proselytization of a new vision of mental
health.[91]

In order to influence public attitudes about the insane, the PUMC first
turned its focus to the municipal police. Although the police no longer managed the psychopathic hospital directly, they still acted as a pivot between the
facility, the families of mentally ill individuals, and Beijing society at large.
More specifically, the police played a role in two-thirds of all admittances to
the psychopathic hospital and were similarly responsible for directing discharged patients back to their families or to other municipal institutions.[92]
Because of their close contact with the local community, the PUMC aimed to
"effect . . . a better understanding of the work of the hospital by the police" by
instructing them in the language, values, and assumptions of contemporary
neuropsychiatry.[93]

In a survey conducted between 1934 and 1935, the psychiatric social worker
Francis Hsü discussed the deficiencies in current police approaches to handling the mentally ill. Hsü noted that the police typically only intervened in
cases of madness when the person had "endangered public safety" or "tres-
passed on [another person's] lawful rights." Those with more subtle tendencies,
however, were frequently overlooked; consequently, many mentally ill people
in need of hospitalization still remained at large. In addition, Hsü pointed out
that the police often used "unclear and ambiguous terms" when reporting the
details of the case to the hospital, thereby obscuring necessary facts that could
be used in the patient's treatment and rehabilitation. And finally, Hsü continued, whenever patients were discharged from the hospital and released to the
custody of the police, they stood a lower chance of recovery than those who
had been released directly to their families. In order to rectify these problems,
Hsü suggested that the PUMC educate the police on "mental illness and its
treatment as well as the ideals of the Psychopathic Hospital." Recommending
that the staff of the facility conduct interviews with police authorities, arrange
police visits to the hospital, and publish "propaganda" for educational purposes, Hsü believed that such actions would enable the police to better align
their work with the mission of the PUMC.[94]

Correspondence between the psychopathic hospital and the Public Security Bureau reveal the PUMC's early attempts to educate the police on the
proper treatment of the mentally ill. In the spring of 1935, for example, the
psychopathic hospital sent a long memorial to the chief of police concerning
a woman who had been rehabilitated after receiving treatment at the facility. Because the police had failed to notify her family for the better part of a
month, however, the woman had relapsed and could no longer be discharged.

"We are very regretful [about this mix-up]," the secretary of the psychopathic hospital wrote. "But honestly speaking, the mentally ill have very weak wills, and various stimuli can easily cause them to fall sick. The patient cannot be returned home, or she will necessarily succumb to vexation and illness." The memorial suggested that in the future, the Public Security Bureau develop protocols that would allow them to notify the patient's family in a timelier manner. Critiquing the dismissive attitude that the police still maintained about the insane, the memorial concluded with the following admonition: "We must cherish and care for [mentally ill] patients. I hope you do not take these words lightly."[95]

Memorials from the psychopathic hospital did not just chide the police when they failed to align their attitudes with the new expectations of psychiatric modernity. In addition, workers at the facility also attempted to redress the high rate of relapse that patients suffered when they were discharged to the custody of the police rather than to their families. "When patients are poverty-stricken or have no family to return to," a memorandum from October 1935 began, "the reason they fall ill [again] often has to do with the fact that their environmental stimuli are poor. If they are discharged from the hospital and take up a roving [lifestyle] with nobody to look after them, the old illness will necessarily return." To that end, the memorial reminded the Public Security Bureau that rehabilitated patients without a family should be transferred to the municipal almshouse rather than left to their own devices. This course of action would certainly "aid in relieving the distress of the patient" while helping to prevent a relapse of the disorder.[96]

In a way, much of the information conveyed in the above memorials was not new. The idea that "environmental stimuli" could induce madness had long been a central component of Chinese medical philosophy, and the expectation that mad people without families should be transferred to other municipal facilities had likewise been the norm throughout the warlord period. What was significant about the above memorials, rather, was the paternalistic tone that the writer had adopted toward the mentally ill. Prior to the 1930s, the police had arguably been more preoccupied with maintaining municipal order than protecting the well-being of the mad person. Even Francis Hsü acknowledged that "the duty of the police is naturally and primarily to maintain the public safety," and anything beyond that responsibility was felt to be the purview of other governmental organs.[97] After the PUMC's takeover of the psychopathic hospital, however, the police were held to a higher standard when it came to the health of the city's insane. As key participants in the new psychiatric welfare apparatus, the police were not only expected to act as guardians of social stability, but also as custodians of the debilitated and dispossessed. The mentally ill, meanwhile, were no longer to be treated as mere delinquents, but rather as genuinely sick individuals in need of appropriate, and compassionate, aid.

In order to streamline and systematize the institutional care of the mentally ill, physicians and social workers at the PUMC worked closely with state organs to craft new legal statutes. By 1935, the Guomindang's revised penal code differed substantially from its 1928 counterpart on matters of mental illness. According to Article 87 of the revised code, "Those who have lost their minds should not be punished, but should be sent to an appropriate facility [*xiangdang chusuo*] and placed under guardianship [*jianhu*]." Unlike the earlier penal code, which stated that the insane should be "incarcerated and penalized [*jianjin chufa*]," the new code purposely relieved the mentally ill of both legal responsibility *and* moral culpability.[98] For the first time since the waning years of the Qing dynasty, the Chinese government had excised the stipulation that mentally ill people be disciplined for their wrongdoings. And while the Guomindang continued to believe that confinement of the insane was legally necessary, the 1935 code was the first to specify that the mentally ill be placed under guardianship within "an appropriate facility" rather than locked in a prison or kept in the home.

The PUMC recognized that this new statute, though constructive, represented a mere "embryo of a system." In an effort to further shape the future of forensic psychiatry in China, the PUMC collaborated with legal scholars at Peking University to create a more specific classificatory mechanism for the adjudication of psychiatric cases. It proposed, for instance, that those with neurasthenia and nervousness be considered fully responsible for their actions, those with light cases of melancholia and traumatic neurosis be eligible for a reduced sentence, and those with more serious disorders such as dementia praecox (schizophrenia) and idiocy be relieved of all legal responsibility. Through this expanded definition of mental illness, the PUMC strove to institutionalize a more nuanced understanding of psychiatric nosology into the Chinese legal system, thereby confirming the need for psychiatric specialists to participate in the adjudication and sentencing of the criminally insane.[99]

Although many of the PUMC's early efforts to achieve psychiatric reform were aimed at government functionaries, physicians at the psychopathic hospital also tried to educate patients' families on the new norms of neuropsychiatric practice. They did so mainly through the use of PUMC-trained social workers. The Social Service Department at the PUMC had been an integral part of the college's rehabilitative program since 1921. Inspired by the Johns Hopkins medical school, which had established a social services department as early as 1912, social workers at the PUMC believed that a patient's full rehabilitation required physical, emotional, and economic support.[100] At the psychopathic hospital, Richard Lyman acknowledged the important role that social workers could play in both the treatment of the mentally ill and the dissemination of neuropsychiatric ideologies. His thinking on the matter derived from his own medical training at Johns Hopkins, where he had been the student of the renowned psychiatrist Adolf Meyer (1866–1950). Meyer was a forerunner in the use of psychiatric social workers in the United States. Believing that mental disorders were the genesis of both biological and social factors, his particular approach to neuropsychiatry involved collecting patients' case histories, compiling records about their familial and social backgrounds, and making home visits.[101]

As head of neuropsychiatry at the PUMC, Richard Lyman spoke openly about the need to incorporate sociologists and social workers into clinical psychiatric services. Unlike his predecessor Andrew Woods, who was far more materialist in outlook, Lyman recognized the benefits of integrating social and physical factors into a "balanced perspective of the whole." As he explained, one of his ambitions in Beijing was to encourage "the training of nonmedical workers as part of the psychiatric unit," which would allow psychologists and sociologists to contribute to neuropsychiatry alongside biomedical physicians.[102] To that end, Lyman employed psychiatric social workers to act as an intermediary between the hospital and the home. For patients whose mental symptoms stemmed from obvious social, familial, or economic causes, social workers were instructed to interview the patient's family, employer, and neighbors about the onset of the condition; take detailed notes about the patient's home environment, income, employment history, and previous medical and social issues; and prepare clinical case files and sociological data based on the information they had collected.[103] Similar to long-standing Chinese beliefs about the social, environmental, and biological nature of madness, PUMC social workers attempted to adjoin these factors into a coherent etiological whole.

In addition to gathering information about individual patients, social workers also transmitted medical knowledge from physicians to families. According to the psychiatric social worker Song Siming, one of his main functions at the hospital was to educate families about the secular (rather than supernatural) origins of mental illness and to convince them that psychiatric disorders should not be stigmatized.[104] On a more routine level, social workers also helped to translate and interpret psychiatric diagnoses, explain the importance of necessary medications, and quell fears about the risks of certain surgical procedures. Since many patients were initially resistant to neuropsychiatric treatments, social workers played a critical role in explaining the logic of the recommended regimen and persuading families to offer their consent.[105]

After the patient had been discharged from the hospital, furthermore, social workers often paid follow-up visits to the familial home. There, they ensured that the patient was continuing to heed the advice of his or her physician and had not reverted to traditional therapies. In this way, social workers helped to disseminate neuropsychiatric ideas to the broader public.[106]

By involving itself in municipal psychiatric work, the PUMC attempted to propagate the values, approaches, and language of "modern psychiatry" to the Beijing populace. While it is difficult to measure the impact they achieved in such a short period of time, the increasing use of psychiatric vocabularies in municipal police files points to the possibility of an incipient epistemological shift. Throughout the mid-1930s, the police progressively replaced the traditional epithet of "madman" with neologisms for "mental illness" and "neurosis," and although some police memorials continued to reference the outdated "asylum," most functionaries had easily made the shift to speaking about the "psychopathic hospital."[107] Through routine interactions with the PUMC, municipal policemen were forced to confront new ideas about the modern provision of mental illness. And through the regular deployment of psychiatric social workers, the PUMC aimed to further disseminate biomedical ideologies beyond the confines of the institution. Though their progress constituted only a "modest accomplishment," it represented, at the very least, "an indication of the emergence of psychiatry in China."[108]

The Adoption of Mental Illness

In January 1934, the Beijing Psychopathic Hospital was removed from the control of the Social Affairs Bureau and placed under the jurisdiction of the Ministry of Health.[109] This shift, though inconsequential to the quotidian management of the facility, was ultimately significant for what it revealed about contemporary government attitudes toward the mentally ill. For the first time since the municipality had become involved in the institutionalization of the insane in the late Qing, the Chinese government had adopted the position that mental illness was a primarily medical, rather than social, concern. As a consequence of this bureaucratic transfer, the final arbiters of insanity changed from agents of social stability to agents of medical expertise, and the municipality—previously held responsible for the mere incarceration of the mentally ill—soon became responsible for their rehabilitation as well.

That this institutional changeover occurred when it did was not a foregone conclusion. To the contrary, the institutionalization of neuropsychiatric medicine in Beijing only transpired as a result of the coincidental intersection between municipal needs and PUMC frustrations. Prior to the municipality's

1933 agreement with the PUMC, neuropsychiatry had remained a marginalized practice—both within the city and within the PUMC itself. Due to the government's earlier lack of interest in the subject, the Beijing asylum continued to perpetuate norms of incarceration and treatment that had been established long before the Guomindang had come to power. Limited funds and unfavorable conditions within the PUMC, meanwhile, had caused the latter's pursuit of neuropsychiatric instruction, research, and treatment to suffer a string of disappointing setbacks. Halfway into the Nanjing Decade, neuropsychiatry remained exceptionally limited as both a medical discipline and a therapeutic practice.

It was not until the PUMC attached itself to the state—and the state, in turn, attached itself to the epistemic prestige of biomedicine—that psychiatric reform began to occur on a substantial scale. Through the legitimizing power of the municipal government, neuropsychiatric practices were institutionalized both within the psychopathic hospital and outside of it. Working with the police, the PUMC began to disseminate new ideas about the adjudication and management of mental illness; collaborating with local scholars, physicians revised long-standing legal statutes relating to the appropriate detention of the criminally insane; and by involving psychiatric social workers in the process of mental rehabilitation, the PUMC attempted to popularize neuropsychiatric ideas while simultaneously discrediting indigenous ones. Through its ties to mechanisms of state power, the PUMC did more to advance its vision of psychiatric modernity in the span of a mere two years than it had over the entirety of the past two decades.

The PUMC was not the only one to benefit from this alliance. Although archival sources do not address the municipality's motivations directly, it is likely that the city government only agreed to work with the PUMC out of a calculated decision that the collaboration would contribute to its own material and political interests. In light of the constant economic and bureaucratic complications at the municipal asylum, the Social Affairs Bureau willingly relinquished oversight of the bothersome institution to the far more enthusiastic management of the PUMC. Yet once the arrangement had gotten under way, the municipality continued to support the expansion of neuropsychiatry for altogether different reasons. By emphasizing the obvious structural changes that differentiated the psychopathic hospital from the earlier warlord asylum, the Guomindang was able to highlight the disparities between its own approach to social welfare and that of the preceding regimes. In so doing, the city government both justified its political legitimacy and solidified the place of neuropsychiatry within the new bureaucratic order.

Over time, neuropsychiatry would come to provide an authoritative rationale for the perpetuation—and expansion—of the municipality's incarceration of errant bodies. As a result of its tacit acceptance of contemporary psychiatric nosology, the municipality sanctioned the broadening boundaries of *who* could be considered mentally ill. By the close of the 1930s, and as the next chapter will discuss, the Ministry of Health would no longer be held responsible for just the institutionalization of the poor, homeless, or violent insane. Instead, as interest in Western conceptions of mental illness continued to grow, Chinese intellectuals gradually came to demand that the state intervene in far more routine instances of behavioral deviance as well—from delinquency and truancy to homosexuality and prostitution. Claiming a concern over the nation's collective "mental hygiene," these intellectuals would advocate for a far more proactive, intrusive, and permanent solution to the problem of mental illness than had ever previously been proposed.

Mental Hygiene and Political Control, 1928-1937

In 1921, half a decade before the Guomindang launched its Northern Expedition to reunify the Chinese nation, the American neurologist Andrew
Woods gave a lecture at Peking University on the "menace of insanity to popular government." "The way most quickly to secure political stability and to
make armies unnecessary," Woods asserted, "is to advance the general level
of mental efficiency . . . among the common people." The implications of this
statement would not have gone unnoticed by those in attendance. At the time
of his speech, China was still embroiled in warlord factionalism and struggling to come to terms with the encroaching forces of Japanese imperialism.
Rather than blaming China's political instability on material or technological
deficiencies, however, Woods suggested that many of the country's difficulties
could be ascribed to the problem of "insanity." Insanity, as he understood it,
did not refer strictly to the "raving maniacs" who required institutionalization. Rather, the category also encompassed those with "dangerously inefficient mental functioning," including "imbeciles, idiots, or morons"; "epileptics
or criminals"; and all sorts of individuals "who are sound but unproductive."
Because these types of people could not "hold their own in the struggle for
existence," they necessarily inhibited the evolutionary progress of the Chinese
nation and race. Woods's speech, in other words, framed insanity in national
terms. Due to the obviously antagonistic relationship between madness and
political stability, Woods urged his Chinese audience to seriously consider
"what [their] government ought to do about the mental health of its people."[1]

Although Woods's lecture did not make a considerable impact at the time
it was given, ten years later his argument would be taken up in a far more serious fashion. By the 1930s, the concept of "mental hygiene" had thoroughly
penetrated Chinese intellectual discourse. An idea that originated in the United

States in the first decade of the twentieth century, mental hygiene embodied two distinct meanings: a humanitarian concern over the welfare of the mentally ill and an authoritarian concern over order and social control.[2] Initially, the movement primarily focused on ameliorating care for the insane and preventing mental disorders from forming. By the end of the First World War, however, supporters of mental hygiene had gradually begun to emphasize a more radical prophylactic approach as well. Fearful that mentally ill people were polluting the gene pool and contributing to social instability, physicians and politicians alike campaigned for laws that would allow for the compulsory segregation or sterilization of "mental defectives." Although the dual aims of mental hygiene might have appeared contradictory to some, they were commonly considered to be complementary facets of the same endeavor: to eradicate the scourge of psychiatric disorders from the face of modern civilization. Indeed, even Andrew Woods spoke explicitly about the need for either "the rehabilitation or the elimination of the mentally diseased."[3]

As the cause of mental hygiene gained international attention, it enabled a mass paranoia on matters of madness. On the brink of the Second World War, madness appeared almost inescapable; as new neuroses were "discovered" by Western psychiatric professionals, a greater swath of people became implicated in their web. A Rockefeller Foundation report, concisely summarizing the state of the field, remarked in 1936 that mental hygiene was concerned with not just the obvious forms of madness but also the "anxieties, phobias, tantrums, complexes, and anomalous or unbalanced behavior of otherwise normal human beings."[4] The belief that psychiatric disorders could affect "normal" as well as "abnormal" individuals blurred the line between sanity and unreason, and enabled psychiatrists to diagnose mental illness whenever a person's behavior deviated from a communally sanctioned norm. Claiming that nonconformity was, in fact, a signal of poor mental health, psychologists, social workers, and other advocates of mental hygiene justified their intrusion into the home, school, and workplace on the grounds that the early identification of psychiatric symptoms could enable the prevention of full-blown madness at a later date. As a consequence of their efforts, fear of mental illness gradually extended from the asylum to the society at large.

When the Chinese intelligentsia began to turn their attention to the problem of mental hygiene in the 1930s, they never treated "madness" as a purely apolitical concern. Just as Andrew Woods had framed insanity as a matter of urgent public interest, Chinese intellectuals interpreted the disorder less as an individual problem than a sociopolitical one; convinced that psychiatric illnesses were contributing to the sluggish advance of Chinese nationhood, they advocated for a more preemptive, systematic, and far-reaching approach to the eradication of madness than had ever previously been suggested. Their motivation for doing so was influenced to a large extent by contemporary Western discourses on eugenics, euthenics, and social engineering. Believing that the elimination of the unfit was a necessary step in the evolutionary progress of mankind, the intelligentsia interpreted mental disease as a barrier to achieving a healthier and more unified citizenry—and hence a stronger and more powerful nation. Throughout the latter half of the Nanjing Decade, the pursuit of mental hygiene was integrated into the Chinese context as a synecdoche for broader concerns with national deficiency and national self-strengthening.

This chapter steps away from Beijing to explore the relationship that was forged between psychology and politics on a national scale. In so doing, it highlights how the concept of mental hygiene was implemented in China toward the ends of achieving social conformity and enabling the authoritarian control of the Guomindang. Although China's preliminary exploration of mental hygiene had just begun to gain momentum when it was prematurely cut short by war with Japan in 1937, the alliance of psychiatry, psychology, and politics that arose over the course of the decade served to reorient the concern over mental illness away from a myopic focus on the psychopathic hospital and toward the broader society. The Chinese mental hygiene movement, short-lived though it might have been, was thus sufficient to signal that the right-wing intelligentsia and the Guomindang both recognized the practical utility of scientific psychology—not simply as a curative mechanism but, more importantly, as a technology of power.

The Origins of Mental Hygiene

In the 1930s, Chiang Kai-shek and his Nationalist Party continued to be plagued by many of the same problems that had haunted the Chinese nation throughout the warlord period. Although Chiang's extensive military apparatus had nominally unified the country in 1928, the perils of warlordism, communism, and Japanese imperialism continually threatened to tear it apart. Chiang, confronted by domestic discontent and external invasion, turned to nationalism as a potential "centripetal force" by which to counter the multiple threats undermining the advance of his regime.[5] If the Chinese people could simply be compelled to sacrifice their individual interests for the grander cause of nationalism, Chiang believed, then the various problems that beleaguered the nation would be no match for the power of a unified Chinese citizenry.

The problem with this line of thinking was that Chiang was fundamentally unable to channel the existing loyalties of the Chinese people into unswerving support for his party. Throughout the Nanjing Decade, he experimented with several strategies—including Leninist organization, military dictatorship, and fascism—in order to redirect preexistent allegiances toward the Guomindang. While he was able to forge a coterie of devoted backers among members of the right-wing intelligentsia, most people remained outwardly resistant to his militaristic rule. As Julia Strauss has noted, "The existing norms of the society in which the regime was embedded . . . [continued to sanction] familialism, cliquism, and the conflation of public interest with private gain."[6] Without a charismatic leader to bring them together, the Chinese people remained atomized and alienated from national politics. Just as Sun Yat-sen had observed many years earlier, they resembled little more than "a sheet of loose sand."[7]

It was against this backdrop that Chinese intellectuals began to give attention to the problems and possibilities of mental hygiene (*xinli weisheng* or *jingshen weisheng*). Although the concept of mental hygiene did not gain traction in China until the mid-1930s, the term—and the international movement it generated—had already been in existence for over two decades by that point. The idea for the movement first developed in the United States through the work of a mental health advocate named Clifford Beers (1876–1943). Throughout his youth, Beers had suffered from a condition that he alternately described as "shattered nerves," "depression," "neurasthenia," a "disordered brain," or a "capitulat[ion] to Unreason."[8] In 1900, after experiencing a mental breakdown and attempting suicide, Beers was committed to a sanatorium. There, he suffered regular abuse at the hands of attendants and physicians, many of whom sought to "profit through the misfortunes of others."[9] When Beers recovered a few years later, he reached out to the psychiatrist Adolf Meyer—the mentor of PUMC physician Richard Lyman—in an attempt to create an organized program for the improvement of mental healthcare. Together, the two established the National Committee for Mental Hygiene (NCMH) on February 19, 1909.[10]

Throughout its existence, the objectives of the NCMH were both poorly defined and constantly shifting.[11] At the time the organization was founded, the goal of mental hygiene was straightforward: to eliminate the stigma of mental illness and improve treatment and care for the mentally ill. Over the course of the next decade, however, the implications of mental hygiene gradually expanded. Due in large part to the discovery of "shell shock" during the First World War, psychiatrists came to the realization that psychoses and neuroses could develop over time in otherwise normal and well-functioning people—particularly if their environmental conditions were unsound.[12] This realization had a profound impact on the future direction of the international mental hygiene movement. If, as the American neuropsychiatrist William White (1870–1937) explained, mentally ill patients simply represented the "end products of many years of bad mental hygiene," then the goal of the movement was not just to treat these individuals retroactively but, more importantly, to determine methods by which to "[cut] off the source of mental disease at its origin."[13] From the late 1910s onward, therefore, the focus of mental hygiene shifted to involve prevention as well as care, with a major emphasis being placed on childhood education and the rearing of psychologically healthy youths.[14]

As the objectives of mental hygiene broadened, psychologists began to participate in the movement alongside psychiatrists. By the 1920s, the two had positioned themselves on opposite, yet complementary, sides of the mental hygiene endeavor. While neuropsychiatry progressively came to be understood as the "negative side of mental hygiene" due to its purely reactive utility, psychologists—alongside educators, sociologists, and lawmakers—attempted to prevent psychiatric symptoms from occurring in the first place.[15] Focusing predominantly on the development of mental hygiene programs in elementary schools, child psychologists aimed to instill in children "habits, ideas, and ideals of order" that would continue to guide their conduct for the rest of their adult lives.[16]

In their frantic search for early indications of mental illness, psychologists became acutely attuned to any type of behavior that could potentially be classified as abnormal. Frankwood Williams (1883–1936), who served as medical director for the NCMH beginning in 1922, pointed out that poor mental health could be evinced not only by the obviously insane but also by more subtle personality types, such as the "domineering, arbitrary father," the "clinging mother," and the "overly modest, overly religious, overly kind individual." The difference between these persons and those with more conspicuous forms of functional psychosis, he argued, "is not so much a matter of kind as of degree."[17] Being mentally ill, in other words, no longer meant the opposite of being mentally healthy; rather, the two were reconceptualized as mere degrees on a continuum. As mental hygienists portrayed "deviant" behaviors as signs of an emerging pathology, socially questionable traits such as criminality, truancy, homosexuality, naughtiness, feeblemindedness, and "all forms of social maladjustment and even unhappiness" came to be seen as distinct markers of an inchoate mental malfunction, and therefore the potential target of medical intervention.[18]

Although the NCMH had originally been established to ensure the welfare of psychiatric patients, over time a more socially oriented strain of thinking began to occupy the attention of its supporters. As mental hygienists continued to conflate mental illness and social deviance, they turned from a narrow focus on the health of the individual to a broader concern over the health of society. Given the growing fear that psychiatric disorders were incurable, degenerative, and ultimately detrimental to the overall fitness of the national body, physicians and lawmakers began to advocate for a more proactive and permanent solution to what they saw as a countrywide crisis. By the 1930s, the NCMH had acknowledged the need for a eugenic approach to the mentally ill, a decision that was widely supported within American politics. Herbert Hoover (1874–1964), the thirty-first president of the United States and an enthusiastic supporter of eugenics, held a conference in 1930 at which he advocated for the "selective" sterilization of the mentally unfit. In conjunction with the 1927 *Buck v. Bell* court ruling, which upheld the right to asexualize mentally defective individuals, thirty American states were compelled to pass sterilization laws over the course of the next decade.[19]

On the eve of the Second World War, mental hygiene encompassed two distinct—yet somehow entirely complementary—views. On the one hand, as Clifford Beers put it, the movement was concerned with the need to foster a "more rational public attitude toward mental illness and the hygiene of mind." Through educational work and the support of neuropsychiatric research, the NCMH aspired to reclaim the mental patient "from a very long period of neglect and inhumanity."[20] On the other hand, and particularly as the cause of mental hygiene gained increased attention within the public at large, the movement simultaneously sought to reduce the threat of mental illness for the general improvement of the nation and race. By applying psychological principles toward the goal of forging socially useful and well-adjusted citizens—and by implementing eugenic measures on those who could not be redeemed—proponents of mental hygiene insisted that their discipline would contribute to the creation of a fitter populace.

When Chinese intellectuals first encountered the concept of mental hygiene, it was this latter interpretation that they found most persuasive: namely, the possibility of preemptively eliminating behavioral deviance to achieve a healthier and more unified society. If scholars in China found these discourses compelling, they were certainly not alone. By this point in the twentieth century, mental hygiene—and its concomitant ideal of racial and national self-strengthening—had become an international phenomenon. From the United States and Canada to Germany and Japan, all "civilized" nations searched for ways to improve their national clout and racial stock through social engineering.[21] When scholars imported these ideas to China in the middle of the Nanjing Decade, therefore, they remained confident that they were at the forefront of a thoroughly scientific movement—one that could save the Chinese nation, once and for all, from the many problems that threatened its continued existence.

Psychology and Society in China

The seeds of mental hygiene began to enter the Chinese imagination in the 1920s, when intellectuals were increasingly traveling to the United States and Western Europe to pursue advanced degrees in the field of psychology. Unlike neuropsychiatry, which remained a relatively understudied discipline in China even throughout the Nanjing Decade, psychology had captured the attention of the intelligentsia from as early as the 1910s. Concerned more with mental processes than mental illnesses, psychology had perhaps appeared less foreign to Chinese sensibilities than scientific psychiatry. Indeed, as many intellectuals were quick to point out, psychology—or the "study of the principles of the heart-mind" (*xinli xue*)—had been extant in China since at least the time of Confucius. The famous thinker Liang Qichao (1873-1929), for instance, argued in 1923 that psychology was a fundamental component of Confucian ideology, while the psychologist Gao Juefu (1896-1993) observed that a strain of psychological thought had emerged in China from as early as the Warring States period (475-221 BC).[22]

Nevertheless, while psychology and Confucian metaphysics may have both interrogated the nature of human consciousness, the type of psychological thinking that existed in imperial China was far removed from the nascent experimental psychology of the twentieth-century Western world. Considered a social science rather than a branch of philosophy, contemporary psychology was less concerned with abstract ontological questions than the empirical study of cognitive and behavioral processes. Situated in the laboratory, experimental psychologists strove to transform their discipline into a rigorous and empirically verifiable science through the close observation of animal and human subjects. They therefore aimed not just to describe behavior, but more importantly to quantify—and perhaps even control—it.[23]

It was scientific psychology's purported ability to explain and manipulate human behavior that quickly attracted the consideration of the Chinese intelligentsia. As the historian Geoffrey Blowers has noted, the earliest Chinese psychologists were drawn to the discipline because they believed that a scientific understanding of human psychology would enable them to foster "correct patterns of behavior" and a "healthy mind."[24] More interested in the practical utility of applied psychology than its philosophical rationale, intellectuals scoured translated texts for insights into social conditioning techniques. The influential educator and president of Peking University Cai Yuanpei (1868-1940), for instance, distinctly noted the relationships between experimental psychology, early education, and the ability to govern the psychological growth of children. Hoping to promote the healthy behavioral

development of Chinese youths, he established China's first psychological laboratory in Beijing in 1917 and chaired the psychological research institute at
the Guomindang's Academia Sinica in 1928.[25] Throughout the 1920s, the popularity of the field continued to grow. The first department of psychology was
founded in Nanjing in 1920, the Chinese Psychological Society was formally
established in 1921, and specialized journals and study groups proliferated in
tandem with the return of psychologists from abroad.[26]

Early Chinese texts on psychology frequently stressed the importance of
proper conditioning in childhood as a means of ensuring social conformity.
The behavioral psychologist Huang Weirong argued that three-fourths of all
cases of abnormal behavior could be attributed to poor training received in
childhood; he logically suggested that psychologists and educators work together to cultivate habits that were "in compliance" with society.[27] Guo Renyuan (1898–1970), also a behavioral psychologist, concurred with this view.
Arguing that "early life is like a blank sheet of paper," Guo insisted that a
proper elementary education was essential for creating "strong and healthy
citizens."[28] And the psychiatrist Gui Zhiliang (1900–1956), who received her
doctorate from Johns Hopkins in 1929 and became the first female psychiatrist to practice in China, asserted that psychiatry should be used for pre-
ventive, rather than simply reactive, purposes.[29] Children who showed signs
of behavioral deviance, she proposed, should be brought to a psychiatrist as
soon as possible. By advising parents on how to "raise the child properly,"
psychiatrists could give children the necessary tools to become "useful social
elements."[30]

Acting in parallel with trends in the United States, Chinese scholars also
began to reinterpret nonconformist behaviors as species of mental illness.
Sun Xiong (1895–1939), a penologist who taught at Fudan University, argued
that mental illness was at play in all types of "abnormal mindsets" (*fanchang
qingtai*); the mentally ill, he continued, thus belonged in the same category
as prostitutes, criminals, and suicidal individuals.[31] A journalist named Si Yi,
writing on the relationship between mental illness and modern society, associated the disorder with homosexuality, adultery, divorce, and any activity
that "jeopardized morals and decency."[32] And as a result of the slow but steady
influx of Freudian thought, a host of sexual behaviors, such as masturbation,
licentiousness, and sexual fetishism, also became linked to psychologically
abnormal states.[33] By categorizing such behaviors as a form of poor mental
health, Chinese intellectuals refashioned previously private activities into a
legitimate target of psychological intervention.

Psychologists and other social scientists justified their intrusion into the personal lives of the Chinese people through appeals to alarming demographic data. The incidence of mental illness, they believed, was rapidly increasing, and if proactive measures were not adopted to halt its spread, then the Chinese nation would soon be overrun with mentally defective individuals.[34] One journalist, citing statistical data from Western psychopathic hospitals, estimated that the entire population of England would be insane within the span of two decades.[35] Some went even further to suggest that "everyone in the civilized world" would soon show symptoms of mental pathology if the rate of insanity continued apace.[36] And others believed that the crisis of mental illness had already reached its apogee. In 1937, an article in the well-known pictorial *Liangyou* (Good companion) declared that 99 percent of people already exhibited some form of mental illness. Simply titled, "Are You Crazy?," the article did little to assuage popular fears of mental degeneration. As the subheadline succinctly summarized, "You might think you're not, but after reading this essay, you'll think again."[37]

Intellectuals perceived mental illness as not only a demographic problem but also an economic one. The psychologist Wu Nanxuan (1893–1980), who will be discussed in more detail later in this chapter, pointed out that hundreds of millions of dollars were spent each year on the institutionalization of the mentally ill and feebleminded in the United States and England alone. In China, too, the government could expect to spend 20,000 to 30,000 yuan on the care of a single individual over the course of his or her lifetime.[38] The psychiatric social worker Song Siming, though relying on different economic data, came to a similarly damning conclusion. Noting that it cost approximately 150 yuan a month to feed and medicate each mentally ill patient, Song surmised that the Chinese government could expect to "waste" at least 150 million yuan on the insane every few weeks.[39] If mental illness did not lead to societal collapse on its own, these scholars cautioned, then the problem would easily bankrupt the country long before then.

The combination of the previous arguments—that mental illness harmed social order, cost exorbitant sums of money, and was relentlessly increasing—convinced psychologists, journalists, and other members of the intelligentsia that mental disorders were a matter of national importance. Sun Xiong warned that psychiatric afflictions implicated "the entire society and race."[40] Song Siming lamented that mentally ill patients "wasted the country's money and could not contribute to society."[41] And Wu Nanxuan declared that mental illness and feeblemindedness were "great racial and social liabilities" that endangered the very future of Chinese civilization.[42] Recognizing that mental disorders constituted a social Darwinist threat to the continuation of the

Chinese nation and its people, psychologists turned from a strictly descriptive preoccupation with madness to an active engagement with the cause of mental hygiene.

Toward a Chinese Mental Hygiene Movement

In the spring of 1930, delegates from fifty-three nations gathered in Washington, DC, to attend the First International Congress on Mental Hygiene. Ernst DeVries, professor of neurology at the PUMC, helmed the Chinese delegation, which consisted of five participants.[43] At the commencement ceremony held on May 5, representatives from each delegation were invited to introduce the current state of mental hygiene in their respective countries. Dr. T. Hsiang Wang (Wang Zuxiang, b. 1897), a public health official with the Guomindang Ministry of Health, was chosen to speak on behalf of the Chinese contingent. Wang readily acknowledged that the scope of mental hygiene in China lagged "somewhat behind" that of other nations. Although there existed a few institutions for the reception of the mentally ill, he explained, most patients who were admitted to these facilities were too impaired to be effectively treated. Over the next few years, however, China was prepared to develop its mental hygiene activities in two ways. First, the Ministry of Health intended to establish examination clinics in all hospitals and health centers for the specific purpose of detecting mental disease at an early stage. Second, the ministry also planned to incorporate mental hygiene into elementary schools, with the aim of both preventing psychiatric disorders and "insuring the optimum mental development in growing children." This brief introduction, optimistic in its tenor, underscored China's support of, and alignment with, the general principles of the international mental hygiene movement.[44]

Prior to the congress, the PUMC had attempted to propagandize the importance of mental hygiene to the Chinese public but had made little headway on its own.[45] Indeed, one of the reasons that the hospital had initiated neuropsychiatric teaching in the first place was because Thomas Salmon (1876–1927), medical director of the NCMH and an affiliate of the Rockefeller Foundation, had suggested that mental hygiene education was indispensable for the complete training of Chinese medical students.[46] Although the subject had fallen to the wayside throughout the 1920s, it was once again revived when the PUMC entered into collaboration with the Beijing municipality in 1933. Richard Lyman, ruminating on the possibility of establishing a mental hygiene clinic at the psychopathic hospital, encouraged social workers to "provid[e] a little unobtrusive education along the lines of mental hygiene" to local families.[47] But outside of his own efforts, Lyman recognized that there was "little actual work" being done to advance the cause within the Beijing community. While sporadic interest was being voiced at nearby universities, none had taken up the concrete task of organizing a national movement.[48]

What Lyman did not know at the time was that a Chinese mental hygiene movement was in fact under way—but was being spearheaded by social scientists with ties to the central government rather than biomedical physicians like himself. Leaders of the movement, concerned more about the social impact of mental illness than its individual repercussions, advocated a two-pronged approach to the pursuit of mental hygiene in China: first, the creation of psychologically healthy and politically conformist citizens, and second, the segregation or elimination of defective individuals through euthenics and eugenics. These dual goals, though shared by a number of participants in the movement, were most clearly articulated by two of the main progenitors of Chinese mental hygiene, Zhang Yinian and Wu Nanxuan.

Zhang Yinian (1904–1960), a psychologist who authored the first Chinese-language monograph on mental hygiene in 1936, received his education at New York University and the University of Michigan. While abroad in the United States, Zhang had been deeply influenced by the international mental hygiene movement and the work of Clifford Beers; upon returning home in the early 1930s, he deemed himself "the Beers of China" and began to teach college courses on the subject at Shanghai's Jinan University.[49] Despite his self-given moniker, however, Zhang's interpretation of mental hygiene had less to do with patient welfare, per se, than with the prevention of psychological disorders for the overall improvement of Chinese society. As he wrote in his monograph, the "worrisome, frightening, and serious problem" of mental illness could easily lead to an increase of criminality; a loss of social order; and economic, moral, and spiritual damage to the Chinese nation as a whole. Yet regardless of the devastation that had already been caused by mental illness, he continued, the Chinese people remained unconcerned about preventing its advance. Although they had generally accepted the utility of public health for the eradication of communicable diseases, they failed to recognize that the elimination of psychological afflictions was equally pressing. Consequently, Zhang bemoaned, epidemics were decreasing while mental disorders were "growing by the day."[50]

For Zhang, the eradication of mental illness and the formation of a psychologically healthy populace were two sides of the same coin. The easiest way to achieve these entwined goals, he believed, was simply to prevent psychological abnormalities from forming in the first place. As he explained in a series of essays, once individuals had begun to exhibit an "eccentric temperament" or "abnormal emotions," this was necessarily a sign that an underlying pathology was afoot; to preserve their mental hygiene, such people would need to develop socially "useful" habits and eliminate behaviors that were "in conflict" with their society.[51] Because healthy and harmful habits were generally established in childhood, Zhang stressed the need for parents and educators to take a prominent role in fostering psychological health. At home, he suggested, parents should set a good example for their children by exhibiting positive marital relations and offering proper discipline, while at school, educators should focus on the cultivation of moral character and the promotion of social norms.[52] The path to achieving mental hygiene was thus forged during childhood; only when children had fully internalized the need to "adapt to the customs of their society" would they be able to lead "fulfilling and successful lives" while thwarting the omnipresent threat of insanity.[53]

Zhang's position represented the more optimistic vein of Chinese mental hygiene. Believing that mental illness could be prevented through proper education and the introduction of healthy social and environmental stimuli, Zhang emphasized the positive role that mental hygienists could play in the development of socially oriented citizens.[54] On the other side of the spectrum, Zhang's contemporary Wu Nanxuan was somewhat less hopeful about the prospects of eradicating mental illness through education alone. Like Zhang, Wu was a psychologist who first learned of mental hygiene while studying abroad in the United States. Upon finishing his doctorate in educational psychology at Berkeley in 1929, Wu returned to China, where he published extensively on the need to implement the principles of mental hygiene domestically. In one of his earliest articles on the subject, Wu lamented that China was the only country that "hadn't devoted special attention to the problem." Describing the current status of mental hygiene in China as "shameful" and "pitiful," he decided to propagandize the content, scope, and necessity of the movement to his fellow citizens.[55]

Wu was particularly fixated on the unique qualities of the German mental hygiene initiative. "There are at least two points that are worthy of our attention," he wrote of the German movement. "Ever since the Socialist Party under the leadership of Hitler has come to power, they have strictly prohibited the procreation of the mentally ill and feebleminded, either by restricting them from marrying or through sterilization." As Wu went on to explain, the German approach to mental hygiene centered less on the slow process of improving environmental stimuli than on the relatively quicker process of eliminating mentally defective people altogether. If German citizens were unable to prove that they were of sound body and mind, then they would be denied the right to marry—and consequently, the right to reproduce. To further protect the gene pool, moreover, Germany had also instituted a sterilization program for the mentally unfit. Sterilization (or "asexualization," as Wu also referred to it) "decisively resolved" the problem of mental illness by eliminating the potential for psychological and degenerative disorders to be passed along to new generations. "The German government's superior attention to the spirit of mental hygiene," Wu positively concluded, "shows clearly in its words and in its actions!"[56]

Inspired by the German model, Wu suggested adopting a dual approach to the eradication of mental illness and feeblemindedness in China: eugenics and euthenics. Claiming that mentally defective people were particularly prone to engaging in crime, vagrancy, and licentious behavior (indeed, he cited a claim that 85–100 percent of all prostitutes could be classified as feebleminded), Wu recommended the preemptive extermination of all classes of "morons," "imbeciles," "idiots," "cretins," and "mongoloids" from the Chinese gene pool. Toward this end, he advocated not only prohibiting the mentally ill and weak-minded from marrying but also sterilizing them to keep them from procreating—a method, he underscored, that had already proven very successful in California. Wu pointed out that more radical procedures were available if these measures proved insufficient, though he doubted most Chinese would allow them: in particular, the possibility of euthanizing the mentally unfit with chloroform to "painlessly exterminate" them in a cost-efficient manner.[57]

The eugenic program, Wu made clear, was an indispensable method by which to defend against the propagation of mentally ill and feebleminded individuals. In this regard, Wu was hardly unique. At the International Congress on Mental Hygiene, a panel devoted to the discussion of eugenics concluded that "every psychohygienist [should] consider himself obligated to give eugenics a chief place in mental hygiene."[58] So widespread was this belief that even Clifford Beers—the very champion of human rights for the mentally ill—refused to have children for fear that he might pass his disorder onto them.[59] Yet the eugenics solution, as Wu recognized, was only useful insofar as it would prevent *future* cases of mental disorder from occurring. For the mental defectives who already existed, a euthenics program would also be necessary to segregate low-functioning or maladjusted individuals from the general population. Introducing a theoretical solution that he referred to as "environmental improvement," Wu suggested that the Chinese government force mentally defective people to register with the state. Once registered, they would be sent to specialized institutions where they would be "socialized" and enjoined to participate in manual labor.[60]

Although Zhang Yinian and Wu Nanxuan represented different poles of the Chinese mental hygiene movement, they both shared the underlying sentiment that psychological disorders were an acute social, racial, and national liability—and therefore required solutions that would primarily serve the interests of the nation rather than just the interests of the individual.[61] As Zhang wrote in an addendum to his monograph on mental hygiene, "The people's hearts and minds are the basis of the nation. If the people's minds are healthy, then the nation will necessarily be powerful and prosperous; if the people's minds are degenerate [duoluo], then the nation will necessarily be in decline."[62] The purpose of mental hygiene, in other words, had less to do with an individualistic orientation toward patient welfare than with a broader concern for the future of Chinese civilization. Although the two were necessarily related—Zhang consistently underscored the indivisible relationships between mental health, social conformity, and national strength—psychologists like Zhang and Wu nevertheless devoted little ink to exploring the more patient-centered aspects of mental therapeutics.[63]

Regardless of how Zhang and Wu approached the task of psychological improvement, their divergent points of view were easily reconciled by their shared goal to achieve social stability and national self-strengthening through the promotion of mental hygiene. Throughout the second half of the 1930s, they collaborated on a variety of projects in order to propagandize the basic values of their cause. Both gave lectures and taught college courses on the subject, both contributed essays to an edited volume on mental hygiene in 1935, and both spearheaded the creation of the Chinese Mental Hygiene Association (Zhongguo xinli weisheng xiehui), which was founded at National Central University in Nanjing in the spring of 1936.[64] At the time of its first meeting, the association boasted a membership of 231 professionals, including psychologists, lawmakers, educators, and social workers. Under the leadership of Wu Nanxuan, who was elected secretary general, representatives of the association gave public lectures and radio broadcasts in major cities like Beijing, Nanjing, and Tianjin; published a quarterly periodical called Xinli weisheng (Mental hygiene); and developed extensive plans for future work. Hoping to collaborate with government organs like the Ministry of Health, the association proposed to survey conditions at psychopathic hospitals, establish specialized classes for feebleminded students, and develop an exam that would determine one's level of mental wellness. Through these various responsibilities, the association ultimately aspired to "promote the mental health of the Chinese people and prevent mental defects and illnesses."[65]

The Chinese Mental Hygiene Association purposely modeled its activities on the example that had been set by similar organizations in the United States and Europe. In particular, it aimed to incorporate government personnel into the cause of mental hygiene as a way to more effectively propagandize its mission. Just as Herbert Hoover had given symbolic credence to the movement by serving as honorary president of the International Congress on Mental Hygiene in 1930, the Chinese association also attempted to find ways by which to integrate its activities into the scope of national politics. Prior to the onset of the Second World War, the association began reaching out to government agencies at both the local and national level to raise financial and logistical support for its cause. Although the effort was cut short by the military conflict, members of the association never gave up the hope that mental hygiene would one day become a matter of national politics—and ultimately a "household name" (*jiayu huxiao*).[66]

Psychological Reconstruction

Writing in 1937, Richard Lyman adopted a tone of cautious optimism about the future of mental hygiene in China. Although he was pleased that the Chinese Mental Hygiene Association had recently been established, he was nevertheless hesitant about overstating its influence, especially since the central government had not yet "invest[ed] extensively in it." Indeed, a full year after the association had been founded, it appeared to have made little concrete headway. Outside of a few Western-managed facilities like the PUMC, no progress had been made to integrate psychiatry into local hospitals or to establish mental hygiene clinics, and the association was still too young to have attracted the serious attention or monetary support of the central government. Yet, despite these setbacks, Lyman remained hopeful. "The near future," he underscored, "holds out the possibility that psychiatry will prove its value and be admitted to official standing in governmental medicine." Achieving this goal, he continued, merely required the "recognition and support" of the Guomindang.[67]

Lyman's summary of the situation was only partially correct. While it was true that the Guomindang had not, as of 1937, taken up the cause of mental hygiene officially, the central government still promoted the underlying thrust of the movement—just in a political capacity rather than an explicitly medical one. For the Guomindang, mental hygiene was intriguing not necessarily for its therapeutic possibilities but, more importantly, for its potential sociopolitical applications. As Yung-chen Chiang has noted, the 1930s was a period in which the social sciences dominated intellectual discourse, particularly insofar as these fields could be used to "control the social, political, and economic forces at work."[68] Under the leadership of Chiang Kai-shek, the Nationalists attempted to harness the utilitarian potential of the social sciences toward the ends of achieving political conformity and social control. The cause of mental hygiene fit well into this objective. As a movement that aimed to produce obedient, compliant, and "useful" citizens, mental hygiene necessarily appealed to the state-building sensibilities of the fledgling regime.

One of the primary means by which the central government showed its support to the cause of mental hygiene was by appointing some of its most vocal advocates to positions of administrative authority in nationalized universities. According to Wen-hsin Yeh, the university system became an important nexus of academic and political power under Guomindang rule. In cities like Beijing, Nanjing, and Guangzhou, college campuses were "given a Party superstructure, put under the command of a new leadership, and propelled in the direction prescribed by the Guomindang," thereby enabling the party to gain immediate influence over the future of higher education.[69] Proponents of mental hygiene figured prominently among the party's early administrative appointments. Wu Nanxuan was assigned to a variety of positions in the Guomindang Party headquarters before taking up a professorship at the Guomindang-controlled National Central University in Nanjing; in 1931, he was appointed chancellor of the newly nationalized Qinghua University in Beijing; and in 1940, he was promoted to the government's Ministry of Control, an agency responsible for monitoring and auditing other governmental units. The psychologists Xiao Xiaorong (1897–1963) and Ai Wei (1890–1955), leading committee members of the Chinese Mental Hygiene Association, were both appointed to National Central University as chairs of the psychology and education departments, respectively. And Guo Renyuan, a behavioral psychologist trained at the University of California, Berkeley, was appointed chancellor of the Guomindang-controlled Zhejiang University in 1933 before being engaged as director of the Guomindang's Institute for Physiology and Psychology in 1940.[70]

What specifically did the Guomindang find appealing about these psychologists, none of whom had overtly expressed their prior allegiance to the regime? For the still nascent party, the allure of psychology lay in its instrumentalist potential as a tool of nation building. From as early as Sun Yat-sen's 1918 proclamation that the "psychological reconstruction" (*xinli jianshe*) of the Chinese people was a prerequisite to achieving political, economic, and social revolution, Chinese leaders had become closely attuned to the relationship between psychological rejuvenation and national self-strengthening. As Sun had argued prior to his death in 1925, "The affairs of the nation are a manifestation of the collective mentality [*renqun xinli*]. . . . The power of the mind is immense." In a way that anticipated Zhang Yinian's comments on the correlation between a healthy mind and a healthy nation, Sun also recognized that the people's minds needed to be rectified in order for the state to realize its modernizing agenda.[71]

The Nationalist Party under the leadership of Chiang Kai-shek internalized and extended this basic supposition. When Chiang ascended to the position of national leader in 1928, he promised to follow in Sun Yat-sen's footsteps by prioritizing the "psychological reconstruction" of the Chinese people. Psychological reconstruction, he recognized, was the "most important factor" in the regeneration of the nation, "without which other kinds of reconstruction [were] of little value."[72] Chiang's right-hand man, Chen Lifu (1900–2001), echoed this point. "From this time on," he wrote in 1930, "psychological reconstruction will be fundamentally attached to political reconstruction as its main program. . . . A revolutionary mentality [geming xinli] must conform to the needs of a revolutionary government."[73] For the Guomindang, then, the mentality of the people and the objective of national progress were inextricably linked; by harnessing the power of the mind and directing it toward a national cause, Chiang hoped to garner absolute loyalty to his regime.

The act of appointing psychologists and mental hygienists to key positions in university administration was therefore not done out of a dispassionate interest in psychological philosophy, but rather out of the belief that psychology could serve as a tool of "partification" (danghua)—that is, the indoctrination of university students with Guomindang ideology.[74] Under the leadership of psychologists like Wu Nanxuan and Guo Renyuan, nationalized universities attempted to regulate the behavior, thoughts, and ideals of the student body by "militarizing, disciplining, and collectivizing" them.[75] At Zhejiang University, Guo implemented a number of reforms that eliminated harmful ideological stimuli and introduced sanctioned habits of body and mind. He enforced daily military training, eliminated leftist political propaganda, dismissed professors who held incorrect political views, and expelled students for such transgressions as missing class, cheating on exams, or dressing improperly.[76] Resonating with his belief that the Chinese people needed to be "organized" and "reformed," Guo aspired to foster an educational environment that introduced socially beneficial stimuli while eliminating detrimental ones.[77] Wu aimed to do the same during his short tenure at Qinghua. Upon being appointed chancellor, Wu stated that he would "scrupulously follow the will of chairman Chiang" in order to "rectify academic discipline" and enforce "political stability."[78] Both Guo and Wu, in other words, sought to strengthen, reform, and unify the behaviors of their students through the adoption of strict codes of conduct. Guo referred to this process as "human engineering" (renlei gongcheng xue).[79]

Psychologists like Guo and Wu were not the only ones to deploy the rhetoric and principles of psychological thought for political ends. Following Sun
Yat-sen's early emphasis on the importance of psychological reconstruction,
military and political leaders also invoked the psychological deficiencies of
the Chinese people as a way to explain the backwardness of the Chinese nation. In 1933, for instance, Li Yuan (b. 1903), an early graduate of Chiang Kai-
shek's Whampoa Military Academy and a general in the Nationalist army,
published a monograph that discussed the adverse relationship between abnormal psychology and Chinese nation building. The book, which he titled
Abnormal Psychology and the Reformation of China (*Biantai xinli yu gaizao
Zhongguo*), illustrated how the mindsets of the Chinese masses were directly
correlated to the stability of the nation. According to Li, China's "current
condition"—which he described as "having fallen deeply into darkness"—
was the product of "the abnormal psychology of its people."[80] Only when the
people "corrected their minds," he argued, would the nation be able to realize
the "glorious revolution" that the Guomindang had set out to achieve.[81]

Li isolated communism, factionalism, and warlordism as some of the many
psychologically abnormal attitudes that had stifled the success of the Nationalist takeover. Despite the fact that Li had never received any formal institutional
training in the principles of Western psychology, he explained his particular
opposition to communism not on theoretical or political grounds but rather on
psychological ones. Believing that a communist revolution was premature and
did not "fit with the times," Li argued that anyone who supported communism
was necessarily displaying the psychological pathologies of "escapism" (*dunbi*)
and "divergence" (*beichi*). Stated differently, Li interpreted communist belief
as a type of mental illness. "The minds of the Chinese people are not correct,
and their thoughts surpass the times," he concluded. In order to save the nation
from extinction, it was imperative to correct the psychological shortcomings
of the Chinese citizenry and compel them to align their thoughts with the demands and conditions of the contemporary political environment.[82]

Perhaps the most obvious incarnation of political psychology during this
period, however, came in the form of the 1934 New Life Movement. A national
campaign that aimed to advance hygiene, discipline, military courage, and
unity of purpose, the New Life Movement was Chiang Kai-shek's crowning
effort to induce the Chinese public to refashion their minds and behaviors to
better align with the revolutionary imperatives of the modern nation. Couching his rationale for the movement in the language of Confucian ethics, Chiang
underscored that "rectifying the mind" and "cultivating the self" were pre-
requisites to "ordering the state."[83] This belief, though ostensibly inspired by
traditional Chinese philosophy, was undoubtedly also influenced by Chiang's

support of "psychological reconstruction." As Chiang asserted at the inauguration of the campaign, "The general psychology of our people today can be described as spiritless." Officials were dishonest, the masses were undisciplined and unhygienic, and adults were corrupt while youths were degraded. It was no wonder that China continued to suffer disorder from within and invasion from without.[84] The only way to solve these problems, Chiang continued, was to completely eradicate old ways of thinking. "Revolution," he claimed, "meant changing everyday patterns of behavior" as well as "habits of thought"—even activities as simple as washing one's face and brushing one's teeth.[85]

Although Chiang claimed to derive inspiration for the New Life Movement from Confucian tradition, the campaign was, in many ways, a thoroughly modern response to problems of a contemporary nature. As scholars like Arif Dirlik and Lloyd Eastman have shown, Chiang's interest in the doctrine of fascism, combined with his desire to extend political control into the quotidian habits of ordinary people, shared little in common with the ideals of the imperial past.[86] More specifically, Chiang's desire to achieve unity of action through the routine modification of human behavior had far less to do with Confucian philosophy than with popularly circulating discourses on social engineering. While previous generations of leaders had certainly stressed the enforcement of normative behaviors as a means by which to ensure stability and order, the New Life Movement represented an unprecedentedly intrusive and regulatory approach to the long-standing problem of civil disobedience.

To contemporary observers, the parallels between the New Life Movement and the more general mental hygiene movement were obvious. Wei Yulin, supervisor of the Beijing Psychopathic Hospital, published an article in 1936 in which he highlighted the similarities between the two campaigns. Both movements, he noted, aspired to reform the "insidious and degenerate minds" of the Chinese people by encouraging ideals of "honesty, sincerity, and simplicity."[87] Richard Lyman made a similar observation. Writing in early 1935, he remarked that the Guomindang's efforts to sponsor mental hygiene had thus far been limited to the "more general influence [of] the New Life Movement," though he remained confident that the regime would extend its support for mental hygiene in the near future.[88]

Lyman's prediction was soon realized. After the Nationalist capital was moved to Chongqing in 1938, the central government became more directly involved in the work of mental hygiene. In 1942, the Guomindang established its first mental hygiene work unit (*xinli weisheng shi*), which consisted of an outpatient clinic and a mental hygiene consultation center. The unit was placed under the leadership of Ding Zan (1910–1968), a psychologist and founding member of the Chinese Mental Hygiene Association. At the clinic, Ding focused the brunt of his attention on "problem children" (*wenti ertong*)—that is, youths who challenged social norms and failed to adhere to proper disciplinary standards. Believing that problem children were simply unable or unwilling to adapt to their environment, Ding stressed the need to "strengthen their social adaptability." Through individual consultations and mental health examinations, he attempted to identify and correct the deviant behaviors of his adolescent patients.[89]

Although the Chinese mental hygiene movement did not gain further momentum due to the conditions of wartime, the underlying imperatives of the movement—including the creation of useful, conformist, and psychologically "healthy" citizens—had incontrovertibly infiltrated the gestalt of contemporary Chinese politics. Concerned with inefficient, irrational, and socially deviant behaviors, mental hygienists in China, like their counterparts in the Western world, sought to employ positivist methods toward the ends of controlling social phenomena and securing national prosperity. Many intellectuals affiliated with the Guomindang therefore perceived abnormal psychology primarily as a transgression against social norms rather than an issue of individual health, and psychology, likewise, came to be seen not just as a therapeutic tool but more importantly as a coercive one. Among the right-wing intelligentsia, in other words, mental hygiene was explicitly remade in the service of state building, political power, and the construction of national fascism—rather than in the service of individual therapeutics.

Strong Minds and Strong Nations

In 1935, the Beijing Ministry of Health began the task of integrating "mental hygiene" into its educational outreach program. The subject was featured in its monthly periodical, which saw a circulation of close to sixty thousand copies over the course of the year, and received attention on the Beijing radio network, where it was featured as part of the ministry's weekly broadcasts.[90] In one broadcast talk, a social worker named Wang Ziming, who was employed at the Beijing Psychopathic Hospital, spoke on the topic of "mental illness and society." The main problem with mental illness, he began, is that it harms social order, jeopardizes societal tranquility, and compromises the race (*zhongzu*); indeed, this was the reason that all the great nations of Europe and the United States had passed legislation preventing the mentally ill from marrying. Yet the disorder, as Wang went on to explain, was not entirely hopeless. Just like physical ailments, mental illness was both preventable and sometimes even curable, as long as the problem was brought to the attention of a psychological or psychiatric specialist. By treating mental symptoms in their early stages, doctors and social workers could stop the disorder from advancing into a far more serious infirmity. Scientific knowledge about mental illness was therefore necessary for two reasons: to correct previous misinformation about the condition itself and to ensure the strength and prosperity of Chinese society in the future.[91]

Wang's radio lecture succinctly captured the essence of mental hygiene discourse in 1930s China. Drawing an explicit parallel between mental illness and societal decay, advocates of mental hygiene emphasized the damage that psychologically unstable individuals could inflict on their social environment. Consequently, while psychiatrists continued to be seen as the proper guardians of the mentally ill within the space of the hospital, various specialists—from psychologists and educators to penologists and social workers—were incorporated into the project of preventing or mitigating the effects of the disorder within the society at large. Emphasizing the utility of proper education, as well as the need to eliminate or isolate defective individuals, psychologists definitively linked the existence of mentally ill people to the instability of public order, the weakening of the economy, the deterioration of the race, and the perpetuation of national ignominy. Mental hygiene in China was thus never strictly oriented toward the health of the pathological patient. Rather, from the time of its earliest inception in China, mental hygiene—like public health as a whole—had consistently been incorporated into the larger project of nation building and national salvation.[92]

What Wang's speech did not convey, however, was the extent to which the pursuit of mental hygiene had enabled an alliance to form between psychology and national politics. Throughout the 1930s, the expanding scope of mental pathology had allowed the Guomindang to co-opt psychological vocabularies and concepts for explicitly political ends. By appointing supporters of mental hygiene to prominent administrative positions in universities and government bureaus, the Guomindang strove to partify education, reinforce sanctioned behaviors, and eliminate heterodox views. Through a stress on "psychological reconstruction," moreover, Chiang Kai-shek sought to reinforce a nationalist ethos that condemned liberalist individualism and privileged conformity and self-sacrifice. And after the establishment of the Chinese Mental Hygiene Association, leaders of the organization received institutional support from the Nationalist government in Chongqing. Although the exigencies of wartime prematurely stifled the momentum of the movement, mental hygiene might have become a more substantial part of the Guomindang political apparatus had history unfolded differently.[93]

The incorporation of nonconformist individuals into the taxonomy of abnormal psychology helped to justify the Guomindang's incursion into the private lives of the Chinese people. In this sense, the discourse of mental hygiene both enabled the increasing scope of state intervention while disabling the ability for individuals to react against it. Claiming scientific authority, psychologists and psychiatrists gave legitimacy to the modern political desire to "incite, reinforce, control, monitor, optimize, and organize" the private behaviors of its citizenry—from their sexual practices and hygienic acts to their ordinary instances of individualistic expression.[94] Believing that they possessed specialized insight into the nature of humanity itself, social scientists aimed to not just correct "abnormal" behaviors, but to encourage their subjects to internalize accepted disciplinary norms. In so doing, they simultaneously helped to bolster the power of the state by pathologizing any activity that strayed from its imagined ideal.

There was one major problem with this objective, however, and that was the Chinese people themselves. Throughout the Nanjing Decade, Chiang's political initiatives were received with only lukewarm enthusiasm—if not outright resistance. Not only was his New Life Movement remembered as an unequivocal failure, but university students also refused to submit to the new disciplinary mandates of administrative appointees like Wu Nanxuan and Guo Renyuan—both of whom were forced out of their positions as heads of Qinghua and Zhejiang Universities following massive student protests in 1931 and 1935, respectively. Referring to Wu and Guo as "fascists" and Guomindang "lackeys," university students pushed back against what they perceived as an authoritarian turn in academic administration, and both men were ultimately pressured to quietly submit their resignations.[95] By the onset of war with Japan, then, Chiang's hopes for the creation of a more obedient, compliant, and deferential populace had repeatedly been denied, often in a very visible and vocal way.

But resistance to new ideologies was not always this blatant, of course. On a more routine level, and as the next chapter will describe, the very assumptions on which scientific psychology were based also failed to displace preexistent beliefs about the nature of madness and psychosomatic health. Taking issue, in particular, with the cleavage that had formed between body and mind, ordinary Chinese people—consciously or otherwise—resisted the imposition of new types of knowledge that did not conform to either their quotidian needs or long-standing systems of belief.

Between the Mad and the Mentally Ill

On the cusp of war, madness remained positioned between two worlds of knowledge. While psychiatry, along with its attendant theories and practices, may have gained support in certain intellectual circles, it remained little more than an unfamiliar interloper in many others. And while the Beijing people may have used the services of the municipal psychopathic hospital, this did not necessarily mean that they had relinquished alternative care-seeking behaviors. "The Chinese soil seems not to resist the growth of psychiatry," Richard Lyman observed in 1937—but he also acknowledged that the Chinese were not ready to accept it unconditionally.[1] Throughout the 1930s, neuropsychiatry existed on a continuum alongside Chinese medicine and religious therapies, and people oscillated between them in ways that reflected their individual needs and beliefs. Regardless of the Nationalist government's efforts to glorify Western psychiatric practices—and despite the intelligentsia's attempts to delineate the boundaries of normal psychological functioning—understandings of madness remained far more a matter of private dominion than public authority.

To certain Western-oriented intellectuals, the stubborn persistence of Chinese medicine necessarily signaled that the triumph of neuropsychiatry was incomplete—and hence, that the Chinese people had not yet concluded their trek to medical modernity. The neurologist Wei Yulin, head of the municipal psychopathic hospital, was one such individual who viewed "modern" and "traditional" forms of medical practice as being lodged in a zero-sum game. Writing in 1936, Wei earnestly implored the Beijing public that "madmen" (*fengzi*) were actually "mentally ill" (*jingshen bing*); that the affliction was caused not by spirits or moral transgression but by a disordered brain; and that the patient should be brought to a hospital and cared for by "specialized men of talent" (*zhuanmen rencai*) rather than managed, to no end, by chains, prayers, or the burning of incense.[2] For Wei, and for many other intellectuals like him, traditional interpretations of madness and biomedical beliefs about mental illness could not be reconciled; where one prevailed, the other necessarily floundered. This position was a logical byproduct of modernist discourse, which viewed "science" and "superstition" as inherently at odds.[3] For scientific psychiatry to truly succeed, Wei's essay seemed to imply, the Beijing people needed to first renounce their traditional views of the pathological body and affirm, in their stead, the unequivocal superiority of biomedicine.

For many others, however, the situation appeared far less stark. Those who were more concerned with the immediate, practical pursuit of health than the distant, ideological pursuit of modernity were not necessarily bothered by the modernist dictum of a zero-sum world. Facing sickness and disease, individuals readily experimented with both forms of medical practice in a far more symbiotic fashion. The Western-trained physician Wu Lien-teh (Wu Liande, 1879–1960), as Bridie Andrews has shown, spurned the use of Chinese medicine in public but kept traditional tonics within the home that his wife employed when their children fell ill.[4] Even the renowned revolutionary Sun Yat-sen, who famously sought treatment at the Peking Union Medical College for his terminal liver cancer, supplemented biomedical remedies with Chinese herbs. The formulas that his doctor prescribed were later published in the Beijing news, alongside the details of his pulse diagnosis.[5] Regardless of the fact that Wu and Sun both denigrated "traditional" medicine in theory, they were far less rigid about discriminating against it in practice. In the quotidian search for the solution to their suffering, both men pivoted between Chinese and Western medicine in ways that belied the supposed epistemological purity of the two conceptual systems.

In contrast to the modernist view that Chinese and Western forms of knowledge were incompatible and irreconcilable, this final chapter will demonstrate how the "mad" body and the "mentally ill" body were ultimately able to find common ground. Composed of a series of vignettes, it focuses on four aspects of this mediating process. The first vignette examines how practitioners of Chinese medicine strove to reconcile the biomedical "brain" with the Chinese "heart" as the locus of mentality. The second vignette turns its attention to matters of translation, and demonstrates how intellectuals made sense of foreign psychiatric neologisms by invoking indigenous theories of madness. Vignette number three illustrates the negotiation between theory and practice in the treatment of the mentally ill, and explains how ordinary people experimented with Western practices of institutional care even when they maintained alternative views about the nature of the mad body. And in the last vignette, I show how neuropsychiatry gradually accommodated itself to the needs of the Chinese people, rather than vice versa. At the PUMC, Chinese social workers challenged biomedicine's view of the body as fundamentally material and mechanistic. Advocating instead for a more holistic approach to psychiatric knowledge and treatment, they persuaded foreign doctors to consider the social and cultural aspects of mental illness as well.

Each of these vignettes illustrates the diverse ways by which intellectuals, medical practitioners, and ordinary people—using the conceptual tools available to them at the time—both contested and appropriated aspects of neuropsychiatric practice in ways that conformed to their personal needs and beliefs. In so doing, they also created new forms of psychiatric knowledge that belonged neither strictly to the world of neuropsychiatry nor to that of Chinese medicine. In the end, Chinese and Western therapies were not inevitably antagonistic. Rather, through the everyday exercise of their prolonged encounter, a final reinvention of madness occurred—one that managed to merge two ostensibly competing systems in a variety of ways.

Vignette 1: Toward a Unified Theory of the Heart and Brain

In 1929, soon after the Guomindang had risen to national power, a biomedical physician named Yu Yan (also known as Yu Yunxiu, 1879–1954) proposed a law that would ban the practice of Chinese medicine in its entirety. Believing it to be ineffective at best and dangerous at worst, Yu claimed that only a total eradication of old-style medicine would enable the Chinese people to achieve both bodily health and national modernity.[6] Although his proposal was met with an unexpected amount of resistance and was soon scrapped, its very existence signaled that Chinese medicine was no longer safe from the modernizing aspirations of the Guomindang state. On the heels of this attempted intervention, proponents of Chinese medicine banded together to defend the legitimacy of their practices. Recognizing that the future of Chinese medicine would require, at the very least, an engagement with the terms of biomedicine, they struggled to find a place for Chinese medical theory within the orbit of scientific epistemology. With this goal in mind, some attempted to codify the effects of herbal therapies or subject their atomized practices to more rigorous empirical testing. These exercises represented the first efforts to streamline and "scientize" (*kexue hua*) the manifold vicissitudes of Chinese medicine.[7]

While changing, in some ways, the outward form of their clinical practice, physicians of Chinese medicine never denied the continuing utility— and perhaps even superiority—of their own medical knowledge. Rejecting the modernist belief that science had obtained a monopoly over truth, they continued to engage with biomedical ideas without surrendering completely to their epistemic power. Some scholars scoured ancient texts for proof that the Chinese had anticipated the basic principles of biomedicine. Others pointed to instances of common ground as confirmation that the two conceptual systems were not as antagonistic as they might have seemed. Spurred both by a desire for self-preservation and by a genuine conviction in the value of their accumulated knowledge, practitioners of Chinese medicine refused to accept the argument that "science" had rendered their own traditions inconsequential.[8]

For matters of madness, intellectuals defended the continuing relevance of Chinese medicine by attempting to assimilate the biomedical role of the brain into indigenous medical theories, which viewed the *heart* as the basis of cognition and a major locus of mental disturbance. As chapter 1 explained, the brain in Chinese medicine played a relatively minor role in bodily function; considered a "sea of marrow," it was thought to be a passive structure that had little relation to cognitive or emotive processes. Due to the increasing authority of biomedicine in 1930s China, however, practitioners of Chinese medicine began to reevaluate their own assumptions about the nature of the brain and its relationship to the body. In a 1933 essay simply titled "Speaking of the Brain," a physician from Jiangsu province named Zong Zihe (1880–1954) posed the following question: "Western medicine states that one's mind, talent, and wisdom [*jingshen caizhi*] are emitted from the brain. Chinese medicine conversely claims that the heart is the master of the intellect [*shenming*], and the brain has nothing to do with it. How are the two so at odds?"[9] One year earlier, Li Jianyi (1891–1967), a doctor from Fujian province, had made a similar statement. "Western medicine says that knowledge and movement are both a product of the brain," he wrote. "Chinese medicine points out that the heart is the clever [one]." Because "nobody had yet meticulously examined which is correct," Li decided to place the two "in dialogue with one another" in order to reach a definitive conclusion.[10]

Despite the different logic by which they responded to this question, the various authors who participated in the debate arrived at a unanimous verdict. The heart, they suggested, was the true source of mental processes, while the brain just served as a repository for thoughts that had been emitted therefrom.[11] Yu Shenchu (1915–2002), a Fujianese practitioner, referenced classic medical texts like *Huangdi neijing* (Yellow emperor's inner canon) to support this line of argumentation. Claiming that the heart was the "root" (*ben*) of cognition while the brain was merely its "tip" (*biao*), Yu insisted that the brain acted as little more than a storage vessel for knowledge that had originally "emanated" from the heart.[12] Zong Zihe reached a similar conclusion when he determined that the heart is the "source" of the brain and the brain simply "stores" the ingenuity and intellect that the heart had produced.[13] And Li Jianyi, applying these basic suppositions to the subject of madness, argued that a disordered brain was the byproduct (*bo*, literally "wave") of imbalances that had developed in the heart; although the symptoms of madness might manifest in the brain, he contended, the *cause* of madness certainly did not originate there.[14]

In seeking to explain why Western medicine had so fundamentally misunderstood the basic relationship between the heart and the brain, participants in the debate traced these errors to the mechanistic, and often myopic, way in which biomedicine conceptualized the human body. Biomedical practitioners, they suggested, focused their gaze too strictly on each organ in isolation; as a result, they failed to see the underlying connections and dialogues that took place between them. This was precisely where Chinese medicine succeeded. Since practitioners of Chinese medicine viewed the body as an intensely integrated organism, they were able to perceive the deeper, more profound patterns of psychosomatic pathology—rather than just their superficial manifestations. "Western medicine only investigates what is close," Li Jianyi definitively concluded, "but does not extend [its investigation] to what is farther away."[15] It was for this very reason that neuropsychiatry remained so fixated on the brain but had failed to see the bigger picture: namely, that the heart was the true "master of the body" (*shen zhi zhu*) and the brain could not function without it.[16]

One of the reasons that practitioners of Chinese medicine remained so confident in their ability to contest biomedical principles was due to the ineffectiveness of contemporary neuropsychiatric practice. Yu Shenchu was forthright in his observation that Western doctors "lacked any fundamental treatment" for mental illness and "could not achieve a complete cure." Relying strictly on sedatives and tranquilizers, psychiatrists could relieve the symptoms of madness only temporarily but could not eradicate them completely.[17] Li Jianyi similarly argued that Western medicine was "unclear" on the foundational causes of madness. While Chinese practitioners recognized the inherent dynamism of the body, Western doctors acted "without regard to changing circumstances." Their basic misconceptions about human physiology necessarily rendered them powerless to treat bodily pathologies; Chinese medicine, he concluded, was thus "sincerely superior" to Western medicine in its curative ability.[18] Regardless of the discursive authority of biomedicine, both writers concurred, the very ineffectiveness of neuropsychiatric treatments enabled a space for Chinese medicine to persist.

Yet, despite these serious critiques, the above authors did not discount biomedical knowledge completely. Even while highlighting its theoretical weaknesses, they simultaneously aimed to integrate neuropsychiatric logic into Chinese medical practice. Zong Zihe, for instance, concluded his essay by acknowledging that Chinese medicine could benefit from biomedical ideas. Although he adamantly upheld his argument that the "basis of the brain is the heart," he also pointed out that Chinese medicine had never satisfactorily researched the role of the brain in psychosomatic functioning. "Chinese medicine knows that the heart is precious," he told his readers. "But it does not know that the magical effects of the heart are stored in the brain."[19] Another practitioner named Wang Qiuyuan came to a similar conclusion. While maintaining the premise that the heart "rules" the body, he nevertheless admitted that the brain played a vital role in motion and cognition. Since the brain was attached to the nerves (*shenjing*),[20] a person's thoughts necessarily had to pass through the brain in order to be diffused to the rest of the body.[21] For both authors, biomedical knowledge filled gaps that Chinese medical theory had not addressed, but did so without nullifying or invalidating the explanatory power of the latter.

In the above analyses, Chinese medicine and biomedicine were framed as complementary rather than antagonistic. The heart and brain, likewise, were not considered discrete or disconnected units, but were instead shown to play reciprocal and interdependent roles within the integrality of the holistic body.[22] And despite the fact that the various authors who participated in the debate each questioned the absolute validity of neuropsychiatric assumptions, they nevertheless recognized the utility of some of its claims— specifically, that the brain *did* play a role in cognition, movement, and the onset of madness, just not the role that biomedical physicians expected. In the end, the debate on the relative functions of the heart and brain did not negate the utility or relevance of Chinese medical theory, but rather enhanced it. Through a conscious engagement with the world of Western medicine, Chinese medicine was both strengthened and redirected toward new lines of inquiry.

Vignette 2: Translating "Mental" Illness into Chinese

While intellectuals were debating the merits and flaws of the biomedical body, they were doing so in a written language that was rapidly evolving.[23] At the same time that writers were making the difficult transition from literary to vernacular expression, they were also forced to assimilate foreign words and unfamiliar scientific concepts into indigenous lexicons. Because these imported calques shared little in common with native terms for medical conditions, translation became a process of mediation—not simply between words, but also between worldviews.[24] Interpreting foreign neologisms through the lens of their own assumptions and beliefs, Chinese intellectuals inevitably (though often unintentionally) transformed the intended meanings of imported biomedical concepts.

Many of the earliest psychiatric neologisms were first developed in Japan and then transmitted to China in the form of translated texts. According to the literary scholar Peng Hsiao-yen, the Japanese had become interested in the study of the mind as early as the mid-nineteenth century, when the intellectual Nishi Amane (1829–1897) first traveled to Holland to study psychology and philosophy. Upon his return, he worked rigorously to devise neologisms for Western metaphysical concepts, a process he accomplished by borrowing liberally from the vocabulary of neo-Confucianism and Chinese medicine. For example, when Nishi first attempted to translate the concept of "psychology" into Japanese, he did so by appropriating the Chinese term *xingli xue* (the study of the principles of human nature) from the famous neo-Confucian scholar Zhu Xi (1130–1200).[25] Sino-Japanese terms for Western concepts therefore consisted largely of preexistent Chinese characters that had simply been placed in new combinations or repurposed to new ends. The shifting meanings of these words left them open to contestation and debate, particularly as scholars invoked seemingly familiar phrases in service of new intellectual objectives.

As psychiatric neologisms gained currency and became more widespread in Chinese texts, their intended meanings were easily distorted and (mis)interpreted through the lens of indigenous systems of knowledge.[26] The Chinese term for "mental illness" (*jingshen bing*), for instance, provides an apt example of how neologisms could unintentionally reinforce traditional understandings of bodily malfunction, thereby perpetuating the very concepts they were meant to supplant. This neologism, originally coined in Japan, made its way to China at the turn of the twentieth century and was ultimately codified as the official name for mental illness in the late Qing and early Republican penal codes, discussed in chapter 2. Although the term was meant to signify the biomedical concept of "mental illness" (*bing* indicated "illness" and *jingshen* was supposed to indicate the "mind" or "psyche"), its intended meaning may have been obfuscated by the fact that the phrase *jingshen* already existed in Chinese medical theory but signified something other than the Cartesian notion of "mind."

In Chinese medicine, *jingshen* is considered a constitutive part of the material body rather than something that transcends or exists apart from it. The phrase itself refers to two interrelated vital forces: *jing* (essence), a material substance formed in the kidneys that is responsible for functions related to growth, aging, and reproduction; and *shen* (spirit), an immaterial concept associated with the heart, which is perhaps best understood as a manifestation of one's vital energies.[27] Both *jing* and *shen* are considered necessary for the creation and persistence of life itself. When male and female *jing* combine through the act of procreation, they produce the animative forces necessary to create life; conversely, when an individual exhausts his or her *jing*, death becomes inevitable. As a consequence of the "seminal" role played by *jing* in the preservation of bodily health, many classical Chinese texts focus on the conservation of *jing* through such practices as sexual and meditative exercises.[28] *Shen*, by contrast, has historically been acknowledged as a far more inscrutable concept.[29] It refers alternately to mysterious, sacred, and magical forces; to the appearance, expression, and complexion of a person; and to the soul, innate talents, intelligence, consciousness, and cognitive processes. When placed alongside one another in the compound phrase *jingshen*, the two characters can express several overlapping ideas. On the one hand, the phrase can signify a sense of the mind, consciousness, or soul—hence its use in the neologism for mental illness. On the other hand, it can also refer to a person's primordial spirit, life essence, energy, or vitality.[30] Thus, while "mental illness" in neuropsychiatry is not inevitably life threatening, an illness or deficiency of the *jingshen* in Chinese medicine can easily prove fatal.

Since the neologism *jingshen bing* was composed of characters and concepts drawn from a non-Cartesian tradition, its interpreted meaning often diverged significantly from the biomedical concept of "mental illness." To illustrate this point, it is useful to return to an individual who was first discussed in chapter 4, the proprietor of a Beijing psychopathic hospital named Wei Hongsheng. As an intellectual who had never left China, did not speak any Western languages, and received his medical training largely on the basis of translated texts, Wei's understanding of *jingshen bing* was naturally inflected with the assumptions and expectations of his own intellectual tradition. In a tract that he published in 1936, Wei explicitly discussed what he meant when he invoked the term. "*Jing* is stored in the kidneys and produces [the associated phase of] water," he wrote, "while *shen* is stored in the heart and produces [the associated phase of] fire."[31] The preservation of health, he continued, required a balanced and reciprocal interaction between the heart and the kidneys. When the two fell into opposition, and when fire (from the heart) and water (from the kidneys) failed to aid one another in the sustenance of bodily health, "this is the origin of *jingshen bing*."[32]

As this explanation illustrates, Wei was not thinking of the Cartesian "mind" when he invoked the neologism for "mental illness." Instead, his conception of *jingshen* remained highly influenced by Chinese medical theory, which positioned *jing* within the kidneys and *shen* within the heart, and attributed the onset of mad behaviors to a bodily imbalance that was not purely "mental" in origin. Wei's proposed treatments for *jingshen bing*, likewise, had little in common with those being used in contemporary neuropsychiatry. As chapter 4 described, Wei insisted that the solution to madness merely involved "opening up the passes, clearing the channels, replenishing blood and *qi*, and making the *jing* and *shen* interact."[33] Wei's writings, in short, invoked old terms for new psychiatric ideas, only to simultaneously imbue these new ideas with alternative meanings than the ones that were intended for them. Through his own "neologistic imagination," to borrow Lydia Liu's words, Wei managed to forge a "middle zone of hypothetical equivalence" between the two conceptual systems of Chinese and Western medicine.[34]

Wei's interpretation of *jingshen bing*, though not unique to him alone, represents a perhaps extreme example of how Western psychiatric concepts could be integrated into the ontological world of Chinese medical theory.[35] Far more commonly, Chinese intellectuals *consciously* strove to domesticate foreign biomedical ideas as a way to demonstrate that Chinese and Western knowledge could potentially be reconciled. One of the ways that they did so was by treating imported neologisms as synonymous with an indigenous medical concept. Yang Huanwen (1897–1966), a practitioner of Chinese medicine who published a lengthy tract on psychiatric nosology in 1933, employed this strategy when he claimed that the Chinese disorder of *kuang* (excited madness) was commensurate with the Western disorder of "paralysis of the insane."[36] Advertisements for the "World's Number One Madness Pill," discussed in chapter 4, proposed that the Chinese condition of "mucous confuses the heart" (*tan mixin*) was simply another term for "what Western doctors refer to as a nervous disease" (*shenjing bing*).[37] And Dr. Williams' Pink Pills for Pale People, a wildly popular proprietary medicine, described the condition of anemia as being "the disorder of thin blood and weak *qi*."[38] By placing a foreign terminology alongside an indigenous one, intellectuals and entrepreneurs attempted to assimilate an otherwise unintelligible concept into the realm of Chinese medicine.

In the process of asserting commensurability between biomedical and Chinese medical ideas, intellectuals effectively eliminated, or at the very least minimized, the conceptual differences between them. To explain what I mean by this point, let us examine a short text by a Chinese medicine practitioner named Wang Runmin. This text, which was published as part of an edited volume on mental illness in 1931, aimed to unpack the inscrutable condition known in English as "hysteria." The topic, admittedly, would have been a difficult one for even the most seasoned of Western practitioners. As "the nosological limbo of all unnamed female maladies," to quote the nineteenth-century neurologist Silas Weir Mitchell (1829–1914), the precise contours of the ambiguous disorder remained utterly perplexing to Freudians and neurologists alike.[39] Perhaps due to the enigmatic and deeply gendered quality of the condition, hysteria did not gain nearly as much attention among the Chinese intelligentsia as neurasthenia did. Nevertheless, periodic texts on the subject began to appear from the 1920s on.[40] Employing the transliteration *xiesideli*—a nonsensical homophone that would have clearly indicated its foreign origins—scholars like Wang Runmin attempted to make sense of the disorder by searching for analogues within the annals of Chinese medical history.[41]

In order to explain the meaning of hysteria to his uninitiated readers, Wang likened it to a condition known in Chinese medicine as *zangzao* (literally, "visceral unrest"). As he claimed in his essay, the two ailments shared much in common. Both affected women, both arose from the uterus, and both caused their sufferers to experience extreme sensitivity to sensory and emotional stimulation. Quoting from the third-century medical text *Essential Prescriptions of the Golden Cabinet* (*Jingui yaolüe*), Wang described *zangzao* in the following way: "Women's visceral unrest [causes them] sadness and makes them want to cry; it is as if [the disorder] has been caused by a ghostly spirit. They stretch and yawn frequently. A decoction of licorice, wheat, and jujube can manage it."[42] Wang then went on to provide his own exegesis of this earlier gloss. "*Zang* refers to the uterus [*zizang*]," he clarified, "and *zao* refers to disharmony of the uterus. The cause of the illness can thus be understood as relating to obstetrics." Hysteria, Wang continued, was also a gendered disorder. As he explained, hysteria arose from the uterus, caused women to feel emotional, and also manifested in physical symptoms such as nausea and constipation. Given the common etiology of the two disorders, Wang concluded that they were synonymous. Indeed, as he asserted quite directly at the outset of his essay, "The illness known as *zangzao* is now referred to as hysteria."[43]

In his effort to forge commensurability between the two disorders, Wang downplayed their fundamental differences. Perhaps most critically, Wang's assertion that hysteria and *zangzao* were both illnesses of the uterus was belied by contemporary medical thought. Although followers of Hippocrates and Galen had originally conceived of the disorder as deriving from the womb—hence the

Greek term *hysterikos*, or "of the uterus"—neurologists had begun to attribute the condition to a malfunction of the *nervous system* from as early as the late seventeenth century. By the time of Wang's writing, hysteria was overwhelmingly being considered a "psychoneurotic disorder" rather than an obstetric or gynecological one.[44] Furthermore, from the second half of the nineteenth century, psychiatrists and neurologists no longer talked about hysteria as an ailment that affected only women. Believed to originate from the nerves rather than the uterus, hysteria was increasingly defined as a condition that could affect both sexes with equal measure.[45] Wang's description of hysteria, which he attempted to align with his understanding of *zangzao*, thereby strayed from the contemporary neurological consensus.

At the same time that Wang was reimagining hysteria, though, he was cleverly manipulating *zangzao* as well. Despite the fact that he referenced the *Essential Prescriptions of the Golden Cabinet* to define the elusive disorder, he also added his own commentary to the original gloss—a commentary that did not necessarily have any hermeneutic basis in previous medical texts. His assertion that *zang* (a generic term for the organs) refers to the uterus was not substantiated by any earlier writings, nor was his contention that *zangzao* was an obstetric affliction; to the contrary, medical practitioners in a later exposition underscored the primary role played by the liver and heart, not the uterus, in the onset of the disorder.[46] According to Charlotte Furth, moreover, the uterus was not believed to play a substantial structural role in Chinese medicine. Thought to be "functionally passive and insignificant," it served few ends outside of gestation.[47] Wang's commentary, therefore, had little basis in Chinese medical theory, and his decision to foreground the uterus was arguably made to underscore the similitude between *zangzao* and hysteria.

By taking advantage of the fact that hysteria and *zangzao* were both historically contingent, dynamic, and ambiguously defined, Wang was able to forge a conceptual space in which Chinese and Western medicine coexisted on an equal footing. Indeed, Wang's assertion that *zangzao* "is *now* referred to as hysteria" signaled that Chinese medicine could not only accommodate Western forms of knowledge, but had perhaps even anticipated them. In Wang's view, then, Chinese and Western medicine were not oppositional systems but rather mutually intelligible ones; having simply employed different words for otherwise comparable concepts, the two had independently arrived at the same conclusions. This revelation was facilitated, to a certain extent, by the malleability of language and the pliancy of its meanings. As a site of negotiation, appropriation, and compromise, translation functioned as a means by which Chinese intellectuals could reimagine and align neuropsychiatric concepts with Chinese medical theory. Thus, mental illness became an affliction of the kidneys and heart, while hysteria was returned to its gendered past. The contingent and mutable nature of medical ideology—negotiated through the unstable medium of the changing Chinese language—enabled, in some ways, the two epistemological systems to achieve at least a temporary reconciliation.

Vignette 3: Mixing Theory and Practice

The process of forging common ground between Chinese medicine and neuropsychiatry was not simply one that was undertaken, consciously or otherwise, by the upper echelons of the Chinese intelligentsia. In the everyday lived experiences of ordinary people, too, aspects of both systems continued to coexist. Specifically, even though Beijing families typically invoked traditional explanations for the onset of madness, they simultaneously began to incorporate biomedical treatments into their preexistent therapeutic regimens. As Hugh Shapiro has rightly observed, mentally ill patients in Beijing "regularly articulated their ideas about mental disorders in the idiom of the received medical canon," yet they did so in new therapeutic spaces and under the gaze of biomedical practitioners.[48] Hopeful that foreign physicians would succeed where native healers had failed, families clung to indigenous *theories* of madness while experimenting with Western *practices* of institutional treatment.

Throughout the 1930s, patients who sought care at local psychopathic hospitals routinely articulated their distress in a relatively traditional vocabulary. At the PUMC, some attributed their disorder to external pathogenic agents, such as cold and heat, while others framed the origins of their affliction in terms of an imbalance of *yin* and *yang*.[49] Many believed that they had gone mad due to a particularly strong bout of emotion, usually rage or fear, which had then affected the corresponding organ of the liver or lung.[50] For instance, one young woman, diagnosed as psychotic and schizophrenic by physicians at the PUMC, attributed the source of her disorder to anger. Furious at her father-in-law for refusing to provide monetary support for her children, she blamed the onset of her condition on domestic angst and pent-up rage. Furthermore, as she explained to the caretaker on duty, her illness had likely been exacerbated by the vengeful influence of her new husband's recently deceased first wife.[51]

Many patients, particularly men, ascribed the source of their madness to psychic stress and mental taxation. Just as scholars in the Qing dynasty had gone mad while preparing for the civil examinations, intellectuals in the Republican period continued to cling to the rationale of cognitive overexertion as a way to explain the onset of their mental symptoms. In 1935, a young soldier named Ma Muzhao, discussed previously in chapter 4, arrived at Wei Hongsheng's psychopathic hospital complaining that he had developed "schizophrenia and nervous tension" as a result of having "overworked his mind" (laoxin).[52] In 1933, similarly, a twenty-three-year-old man named Fan Huanbi checked himself into a private mental hospital in Shanghai, explaining to the attendants that he had developed disordered nerves "because he had thought too much."[53] The popularity of neurasthenic discourses, moreover, both solidified and perpetuated the perceived etiological relationship between cogitation and madness; since neurasthenia was known to be caused by "mental overwork" (jingshen guolao) and "morbid introspection," the disorder provided sufferers with a culturally sanctioned rationale for their psychosomatic distress.[54]

Despite biomedicine's antipathy to supernatural explanations for disease, Chinese patients continued to insist that their madness was caused by spirits, ghosts, and deceased ancestors. Andrew Woods noted how a coolie woman, whom he diagnosed as hysterical, had convinced herself that "a chicken had 'taken possession' of her."[55] Richard Lyman discussed a schizophrenic patient whose interview involved the "loose mention of ghosts and spirits."[56] And the psychiatrist James Lincoln McCartney (1898–1969) remarked that supernatural forces inevitably pervaded the ideations of the mentally deranged; the Chinese patient, he claimed, "sees devils; he hears them; he feels them; he is possessed by them, and is tormented by them in every conceivable manner."[57] Although social workers at the Beijing Psychopathic Hospital noticed that upper-class patients tended to spurn this view, those with "an absence of education" often believed in the existence of ghosts and saw them in their hallucinations.[58] One twenty-six-year-old man, for example, went mad out of fright after he was forced to "curse a spirit" in writing (xie yinzhuang), while a thirty-seven-year-old woman claimed to have gone mad after "seeing ghosts and specters."[59]

Sufferers of mental illness also drew on long-standing cultural repertoires to frame the ways in which they articulated and experienced their "psychic" distress. As the anthropologist Arthur Kleinman has argued, mental illness in non-Western societies is often experienced somatically, rather than existentially; consequently, Chinese patients typically articulate their suffering in a somatic idiom rather than a psychological one.[60] At the PUMC, social workers observed that their charges tended to endure physical symptoms for problems that otherwise seemed emotional or intrapsychic. The social worker Ida Pruitt (1888–1985), for instance, described a female patient who suffered from chronic epigastric pain but whose tests revealed no organic basis for the affliction. Investigating the woman's background, she determined that her patient's psychosomatic distress derived from her "unhappy" family life, where she was frequently beaten by her father-in-law and harassed by the family matriarch. To resolve the situation, Pruitt simply proposed that the woman and her husband move away from his family's compound, a suggestion with which they happily complied.[61]

In other cases, patients referenced the traditional concept of mucous stagnation to describe their experience of the disorder. As they told the intake officers who received them, they suffered not from "madness," per se, but from "mucous confusion," "mucous fire," "mucous illness" (*tanji*), and "mucous *qi*" (*tanqi*).[62] Cultural beliefs about the pathological influence of mucous also conditioned patients to interpret their disorder in a somatic register. When explaining the symptoms of their suffering to neuropsychiatric practitioners, they often referenced the thick phlegm that had accumulated in their chest and abdomen. James McCartney noted how his psychotic patients isolated the physical roots of their disorder within the internal organs of the torso, which they believed had been stopped up with sputum.[63] One such patient, whom the police had found unconscious in the middle of the street, confirmed that he had "felt confused" and his "mouth had filled with a whitish liquid" just prior to fainting. He was briefly detained under suspicion of madness before being discharged to the care of his brother.[64]

Indeed, despite neuropsychiatry's attempts to reframe mental illness as a disorder of the brain, psychiatric patients insisted that the somatic roots of their ailment lay elsewhere, namely within the heart and chest. Mad people claimed that their heart felt "busy," "confused," "muddled," "sick," or "tugged upon" (*jiu*).[65] At the psychopathic hospital, they experienced physical symptoms including heart palpitations, a sense of obstruction within the chest, and difficulty breathing.[66] At least partially, the widespread emphasis on the heart as the site of "mental" distress was bolstered by the Chinese language itself. Not only did the word *xin* refer to both the physical heart and the metaphysical mind, but the term was often employed analogically to describe a range of other emotions. In 1934, a social worker at the Beijing Psychopathic Hospital named Yao Tzu-ai conducted a survey of 316 patients in order to determine how the Chinese under her care expressed emotion. Many, she concluded, fixated on the heart as the biological anchor of emotional pain. "Heart death" (*xinsi*) described a complete loss of hope, "cold heart" (*saixin*) denoted loss of interest and disappointment, "discomforted heart" (*exin*) referenced abhorrence or disgust, and "burning heart" (*xinjiao*) signified great anxiety, as if the heart "were being consumed by fire."[67] Since the relationship among cognition, emotion, and the heart was reinforced both etiologically and linguistically, it was only natural for "mental" patients to experience the locus of their suffering within the chest.[68]

Because these expressions of madness were being voiced within the space of the psychopathic hospital, it was inevitable that biomedical physicians and their Chinese patients would experience miscommunications and misunderstandings. Hugh Shapiro has previously described the case of one mentally ill woman who arrived at the PUMC with her nose plugged with paper. When she expressed her fear that polluted air would enter her body and cause her abdomen to distend, physicians diagnosed her as schizophrenic. What her Western doctors failed to realize, however, was that such concerns were not uncommon among the lower classes; as an opening onto the outside world, the nostrils were often interpreted in Chinese medicine as an entryway through which miasmatic poisons could penetrate the body and cause disease.[69] Once Chinese configurations of illness entered the psychopathic hospital, in other words, Western physicians deprived them of their independent meaning and absorbed them into the ontology of neuropsychiatry. Chinese patients, meanwhile, attempted to resist these partisan interpretations by underscoring the validity of their own medical knowledge.[70]

These sorts of interactions, though likely frustrating at the time, should not be read as evidence that Chinese medicine and biomedicine were inherently antagonistic. I suggest, to the contrary, that they serve as proof of their very reconciliation. Although Chinese patients may not have accepted the underlying premises of neuropsychiatric *theory*, they were nevertheless open to experimenting with neuropsychiatric *practice*. The psychopathic hospital thus became a place of encounter between Chinese beliefs and Western therapies. In the search for a solution to their suffering, patients and families approached the curative technologies of biomedicine as simply one possibility among many, and they experimented with a range of solutions without necessarily conceding ideological allegiance to any one in particular. But precisely because they did not consider theory and practice to be irreconcilable, neuropsychiatry was able—at least in a curative capacity—to penetrate their existent worldview. In this way, too, did Chinese medicine and neuropsychiatry ultimately converge within the everyday lives of the Beijing people.

Vignette 4: The Patient as Person

Although Chinese and Western medicine may have retained largely divergent views on the etiology of madness, one of the ways they overlapped was in their shared belief that personal trauma could lead to psychosomatic distress.

As Richard Lyman observed in 1934, "The factors which are dominant precipitating influences [of mental illness] in America (such as work, sex, resentment against the social order, etc.) are also to be found here in China."[71] Yet, despite the acknowledgment that mental disorders could be linked to social causes, most neurologists at the PUMC expressed little interest in treating patients with purely psychogenic complaints. Concerned more with organic, material diseases than functional neuroses, physicians often dismissed or ignored patients whose illnesses had no obvious biological basis. To them, the only disorders worth investigating were strictly somatic ones.[72]

This final vignette will show how Chinese medicine was able to influence the contemporary biomedical construction of mental illness, which upheld a mostly mechanistic and materialist view of bodily structure and malfunction. Insisting instead that the patient be treated as a unified, integrated entity— one who was not divided, in a dualist fashion, between his mental and physical aspects—Chinese social workers at the PUMC and Beijing Psychopathic Hospital proposed that mental illness be understood in emotional, social, and cultural terms, rather than exclusively somatic ones. Through an emphasis on approaching the patient as a *person*, rather than as a purely biological entity, Chinese social workers sought to fundamentally alter the ways in which PUMC physicians—and materialist neuropsychiatry as a whole—interpreted the causes and solutions of mental disorders. As a result of their efforts, biomedicine at the PUMC tentatively entered the epistemic space of Chinese medical theory.

According to a study conducted in 1935, over two-thirds of patients who visited the neurological clinic at the PUMC demonstrated no organic disease.[73] Although it was clear that they suffered from severe psychological distress, physicians could pinpoint no material cause for their complaints; surmising that the source of their suffering was psychosocial rather than biological, many physicians concluded that such people did not require medical assistance. Andrew Woods, for instance, opined in 1924 that "a troublesome proportion of general hospital patients complain of symptoms which are exaggerated and misleading, or which are in toto built upon a psychical basis."[74] Other internists estimated that as many as 70 percent of their patients presented no organic symptoms, and therefore had no need to receive medical treatment.[75] And despite the fact that Richard Lyman had incorporated psychiatric social workers into the daily management of the municipal psychopathic hospital, physicians at the PUMC itself remained generally uninterested in psychogenic complaints. Finding such cases to be a "nuisance" and not epistemologically useful, they typically discharged or refused to admit patients without any obvious neurological damage.[76]

Reports from clinicians and social workers confirm that a large proportion of Chinese patients attributed their distress to socioeconomic circumstances, many of which were gendered. While psychotic women complained of domestic adversities, men complained of business failures and economic pressures.[77] The American sociologist Herbert Day Lamson (1899–1954) observed that women "became deranged" when their husbands took concubines or their mothers-in-law mistreated them.[78] Andrew Woods similarly noted how female madness arose when women were "cruelly overworked and imposed upon" or feared that their "sexual attractiveness [had] waned."[79] Men, meanwhile, tended to frame the source of their madness in terms of financial hardship or the inability to perform an expected social role. The psychiatric social worker Song Siming, who was employed at the Beijing Psychopathic Hospital, claimed that loss of face, belittlement, and being unable to fulfill an expectation or demand most frequently led to mental illness in his male patients. Among these, he cited the example of a thirty-two-year-old man from Shandong province, who went mad and "saw ghosts and spirits" because he could not afford to pay his rent and care for his wife and sickly daughter.[80] In Shanghai, too, patients like Wu Shaozhang, aged thirty-seven, became unhinged because they "thought too much" about their economic straits, while Zhang Jinsheng, aged forty-four, "tore off his clothes and spoke crazy words" after having lost his position at work.[81] Overcome by the desires and disappointments of their social reality, ordinary people retreated into the solitary world of madness.

Although it was undeniable that most of these men and women had experienced genuine mental breakdowns, some prospective patients strategically adopted the language and behaviors of mad people as a means of both contesting the domination of the patriarchal system and achieving refuge from its unattainable expectations. One woman, for instance, feigned madness and fled to the PUMC to escape the mistreatment of her abusive in-laws,[82] while another registered at the local psychiatric ward to avoid the tyranny of her husband's jealous concubine.[83] Within this context, the psychopathic hospital became a place of refuge: a site where individuals could receive respite from the obligations of their ordinary existence, as well as care, support, and official legitimation for their psychosomatic suffering.[84] Yet, precisely because such people exhibited a form of psychic distress that did not align with the neurological materialism of the PUMC, they were often denied the attention they so desperately sought. Throughout the 1920s, the PUMC maintained a strict policy that psychogenic cases be turned away or transferred to alternate institutions.[85] Consequently, individuals with no organic basis for their complaints were left with little recourse for their suffering.

This approach to the treatment of the mentally ill would not begin to change until the mid-1930s, following the hiring of Richard Lyman and his recruitment of a Chinese sociologist named Dai Bingham (1899–1996). While pursuing a doctorate in sociology at the University of Chicago, Dai was hired to work as a psychotherapist at the PUMC, a role he performed between 1935 and 1939.[86] A short period into his tenure, he lambasted the cavalier way that his PUMC colleagues dispensed with the mentally ill:

> To say that patients who have no organic disease have no business to come to the hospital and take up their valuable time, or to ridicule these patients for their stupidity, or get disgusted with them for their supposed maliciousness when they keep returning to the hospital, in spite of orders to the contrary, should certainly not be the attitude of the representatives of a responsible medical profession, although it is a lamentable fact that such seems to be the attitude of many practitioners.

Recognizing that people who were denied treatment at the PUMC would have few alternatives outside of "quack doctors and witchcraft," Dai emphasized the need for a "new orientation as regards the concepts of health and disease" at the hospital. He therefore advocated for an improved set of regulations concerning the intake and discharge of mentally ill patients, alongside a fundamentally different approach to the treatment of psychiatric disorders.[87]

In Dai's view, biomedicine had several flaws when it came to the provision of mental illness. On the one hand, Western physicians tended to think of the patient as little more than a "biological organism." Conditioned by their materialist outlook, they rarely considered the person's life history or individual experiences when investigating the nature of the disease. Even when they did, though, the patient's perspective was necessarily considered secondary to his or her physical symptoms, which were believed to be more objective and empirically reliable. On the other hand, Dai also disavowed the dualist rift between body and mind. "In life," he argued, "such a dichotomy does not exist." By ignoring the "unitary nature of the human organism," and by focusing strictly on eradicating the *disease* rather than treating the *patient*, biomedicine, he argued, would inevitably be frustrated in its attempts to effect a complete cure.[88]

In contrast to the biological point of view, Dai advocated for a more integrated approach to the treatment of psychiatric patients. Convinced that humans were more than just the sum of their material parts, he suggested that biomedical physicians consider the role that culture and socialization play in the onset of disease. As he explained, human life was inextricable from its environment and social context; the preservation of health and the eradication of illness therefore required an attention not simply to conditions at the cellular level, but also to the state of one's interpersonal relationships and emotional well-being. In a series of essays, he urged his colleagues to think of the patient as a multifaceted *person* rather than a mere "physico-chemical reactive system." Only when physicians accepted the indivisible relationship between body and mind, soma and society, would they be able to overcome their "impasse" in understanding the causes and cures of psychiatric disorders.[89]

Although Dai referred to the above position as the "sociological point of view," his perspective was deeply interwoven with ideas borrowed from Chinese medicine and philosophy. Indeed, over the course of his career, Dai became more explicit about the ways that Chinese systems of knowledge could contribute to psychotherapeutics. In his own practice, he often incorporated aspects of Daoist doctrine into his counseling sessions. Adopting a "non-action" (*wu wei*) approach to therapy, Dai believed that "the best therapist is no therapist" and that patients ultimately made the best recovery when they could rely on their own intuitions.[90] He claimed, moreover, that psychiatrists could benefit from integrating the practices of Zen (Chan) Buddhism into their approach to patient counseling. Through meditation or the recitation of koans, patients could alleviate their suffering and become "empty in the sense of freedom from all kinds of preoccupations."[91] Finally, Dai also experimented with the therapeutic applications of Confucian philosophy. One patient, who suffered from severe headaches—a problem that would have been considered purely neurological at the PUMC[92]—attributed his condition to a constant sense of competition with his classmates at school. Dai, inspired by the Confucian principle of *ren* (which he defined as the quality of "being human"), suggested to his patient that he rejoice in the success of other people rather than compete against them for praise and recognition. The patient, upon putting this principle into action, remarked that he was able to feel "liberated" for the first time in his life.[93]

At the PUMC, Dai vigorously promoted the importance of adopting an integrated, patient-centered approach to mental health. To that end, he provided psychotherapeutic training to Western-educated physicians and staff. Referring to his technique as "personality study," Dai encouraged his colleagues to become more cognizant of the close connection between the pathological body, its sociocultural context, and the person's subjective experience of illness; in so doing, he aspired to increase his colleagues' awareness of the utility of psychotherapeutics while also encouraging them to integrate these techniques into their own practice.[94] In Beijing, furthermore, Dai was vocal about his multiculturalist view of mental health. Anticipating the position now held by most medical anthropologists, he argued that different cultures maintain different ideas about what constitutes "madness." In China, he noted, shamanistic trances were considered perfectly normal, a view that contrasted with the received biomedical position. By acknowledging the idiomatic nature of mental wellness and illness, Dai concluded, physicians could develop a deeper understanding of the types of issues they might confront among non-Western populations.[95]

For Dai, then, the problem of "mental illness" was, at root, the problem of "being human."[96] Condemning neuropsychiatry's tendency to turn the person into a "physiological machine," he instead recommended an approach to psychiatric therapeutics that took into consideration the life history, human relationships, cultural assumptions, and social position of each respective patient. His beliefs were inspired to a large extent by Chinese philosophy and medical theory. Recognizing the integrated nature of body and mind, he advocated for a unitary view of the "person" rather than a mechanistic view of the "organism." Dai's efforts, which ultimately aimed to enhance the "conceptual equipment of the average physician," provide witness to the dynamism of the East-West encounter.[97] Indeed, it was not simply Chinese medicine that evolved through its interactions with the West. Western physicians, too, stood to benefit profoundly from their experiences among the Chinese.[98]

Between East and West

In the four vignettes above, neuropsychiatry did not so much displace preexistent views about madness as it complemented, augmented, and sometimes even reinforced them. Chinese medicine practitioners were able to systematically integrate the Chinese "heart" and the biomedical "brain" into a single conceptual system, thereby retaining the epistemic utility of both. Intellectuals invoked Chinese medical concepts to explain neuropsychiatric neologisms, blurring their respective boundaries in the process. Patients experimented with new care-seeking behaviors while continuing to articulate their illness narratives in a traditional vocabulary. And biomedicine, too, was forced to reconsider its vision of the mechanical body, divided neatly between its somatic and psychic halves. Despite the fact that neuropsychiatry had become institutionalized in Beijing by the 1930s, its existence and official sanction did not undermine the persistence of preexistent assumptions about the nature of the body and the essence of the mad condition.

This is not to say that Chinese medicine and neuropsychiatry were always able to so comfortably coexist. Just as Wei Yulin, who began this chapter, endeavored to replace Chinese beliefs about madness with Western views on mental illness, other medical modernizers—often having trained in Japan or the West—found little of use in the conceptual doctrines of Chinese medical theory. Promoting instead the "absolute superiority of modern medicine," they uniformly supported the abolition of "backward" Chinese practices.[99] But this viewpoint, I would suggest, constitutes a small, albeit vocal, extreme. Ordinary people, moved less by ideology than expedience, remained flexible in their approach to health; what worked could be used and what did not could be discarded. Some practitioners of Chinese medicine also responded to the confrontation with biomedicine less out of opposition than genuine intellectual interest. Recognizing that the two systems were merely trying to achieve the same end—to understand the body and to eradicate its diseases—they integrated useful words and principles into their preexistent repertoires while retaining the tried-and-true theories that underlay their own medical regimens. And in the case of Dai Bingham, dissatisfaction with the limits and biases of contemporary neuropsychiatric practice compelled him to emphasize the benefits of an integrated approach to psychiatric therapeutics.

In the ongoing search for the cure to madness, then, "science" and "superstition" were not at the forefront of most peoples' minds, nor was the elusive aspiration to achieve medical modernity and national self-strengthening. Far more frequently, quotidian concerns begot quotidian desires: to make sense of suffering, to alleviate pain, and to restore the individual to a state of productivity and health. It was in the pursuit of these goals that families, intellectuals, and medical practitioners oscillated between Chinese and Western medicine, thereby creating new forms of medical knowledge along the way. Thus madness was not only remade but also dispersed, pivoting (once again) between the various words, theories, and bodily morphologies that sought to contain it.

Conclusion

On August 8, 1937, Beijing fell to Japanese forces. When the Guomindang army retreated, those with the means and the motivation followed alongside to the southwest. Most, however, remained in the city to eke out a life under the watchful eye of the Japanese. In December of that year, Japan established the Provisional Government of the Republic of China, a puppet regime that operated, at least ostensibly, under the leadership of a Chinese bureaucrat named Wang Kemin (1879–1945). Supported by a coterie of Chinese intellectuals—including Zhou Zuoren, the neurasthenic essayist whom we first met in chapter 4—the regime sought to return Beijing to an imagined status quo. Hardly anyone believed that the puppet government was acting on its own power. But for the sake of maintaining a modicum of normalcy, many chose to overlook that the city no longer belonged to them.

Despite the war, the Guomindang's earlier provision of madness continued apace for a time. The Peking Union Medical College maintained its operations in the city for a few years, and even persisted in its arrangements with the municipal Ministry of Health, now under the supervision of the Chinese puppet government.[1] The psychopathic hospital, enlarged and relocated to the Temple of Earth (*Ditan*) in northeastern Beijing, continued to be overseen by Wei Yulin.[2] But as the United States declared war on Japan in 1941, and as the foreigners still living in the city were pulled into the global conflict, the situation at the psychopathic hospital slowly began to change for the worse. The next year, the Peking Union Medical College closed down entirely.[3] As its personnel scattered to other parts of the country, and as the budget of the psychopathic hospital was unceremoniously slashed in half, a steady stream of nurses, staff, and social workers decided to put their talents to use in other places. By 1942, a total of sixteen individuals had quit.[4] Two years after that, Wei tendered his resignation as well, and the hospital was subsequently turned over to the care of the Japanese.[5]

By the time the Second Sino-Japanese War (1937–1945) and the ensuing civil war (1945–1949) concluded, it is estimated that only a handful of psychiatrists—somewhere between thirty and sixty in total—remained in the country.[6] Most, having either become weary of the incessant warfare or fearful of the impending communist victory, chose to pursue their careers elsewhere. Some moved to Taiwan or Hong Kong, while others reignited connections in the United States. Dai Bingham, for instance, followed Richard Lyman to Duke University, while the psychiatric social worker Francis Hsü pursued a doctorate in anthropology and was later hired at Northwestern University in Chicago.[7] Although a few of the people who had previously worked at the psychopathic hospital decided to stay on in China, the future of their field would be dramatically—and in some ways irreparably—altered by the rapidly changing political context.

Under the leadership of the Chinese Communist Party (CCP), which rose to power in 1949, the contours of madness were once again redefined. Seeking to distance itself from Western forms of psychological epistemology, which were deemed subjective and idealist, the CCP pressured psychiatrists and psychologists to reframe their work in accordance with the conditioned response model of Pavlovian materialism.[8] At the First National Conference of Psychiatric Specialists, held in Nanjing in 1958, attending members condemned the earlier reliance on foreign psychiatric theories and urged, in their stead, the development of indigenous techniques; these included strategies such as the reading of Maoist texts and the cultivation of "revolutionary optimism"—that is, the conviction that patients could consciously will themselves back to health for the greater good of the communist movement.[9] During the Cultural Revolution (1966–1976), in tandem with the radicalization of domestic politics, the mentally ill occasionally became targets of attack. Conflating ideological deviance with madness, authorities deployed the language of forensic psychiatry as a pretext to institutionalize those who espoused heterodox or counterrevolutionary views. Treatment for the mentally ill consisted largely of political study and self-criticism sessions, while the most extreme offenders were publicly persecuted, jailed, or sometimes even executed.[10]

It was not until the death of Mao Zedong (1893–1976), and the subsequent reopening to the Western world in the decades that followed, that psychiatric practices in China would return to a version akin to the ones that were slowly being established in the 1930s. By that time, however, "mental illness" in the West no longer looked quite the same as it had half a century earlier. Psychiatrists had long since abandoned classifications like "hysterical" and "neurasthenic." (Although neurasthenia has been retained in Chinese psychiatric taxonomy, it is now considered a "culture-bound syndrome" in American medicine.)[11] Masturbation and homosexuality were no longer regarded, at least officially, as evidence of mental pathology.[12] And the pursuit of mental hygiene had also been renounced, along with its concomitant interest in the sterilization and forced segregation of the feebleminded and mentally ill. Meanwhile, psychiatry and neurology were progressively cleaved in two, once again reflecting changing assumptions about the relationship between brain and mind, body and soul. As madness in China had evolved, so too had it evolved in the West. And just as in the early twentieth century, when the Chinese on the cusp of revolution had to make sense of the (often conflicting) psychiatric discourses that confronted them, reformers in the late twentieth century would be forced to do the same.[13]

Beyond Beijing

In tracing a genealogy of madness from the late Qing to the Second World War, this book has argued that psychiatry in China underwent a continual process of meaning making. This was a dialogical, not unidirectional, process. Rather than simply mirroring structures of Western psychiatric modernity (which were themselves contested and being constantly redefined), new meanings and practices of madness in Beijing were actively forged by a variety of actors in ways that reflected their own needs, ideals, and interests. Even though foreign physicians sought to impose their respective visions of mental illness onto the Chinese people, and even though subsequent government regimes desired to attain the legitimacy that psychiatric "modernity" would bestow on them, the discourses and institutions that they introduced to the public took on new lives of their own. As individuals at different levels of society appropriated, transformed, or simply ignored different aspects of these imported ideologies, psychiatry—and, indeed, the very state of scientific modernity itself—was continually remade and reinvented in their own image.

Modernity, in this sense, appeared as a modular rather than a monolithic condition. Far from the "final stable structure" described by the historian Benjamin Schwartz,[14] scientific modernity was at once insecure and continually in flux, composed not of a single ideology but a variety of component (and often competing) parts. It was its very modularity, at least to a certain extent, that enabled the Chinese people to pick apart, selectively repurpose, and redefine psychiatric ideas in ways that suited their own agendas—thereby transforming their meanings and uses in the process. Even in the face of the Western influence, then, the provision of mental illness in early twentieth-century China remained largely a product of the Chinese imagination.

Having situated this narrative in Beijing—a place that, as noted at the beginning of this book, experienced a historically peculiar relationship to the forces of Western imperialism and industrial capitalism—one might be moved to question how representative it is to the rest of China. Could similar circumstances, actuated by similar actors, have unfolded outside of Beijing, as well? The answer to this question is both no and yes. On the one hand, the exact elements that comprised this story are, to a certain degree, historically unique. Although a handful of foreign-managed asylums had sprung up throughout urban China beginning in the late Qing and early republic, Beijing was the only city in the country that boasted a public asylum managed entirely by the municipality itself. And although foreign physicians, like those at the Peking Union Medical College, had begun to throw themselves more heartily into psychiatric work by the middle of the Nanjing Decade, none had orchestrated the same type of arrangement with the local Ministry of Health as Richard Lyman had successfully done. Outside of major urban areas, moreover, the status of the insane at the end of the republic likely differed little from how it had appeared at the beginning. Insulated from many of the discourses that were taking shape in the coastal cities, rural dwellers continued to employ vocabularies and modes of treatment that had been the norm throughout much of the late Qing.[15] Comparatively speaking, the specific details and circumstances that animated this account are, on a whole, particular to Beijing itself.

On the other hand, the thread that underlies my more general narrative—that psychiatric knowledge and practices have continuously been remade in a way that serves the needs and interests of a range of domestic actors—is arguably generalizable both to China writ large and to other colonial contexts.[16] Though situated primarily in Beijing, this book has occasionally extended its orientation outward to other locations, including the treaty ports of Shanghai and Guangzhou. In both places, psychiatric practices were forced to accommodate the contingent demands and desires of the local people, and the geography of madness and its treatment was inevitably changed as a result.

In Shanghai, despite the existence of foreign-managed and self-proclaimed "modern" psychopathic clinics, biomedicine could hardly be said to monopolize the provision of mental disorders.[17] Instead, Chinese-run facilities, like the Shanghai Specialized Hospital for the Insane (Shanghai fengdian zhuanmen yiyuan), combined an institutional approach to psychiatric treatment with a decidedly nonbiomedical therapeutic methodology—one that continued to reference pathological processes like "mucous confusion" (*tanmi*) and "*qi* obstruction" (*qiyu*). By couching their treatments in a familiar vernacular, and by only employing native medical techniques like acupuncture and *tuina* massage, physicians at the Shanghai Specialized Hospital claimed that they could serve the needs of their Chinese clientele more effectively than a facility built on the precepts of neuropsychiatry.[18] In Guangzhou, similarly, the John G. Kerr Refuge for the Insane may have attracted the interests of local patrons, but it was scarcely effective at persuading them to accept a biomedical rationale. Given that the refuge provided religious counsel, vocational training, and long-term managerial care alongside treatment, families and patients alike patronized the facility not necessarily on account of its neuropsychiatric orientation, but rather because it offered services that they could otherwise not attain: specifically, reprieve from the emotional and financial burdens of madness, as well as relief from the existential hardships of everyday life.[19] Records from the refuge therefore reveal a latent ambivalence toward biomedicine itself, one that manifested in families' repeated efforts to enhance Western remedies with Chinese ones.[20]

Just as in Beijing, individuals in Shanghai and Guangzhou viewed Western psychiatric services as a strategic resource, one that could supplement—though not necessarily replace—preexistent ideas about the nature and treatment of madness. While families and local communities may have taken advantage of the charity provided by foreign psychopathic hospitals, this did not mean that they were entirely committed to its underlying ideologies.[21] And while Chinese-managed clinics may have appropriated the institutional format of the psychopathic hospital, they simultaneously imbued these foreign spaces with an indigenous therapeutic content. In all three locations, psychiatric methodologies enabled new remedial and managerial possibilities to arise. Nevertheless, the specific ways that these ideologies were put into practice were ultimately determined by the needs of the Chinese people themselves.

Looking Forward

When it comes to matters of mental illness, the concerns of the past have not necessarily diminished in the present but have simply taken a different form. This is particularly true for the ways that the Western world has continued to monitor psychiatric treatment in China—as well as the ways that the Chinese people have responded to the critiques that have been raised. Beginning in the early 2010s, the American news media became closely attuned to ongoing problems in Chinese psychiatric care, especially following a series of stabbings at rural elementary schools that were perpetrated by individuals suspected of being psychologically unstable. Claiming that the mentally ill in China are "invisible"[22] or "in the shadows,"[23] and that psychiatric treatment is "inadequate,"[24] "unaddressed,"[25] "lacking,"[26] and a "medical backwater,"[27]

foreign pundits and physicians have championed more aggressive government intervention into matters of treatment, prevention, and access to professional care.

The Chinese Ministry of Health has responded in turn. As early as 2004,
the government set in motion an initiative that would train thousands of
additional mental health professionals and establish numerous community
mental health centers across the country.[28] In 2012, furthermore, the Ministry of Health passed China's first National Mental Health Law (Jingshen
weisheng fa), which aimed to expand mental health services into rural areas,
improve quality of care, and provide patients with increased rights to deny
unwanted treatment.[29] Taking these steps, the government has proclaimed,
will enable the Chinese to achieve "psychological harmony" (*xinli hexie*)—a
turn of phrase that distinctly recalls the "psychological reconstruction" of the
Republican era.[30]

Despite the rhetoric and efforts of the Chinese government, however, the
treatment of mental illness in contemporary China looks strangely little like
it does in the West. Although highly sophisticated psychopathic hospitals
exist in large urban centers, institutional and professional care is typically
considered a supplemental strategy rather than an option of first resort. Consequently, an estimated 90 percent of people with mental illness live with
their families (as opposed to 40 percent in the United States),[31] and only
5 percent of people with a diagnosable mental illness have ever seen a mental health professional.[32] In seeking to explain these disparities, researchers
have pointed to three main causes: the high costs of psychiatric services, geographical unevenness in access to care, and an absence of knowledge about
mental illness and scientific psychiatry. For instance, in a recent survey about
attitudes toward schizophrenia in a rural township outside of Chengdu, researchers concluded that most respondents "had no knowledge of mental illness." When their relatives exhibited behavioral, cognitive, or emotional difficulties, families instead attributed these problems to supernatural influences,
an underlying physical imbalance, or simply thinking too much. The types of
treatments that they pursued were subsequently informed by their perceived
etiology of the disorder.[33]

While the above explanations are certainly valid, I would also suggest that
they are incomplete. Rather than frame Chinese responses to mental illness
entirely in negative terms (that is, lack of monetary support, lack of access,
and lack of knowledge), it is perhaps equally useful to view the current status
of mental healthcare in China at least partially as the product of a deliberate
strategy, one that has been determined by local needs and beliefs. For example, the anthropologist Zhiying Ma, who has observed patient-physician

interactions in a Guangzhou psychopathic hospital, has shown how families frequently challenge the advice of biomedical physicians even after having chosen to pursue institutional care. Believing that Chinese medicine is equally, if not more, advantageous to the patient, families pursue a range of therapeutic strategies concurrently: they prepare homemade broths to counteract the negative side effects of psychotropic drugs, they confer with other families about the efficacy of local healers, and they narrate the symptoms of mental illness in the language of Chinese medical epistemology. Criticizing biomedicine as only "treating the branches but not the root" of the disorder—that is, alleging that it only alleviates the symptoms of mental illness but not its underlying cause—families experiment with neuropsychiatric models while also resisting their biological reductionism.[34]

At the level of the state, moreover, the CCP has taken initiatives to advance the cause of psychotherapy and diminish the stigma of mental illness, but it has done so in ways that might appear unconventional or problematic to Western audiences. As Hsuan-Ying Huang has pointed out, recent increases in the number of psychological counselors can be attributed to a longer-term strategy engineered by the Chinese government. Following the dismantling of collectivization and the end of state-ensured job security, the Ministry of Labor and Social Securities attempted to create new forms of employment as a means of stimulating economic development. Psychological counseling was one such vocation that the ministry promoted through the creation of short-term and part-time training courses, all of which were geared toward non-professionals rather than medical specialists. The field was then popularized through primetime television programs that featured therapists miraculously "solving" their patients' problems in twenty-minute intervals. It was not just a spontaneous demand for psychotherapy that led to the emergence of the "psycho-boom" in urban China, Huang concludes, but rather the result of the state hoping to achieve continued economic growth.[35]

Watching these developments occur, I cannot help but be reminded of the situation in China one hundred years ago, when missionaries and physicians set in motion the beginnings of what would become a much longer process of psychiatric development in Beijing. Accusing the Qing government of failing to provide adequate support for its insane people, foreign observers derided what they saw as inhumane and superstitious practices involving the mentally ill. Over the course of the next three decades, different segments of Beijing society responded to these accusations directly—but did so in unexpected ways. The municipal police recognized the need to adopt a more proactive response to the insane but conflated madness with deviance and subversive activity in the process. When ordinary people took advantage of the social services offered by the state, they not only legitimized the burgeoning police presence in their lives but also tied madness more closely to poverty and vice. In the pursuit of profit, meanwhile, psychiatric entrepreneurs insisted on the medicalization of "mental" illness and "nervous" disease. And while Guomindang bureaucrats appropriated psychiatric discourses in the interests of financial expedience and political legitimacy, the right-wing intelligentsia sought to eradicate poor mental hygiene as a means of attaining political conformity and national strength. Throughout this process, a range of actors merged Chinese medicine and neuropsychiatry in ways that belied their apparent incongruities.

Each of these groups internalized the need for new responses to madness but did so on their own terms and in ways that appealed to their own interests. In the process, they created new forms of psychiatric knowledge that may or may not have had any resonance to the types of discourses being supported in the West. The situation today, I would argue, is little different. As in the early twentieth century, care for the mentally ill in China has again become a cause to be championed and a movement worthy of international attention. And just as one hundred years ago, the Chinese have responded to these calls in ways that satisfy their own sensibilities and agendas—agendas that may intersect with those of the West but do not necessarily align with them completely. This is not to deny that there remains considerable room for improvement when it comes to issues of Chinese (as well as global) mental health. But while it is noble and just to hope for a better future for the mentally ill (in China, in the West, and elsewhere in the world), we must also be reminded that divergence from Western norms does not always equal failure, and that what is appropriate in one context may be considered unsuitable in another. Disparities in treatment should therefore not automatically be considered "inadequacies," but must also be evaluated through the lens of Chinese values, epistemologies, and contemporary desires.

*

By using madness as a pivot around which "modernity" is circumscribed, this book has endeavored to show that modernity (broadly construed) and psychiatric modernity (more narrowly) are not just ready-made conditions waiting to be achieved by non-Western populations. Rather, modernity is better conceived as an ongoing process of *becoming*: one that does not so much exist "out there" in any sort of objective capacity, but requires instead the agential participation of individual actors who give it meaning through the very act of going about their lives. Thus conceptions of madness reflect and refract the subjectivities of specific populations, and articulating what it means to be "mad"—in much the same way as articulating what it means to be "modern"—requires a deep engagement with the moral life of a particular society and its people.

The philosopher Ian Hacking once argued that mental illnesses require a specific "ecological niche" in which to "thrive."[36] To this I would add that the niche itself could not exist without the individual tillers who cultivate it—those who not only plant its seeds, but also thresh the earth and water its soil. In China, as in the West, these actors have continually transformed the shape of the psychiatric environment both in response to historical conditions and in the pursuit of their own needs. And just as the ecological conditions of the Western world have diverged considerably from those in China, so too have the meanings of madness that have germinated in their midst. We should not be surprised, then, when those meanings continue to be invented and reinvented inexorably into the future.

Glossary of Chinese Terms

Ai Wei 艾偉
anzhi 安置
Bao Fangzhou 鮑芳洲
baojia 保甲
beichi 背馳
ben 本
biao 標
bufa 不罰
buwei zui 不為罪
Cai Yuanpei 蔡元培
chanhou diankuang 產後癲狂
Chao Weifang 巢渭芳
Chen Lifu 陳立夫
Chiang Kai-shek (Jiang Jieshi) 蔣介石
chubing 除病
chufen 處分
Dai Bingham 戴秉衡
dian 顛 / 癲
dianji 癲疾
diankuang 癲狂
dianxian 癲癇
Ding Ganren 丁甘仁
Ding Zan 丁瓚
Ditan 地壇
douliu 逗留
dunbi 遁避
duoluo 墮落
exin 惡心
fakuang 發狂
fan 犯

fanchang 反常
fannao 煩惱
fanzao 煩躁
fengbing 瘋病
fengbing sharen 瘋病殺人
fengbing zhiren 瘋病之人
fengdian 瘋癲
fengfu 瘋婦
fengke zhuanjia 瘋科專家
fengmi 瘋迷
fengren 瘋人
fengren yuan 瘋人院
fengzi 瘋子
fenluan 紛亂
fu 腑
funü ganhua suo 婦女感化所
fushe 附設
ganqi 肝氣
Gao Juefu 高覺敷
Gong'an ju 公安局
Gu Jiegang 顧頡剛
Gui Zhiliang 桂質良
Guo Renyuan 郭任遠
Hong Xiuquan 洪秀全
huadian 花癲
huan 患
Huang Chujiu 黃楚九
Huang Weirong 黃維榮
Huangdi neijing 黃帝內經
huatan 化痰
hun 魂
Ishikawa Hanzan 石川半山
jianhu 監護
jianjin 監禁
jiannao wan 健腦丸
jiaoyang yuan 教養院
jingshen bing 精神病
jingshen bing liaoyang yuan 精神病療養院
jingshen guolao 精神過勞
jingshen huanghu 精神恍惚
jingshen weisheng 精神衛生
Jingshen weisheng fa 精神衛生法
jingshen xiuyang yuan 精神修養院
Jingui yaolüe 金匱要略
jingzhi 精志
jiuji yuan 救濟院

juexing 覺性
jujin 拘禁
kaishi 開釋
kang 炕
kanya 看押
Kawashima Naniwa 川島浪速
kexue hua 科學化
kouliu 扣留
kuang 狂
kuangtai 狂態
Lao She 老舍
laoxin 勞心
leiyou fengji 類有瘋疾
Li Jianyi 李健頤
Li Yuan 李園
Li Yuanhong 黎元洪
Liang Qichao 梁啟超
Lin Chuanshu 林傳樹
lingpian 靈片
lingxing 靈性
lingyi 鈴醫
Liu Changyou 劉長佑
Liu Na'ou 劉吶鷗
liumen 六門
Lu Xun 魯迅
Ma Peizhi 馬培之
Mao Zedong 毛澤東
mixin 迷信
mousheng yingye 謀生營業
mu 畝
Mu Shiying 穆時英
nanyu 難愈
Natsume Sōseki 夏目漱石
nilun 逆倫
Nishi Amane 西周
panxuan 盤旋
po 魄
qi 氣
Qinding da Qing xin xinglü 欽定大清新刑律
qiyu 氣鬱
ren 仁
renlei gongcheng xue 人類工程學
ruchang 如常
ruyi 儒醫
Shanghai fengdian zhuanmen yiyuan 上海瘋癲專門醫院
Shehui ju 社會局

shen 神
Shen Jiaben 沈家本
shenji 神機
shenjing 神經
shenjing bing 神經病
shenjing jinzhang 神經緊張
shenjing shuairuo 神經衰弱
shenming 神明
shenren 神人
shenxin 身心
shenzhi 神志
Shi Sunzhi 史損之
shifang 釋放
shouyang pinmin suo 收養貧民所
si 思
Song Jiaoren 宋教仁
Song Siming 宋思明
Sun Xiong 孫雄
Sun Yat-sen (Sun Zhongshan) 孫中山
Tang Erhe 湯爾和
tanhuo 痰火
tanji 痰疾
tanmi 痰迷
tanmi xinqiao 痰迷心竅
tanqi 痰氣
Wang Baohua 王保華
Wang Chengxun 王承勳
Wang Kemin 王克敏
Wang Jiaxiang 王嘉祥
Wang Qiuyuan 汪秋元
Wang Runmin 王潤民
Wang Shixiong (Mengying) 王士雄 (孟英)
Wang Zuxiang (T. Hsiang Wang) 王祖祥
Wei Hongsheng 魏鴻聲
Wei Hongsheng jingshen bingyuan 魏鴻聲精神病院
Wei Yulin 魏毓麟
Weisheng bu 衛生部
Weisheng ju 衛生局
Weng Zhilong 翁之龍
wenti ertong 問題兒童
Wu Lien-teh (Wu Liande) 伍連德
Wu Nanxuan 吳南軒
wu wei 無為
wuxing 無形
xian 癇 / 痫
xiangdang chusuo 相當處所

xiao shimin 小市民
Xiao Xiaorong 蕭孝嶸
xie yinzhuang 寫陰狀
xin 心
xinbing 心病
xingli xue 性理學
xinji 心疾
xinjiao 心焦
xinli fenlie 心理分裂
xinli hexie 心理和諧
xinli jianshe 心理建設
xinli weisheng 心理衛生
xinli weisheng shi 心理衛生室
xinli xue 心理學
xinshen jiankang 心身健康
xinshen sangshi 心神喪失
xinshen yumen 心神鬱悶
xinsi 心死
xiyi gongchang 習藝工廠
Xu Langguang (Francis Hsü) 許烺光
Xu Zhimo 徐志摩
Xu Zhuodai 徐桌呆
xueshu 學術
yang 陽
Yang Huanwen 楊煥文
yanyi qiushen 延醫求神
yi'an 醫案
yidao 醫祷
yin 陰
yinfeng shangren 因瘋傷人
yizhi 醫治
yongyi 庸醫
yongyuan jiangu 永遠監錮
youmin 游民
Yu Shenchu 俞慎初
Yu Yan (Yunxiu) 余巖 (雲岫)
Yuan Shikai 袁世凱
zang 臟
zangzao 臟躁
Zhang Mengxiong 張夢熊
Zhang Yinian 章頤年
Zhao Jiyuan 趙吉元
zheng 症
Zhongguo xinli weisheng xiehui 中國心理衛生協會
zhongzu 種族
Zhou Xiaonong 周小農

Zhou Zuoren 周作人
zhu 主
Zhu Xi 朱熹
Zhu Zhenheng (Danxi) 朱震亨 (丹溪)
zhuangre hunkuang 壯熱昏狂
zhuanmen rencai 專門人才
Ziran zhiliao yiyuan 自然治療醫院
zizang 子臟
Zong Zihe 宗子和
zuodao 左道

Notes

Introduction

1. Beijing Municipal Archives (hereafter, BMA) J181-019-32402.

2. Michel Foucault, *Power/Knowledge* (New York: Pantheon Books, 1972), 97.

3. On chemistry, see James Reardon-Anderson, *The Study of Change: Chemistry in China, 1840–1949* (Cambridge: Cambridge University Press, 1991); on the social sciences, see Yung-chen Chiang, *Social Engineering and the Social Sciences in China, 1919–1949* (Cambridge: Cambridge University Press, 2001).

4. Leo Ou-fan Lee, *Shanghai Modern: The Flowering of a New Urban Culture in China, 1930–1945* (Cambridge, MA: Harvard University Press, 1999), 43.

5. For example, D. W. Y. Kwok, *Scientism in Chinese Thought, 1900–1950* (New Haven, CT: Yale University Press, 1965); Tse-tung Chow, *The May Fourth Movement: Intellectual Revolution in Modern China* (Cambridge, MA: Harvard University Press, 1960); Vera Schwarcz, *The Chinese Enlightenment: Intellectuals and the Legacy of the May Fourth Movement of 1919* (Berkeley: University of California Press, 1986).

6. Shu-mei Shih, *The Lure of the Modern: Writing Modernism in Semicolonial China, 1917–1937* (Berkeley: University of California Press, 2001), 49.

7. Liping Bu, "Social Darwinism, Public Health, and Modernization in China, 1895–1925," in *Uneasy Encounters: The Politics of Medicine and Health in China, 1900–1937*, ed. Iris Borowy (New York: Peter Lang, 2009), 115.

8. Bridie Andrews, *The Making of Modern Chinese Medicine, 1850–1960* (Honolulu: University of Hawaii Press, 2014), 11.

9. Ralph Croizier, *Traditional Medicine in Modern China: Science, Nationalism, and the Tensions of Cultural Change* (Cambridge, MA: Harvard University Press, 1968).

10. Ruth Rogaski, *Hygienic Modernity: Meanings of Health and Disease in Treaty-Port China* (Berkeley: University of California Press, 2004), chapter 6; Sean Hsiang-lin Lei, *Neither Donkey nor Horse: Medicine in the Struggle over China's Modernity* (Chicago: University of Chicago Press, 2014), chapter 2; Carol Benedict, *Bubonic Plague in Nineteenth-Century China* (Stanford, CA: Stanford University Press, 1996), chapter 6.

11. David Arnold, *Colonizing the Body: State Medicine and Epidemic Disease in Nineteenth-Century India* (Berkeley: University of California Press, 1993); Warwick Anderson, *Colonial*

Pathologies: American Tropical Medicine, Race, and Hygiene in the Philippines (Durham, NC: Duke University Press, 2006).

12. Ari Heinrich, *The Afterlife of Images: Translating the Pathological Body between China and the West* (Durham, NC: Duke University Press, 2008).

13. Which is not to say that previous dynasties did not become involved, to some extent, in adopting and enforcing public health measures. For instance, T. J. Hinrichs and Linda Barnes, eds., *Chinese Medicine and Healing* (Cambridge, MA: Harvard University Press, 2013), 97–128 and 161–208.

14. Vivien Ng, *Madness in Imperial China: From Illness to Deviance* (Norman: University of Oklahoma Press, 1990); Fabien Simonis, "Mad Acts, Mad Speech, and Mad People in Late Imperial Chinese Law and Medicine" (PhD diss., Princeton University, 2010); Hsiu-fen Chen, "Medicine, Society, and the Making of Madness in Imperial China" (PhD diss., University of London, 2003).

15. See, for instance, Madeleine Yue Dong and Joshua Goldstein, eds., *Everyday Modernity in China* (Seattle: University of Washington Press, 2006), 4; Timothy Mitchell, ed., *Questions of Modernity* (Minneapolis: University of Minnesota Press, 2000), xii.

16. The idea of China "awakening to a new world order" can be found in John Fitzgerald, *Awakening China: Politics, Culture, and Class in the National Revolution* (Stanford, CA: Stanford University Press, 1996), 6.

17. Lu Xun, "Kuangren riji" [Diary of a madman], in *Selected Stories of Lu Hsun* (Beijing: Foreign Languages Press, 1960 [1918]).

18. Xiaobing Tang, "Lu Xun's 'Diary of a Madman' and a Chinese Modernism," *PMLA* 107, no. 5 (October 1992): 1222.

19. Xu Zhuodai, "Xurong fengzi" [The vain lunatic], *Hong zazhi* 2, no. 60 (1923): 1–9; Lao She, "Xisheng" [Sacrifice], in *Yinghai ji* [Cherries and the sea] (Shanghai: Renjian shuwu, 1935).

20. Lillian Feder, *Madness in Literature* (Princeton, NJ: Princeton University Press, 1980), 3–5.

21. Birgit Linder, "Trauma and Truth: Representations of Madness in Chinese Literature," *Journal of Medical Humanities* 32, no. 4 (2011): 291–303.

22. I have borrowed this turn of phrase from Roy Porter, *Mind Forg'd Manacles: A History of Madness in England from the Restoration to the Regency* (Cambridge, MA: Harvard University Press, 1987), 2.

23. David Der-Wei Wang, *Fictional Realism in Twentieth-Century China* (New York: Columbia University Press, 1992), 6.

24. For example, Sloan Mahone and Megan Vaughan, eds., *Psychiatry and Empire* (New York: Palgrave Macmillan, 2007); Jock McCulloch, *Colonial Psychiatry and 'the African Mind'* (Cambridge: Cambridge University Press, 1995); Jonathan Sadowsky, *Imperial Bedlam: Institutions of Madness in Colonial Southwest Nigeria* (Berkeley: University of California Press, 1999).

25. Michel de Certeau, *The Practice of Everyday Life*, vol. 1 (Berkeley: University of California Press, 1984), xiv.

26. Only two monograph-length studies of madness in the Republican period have been written: Hugh Shapiro, "The View from a Chinese Asylum: Defining Madness in 1930s Peking" (PhD diss., Harvard University, 1995), and Peter Szto, "The Accommodation of Insanity in Canton, China: 1857–1935" (PhD diss., University of Pennsylvania, 2002).

27. Even when they do exist, they are not necessarily accessible. Hugh Shapiro, for instance, relied to a large extent on clinical records from the Peking Union Medical College in his 1995

dissertation. When I did my fieldwork in China, however, these sources were no longer available to researchers.

28. In Japan, the first public psychiatric hospital was opened in 1875. Although psychopathic wards were not established in Korea until the colonial period, Western missionary hospitals had begun to accept psychiatric patients throughout the last quarter of the nineteenth century.

29. Arthur Kleinman, *The Illness Narratives: Suffering, Healing, and the Human Condition* (New York: Basic Books, 1988), 3–6. See also Eric Cassell, "Illness and Disease," *Hastings Center Report* 6, no. 2 (April 1976): 27–37; Cecil Helman, "Disease versus Illness in General Practice," *Journal of the Royal College of Medical Practitioners* 31 (September 1981): 548–552.

30. Byron Good, *Medicine, Rationality, and Experience: An Anthropological Perspective* (Cambridge: Cambridge University Press, 1994), 2.

31. Liah Greenfield has recently argued that schizophrenia is a modern condition, appearing only in tandem with the rise of nationalism. Other researchers have also interrogated the relationship between schizophrenia and culture by showing how the disorder manifests differently around the world. Liah Greenfield, *Mind, Modernity, Madness: The Impact of Culture on Human Experience* (Cambridge, MA: Harvard University Press, 2013); T. M. Luhrmann et al., "Differences in Voice-Hearing Experiences of People with Psychosis in the USA, India and Ghana: Interview-Based Study," *British Journal of Psychiatry* 206, no. 1 (June 26, 2014): 41–44.

32. Michael MacDonald, *Mystical Bedlam: Madness, Anxiety, and Healing in Seventeenth-Century England* (Cambridge: Cambridge University Press, 1981), 1.

33. Porter, *Mind Forg'd Manacles*, 31.

34. Thomas Szasz, *The Myth of Mental Illness: Foundations of a Theory of Personal Conduct* (New York: Harper & Row, 1961); Thomas Szasz, *The Manufacture of Madness: A Comparative Study of the Inquisition and the Mental Health Movement* (New York: Harper & Row, 1970). The sociologist Thomas Scheff has likewise hypothesized that symptoms of mental illness are merely "violations of culturally particular normative networks." Thomas Scheff, *Being Mentally Ill: A Sociological Theory* (Chicago: Aldine, 1966), 38–39.

35. Arthur Kleinman, *Rethinking Psychiatry: From Cultural Category to Personal Experience* (New York: Free Press, 1988), 3; italics in original. See also Janis Jenkins, *Extraordinary Conditions: Culture and Experience in Mental Illness* (Berkeley: University of California Press, 2015).

36. On the history of this historiography, see Mark Micale and Roy Porter, eds., *Discovering the History of Psychiatry* (Oxford: Oxford University Press, 1994).

37. David Roberts, *Victorian Origins of the British Welfare State* (New Haven, CT: Yale University Press, 1960), 63. See also Albert Deutsch, *The Mentally Ill in America: A History of Their Care and Treatment from Colonial Times* (New York: Doubleday, 1937).

38. Though it has not been put to rest completely. Edward Shorter, for instance, has remained optimistic about the progress of the biological sciences and their ability to interpret mental illness within a purely somatic lens. Edward Shorter, *A History of Psychiatry: From the Era of the Asylum to the Age of Prozac* (New York: Wiley, 1997).

39. Andrew Scull, *The Most Solitary of Afflictions: Madness and Society in Britain, 1700–1900* (New Haven, CT: Yale University Press, 1993), 5; see also David Rothman, *The Discovery of the Asylum: Social Order and Disorder in the New Republic* (Boston: Little, Brown, 1971).

40. Scull, *Most Solitary of Afflictions*, 381.

41. In addition to Scull and Rothman, see Gerald Grob, *Mental Institutions in America: Social Policy to 1875* (New York: Free Press, 1972).

42. William Parry-Jones, *The Trade in Lunacy: A Study of Private Madhouses in England in the Eighteenth and Nineteenth Centuries* (London: Routledge & Kegan Paul, 1972).

43. Jan Goldstein, *Console and Classify: The French Psychiatric Profession in the Nineteenth Century* (Cambridge: Cambridge University Press, 1987).

44. Andrew Abbott, *The System of Professions: An Essay on the Division of Expert Labor* (Chicago: University of Chicago Press, 1988), 16.

45. On gender and psychiatric medicine, see Elaine Showalter, *The Female Malady: Women, Madness, and English Culture, 1830–1980* (New York: Penguin, 1987). On race and colonialism, see Frantz Fanon, *The Wretched of the Earth* (New York: Grove Press, 1963 [1961]), and Richard Keller, *Colonial Madness: Psychiatry in French North Africa* (Chicago: University of Chicago Press, 2007).

46. George Makari, *Revolution in Mind: The Creation of Psychoanalysis* (New York: Harper Collins, 2008), 4.

47. Theodore Jun Yoo, *It's Madness: The Politics of Mental Health in Colonial Korea* (Berkeley: University of California Press, 2016), 64.

48. See, for instance, Ian Dowbiggin, *Keeping America Sane: Psychiatry and Eugenics in the United States and Canada, 1880–1940* (Ithaca, NY: Cornell University Press, 1997).

49. For a discussion of the emergence of psychiatry as a professional field, see Andrew Scull, Charlotte MacKenzie, and Nicholas Hervey, *Masters of Bedlam: The Transformation of the Mad-Doctoring Trade* (Princeton, NJ: Princeton University Press, 1996).

50. Porter, *Mind Forg'd Manacles*, 1.

51. In Beijing, the population grew immensely between 1912 and 1949. In 1912, approximately 725,000 people lived within the city; by 1948, the population had more than doubled. Lillian Li, Alison Dray-Novey, and Haili Kong, *Beijing: From Imperial Capital to Olympic City* (New York: Palgrave Macmillan, 2007), 149–150. On the transformation of the city in China, see Joseph Esherick, ed., *Remaking the Chinese City: Modernity and National Identity, 1900–1950* (Honolulu: University of Hawaii Press, 2000).

52. On municipal governance throughout this period, see Shi Mingzheng, "Beijing Transforms: Urban Infrastructure, Public Works, and Social Change in the Chinese Capital, 1900–1928" (PhD diss., Columbia University, 1993).

53. David Strand, *Rickshaw Beijing: City People and Politics in the 1920s* (Berkeley: University of California Press, 1989), 5.

54. Madeleine Yue Dong, *Republican Beijing: The City and Its Histories* (Berkeley: University of California Press, 2003), 108–109, 215.

55. Janet Chen, *Guilty of Indigence: The Urban Poor in China, 1900–1953* (Princeton, NJ: Princeton University Press, 2012).

56. As Zhao Ma has pointed out, legal authorities progressively replaced case summaries with transcriptions in twentieth-century criminal records. Although they did so to make them appear less subjective, such transcripts were not unmediated. In the police records used here, functionaries tended to ask the same questions of each witness in the same order (name, age, place of birth, family members, etc.), and so individual testimonies often appeared formulaic. While these testimonies were not always recorded verbatim, the overall gist of such statements, I believe, was still conveyed accurately. See Zhao Ma, *Runaway Wives, Urban Crimes, and Survival Tactics in Wartime Beijing, 1937–1949* (Cambridge, MA: Harvard University Press, 2015), 30–32.

Chapter One

1. Following Nathan Sivin and Volker Scheid, I translate *zheng* as "symptoms" or "signs" of illness, *bing*. See Nathan Sivin, *Traditional Medicine in Contemporary China* (Ann Arbor: University of Michigan, 1987), 99; Volker Scheid, *Chinese Medicine in Contemporary China: Plurality and Synthesis* (Durham, NC: Duke University Press, 2002), 201.

2. *Xie*, which is often translated as "evil" or "pathogenic" in Chinese medical texts, represents the antithesis of *zheng*, or correct, bodily functions. As Elisabeth Hsu points out, the term *xie* can sometimes carry a moral connotation, since the opposition between *xie* and *zheng* mirrors the Confucian distinction between orthodox values (*zheng*) and heterodox ones (*xie*). Elisabeth Hsu, *The Transmission of Chinese Medicine* (Cambridge: Cambridge University Press, 1999), 68–69.

3. Academia Sinica Institute of Modern History Archives (hereafter, AS) 01-12-035-01-024. At the time, the Qing legal code specified that mad people who had committed homicide must be "permanently confined" (*yongyuan jiangu*). However, because Shuqin did not actually kill the Catholic priests, it is uncertain whether he would have been forced into permanent confinement.

4. This was because Qing law likened "killing because of madness" to "accidental killing." Geoffrey MacCormack, "The Legal Treatment of Insane Persons in Late Imperial China," *Journal of Legal History* 13, no. 3 (1992): 251–269.

5. In instances when there was no family to care for the mad person, local leaders would be punished with an administrative sanction. Simonis, "Mad Acts," 453–458; Ng, *Madness in Imperial China*, 66–67.

6. Charles Selden, "Work among the Chinese Insane and Some of Its Results," *China Medical Missionary Journal* 19, no. 1 (January 1905): 3–4.

7. Fabien Simonis discusses four reasons why "people with the madness illness" were not automatically confined: families distinguished between temporary/intermittent insanity and long-term insanity; families retained faith in the potential to cure the mad person; they pitied his or her condition; and families did not want to lose a contributor to the household economy. "Mad Acts," 465–467. Vivien Ng similarly observed that families were often resistant to letting the government intervene in their private affairs. *Madness in Imperial China*, 75–78.

8. Selden, "Work among the Chinese," 3.

9. Robert Fortune, *Yedo and Peking* (London: J. Murray, 1863), 361.

10. Selden, "Work among the Chinese," 3–4.

11. AS 01-12-141-01-001.

12. Simonis, "Mad Acts," 467–468.

13. On the history of this penal denomination, see Su Yigong, *Ming Qing lüdian yu tiaoli* [Laws and ordinances in the Ming and Qing] (Beijing: Zhongguo zhengfa daxue chubanshe, 1999), 146–154. For examples of cases related to "homicide due to madness," see Yu Guojuan, *Qingchao xingbu tongxing tiaoli* [Regulations of the Qing dynasty Board of Punishments] (Zhejiang: Zhejiang guji chubanshe, 2012), 38–42.

14. AS 01-12-141-01-001.

15. Selden, "Work among the Chinese," 4. See also Charles Selden, "Treatment of the Insane II," *China Medical Journal* 23, no. 4 (July 1909): 224–225; J. L. McCartney, "Neuropsychiatry in China," *Archives of Neurology and Psychiatry* 18, no. 1 (1927): 88; Simonis, "Mad Acts," 462–463.

16. J. H. Ingram, "The Pitiable Condition of the Insane in North China," *China Medical Journal* 32, no. 2 (March 1918): 153.

17. John Kerr, the founder of the Kerr Refuge for the Insane in Guangzhou, remarked that the father "holds the power of life and death over his family" and that "death has been hastened among the poorer classes by the want of care and ill-treatment." Although Charles Selden acknowledged that homicide did occasionally take place, he believed that such an extreme action "probably seldom occurs." See J. G. Kerr, "The 'Refuge for the Insane,' Canton," *China Medical Missionary Journal* 12, no. 4 (December 1898): 177; Selden, "Work among the Chinese," 5.

18. Selden, "Work among the Chinese," 5.

19. "Yinjing chengbing" [Becoming sick due to a scare], *Wushen quannian huabao*, no. 23 (spring 1908). On the relationship between natural medicine and demonic belief, see Chen Hsiu-fen, "Dang bingren jiandao gui: shilun Ming-Qing yizhe duiyu 'xiesui' de taidu" [The patient sees a ghost: The attitude of Ming-Qing physicians on evil spirits], in *Zongjiao yu yiliao* [Religion and medicine], ed. Lin Fushi (Taibei: Lianjing, 2011), 329–364.

20. On madness prior to the English Revolution, see MacDonald, *Mystical Bedlam*. On supernatural accounts of madness in eighteenth-century England, see Jonathan Andrews and Andrew Scull, *Customers and Patrons of the Mad Trade: The Management of Lunacy in Eighteenth-Century London* (Berkeley: University of California Press, 2003), chapter 6.

21. The meanings of these terms shifted over time. In *Nan Jing* (Classic of difficult issues, compiled in the second century), *kuang* and *xian* are paired; while *kuang* is characterized by an excess of *yang*, *xian* is characterized by an excess of *yin*. See Paul Unschuld, *Nan Jing: The Classic of Difficult Issues* (Berkeley: University of California Press, 2016 [1986]), issue 59. In *Zhubing yuanhou lun* (Origins and signs of the various illnesses, compiled in 610), *dian* was characterized as a seizure illness. By the early twentieth century, however, *dian* had come to be seen as the opposite of *kuang*. For example, see Chen Zhongquan, "Diankuang zhi fenxi yanjiu" [Research into the difference between dian and kuang], *Zhongyi shijie* 2, no. 11 (1931): 34–35.

22. In particular, debates continued into the twentieth century as to whether *dian* and *xian* referred to different behavioral patterns or the same condition. The medical reformer Yu Yan (also known as Yu Yunxiu), for instance, argued that the two were interchangeable. There is some historical basis to this argument. As Fabien Simonis has shown, early articulations of *dian* in the medical canon conceptualized the disorder as a "falling sickness" or "seizure sickness." Colloquially, however, *dian* was often paired with *kuang* to refer to a general "madness" (*diankuang*), hence its later appropriation as a variant typology of madness. Because most scholars agree that a tripartite distinction between *dian-xian-kuang* had coalesced by the nineteenth century, I will retain this triad throughout the rest of the monograph. For more on the history of these terms, see Chen, "Making of Madness," 77–121, and Simonis, "Mad Acts," 47–54.

23. For a longer discussion, see Hsiu-fen Chen, "Articulating 'Chinese Madness'" (paper presented at the first annual Asian Society for the History of Medicine meeting, 2003).

24. In her dissertation, Martha Li Chiu argues that there was no mention of "an explicit higher-order category of mental illness" in the Chinese medical canon; Fabien Simonis similarly refers to the "disunity" and "dispersion" of madness in Chinese medical history. Martha Li Chiu, "Mind, Body, and Illness in a Chinese Medical Tradition" (PhD diss., Harvard University, 1986), 284; Fabien Simonis, "Medicaments and Persuasion: Medical Therapies for Madness in Nineteenth-Century China," in *Psychiatry and Chinese History*, ed. Howard Chiang (London: Pickering & Chatto, 2014), 55–70.

25. For an in-depth study of one medical lineage, see Volker Scheid, *Currents of Tradition in Chinese Medicine, 1626–2006* (Seattle, WA: Eastland Press, 2007).

26. Andrews, *Making of Modern Chinese Medicine*, 9.

27. John J. Kao, *Three Millennia of Chinese Psychiatry* (New York: Institute for Advanced Research in Asian Medicine, 1979); T'ien Ju-k'ang, "Traditional Chinese Beliefs and Attitudes toward Mental Illness," in *Chinese Culture and Mental Health*, ed. Wen-shing Tseng and David Wu (Orlando, FL: Academic Press, 1985), 67–81; Chen, "Making of Madness"; Simonis, "Mad Acts."

28. Paul Unschuld and Hermann Tessenow, *Huangdi neijing suwen: An Annotated Translation of Huang Di's Inner Classic—Basic Questions* (Berkeley: University of California Press, 2011), 72.

29. Shigehisa Kuriyama, *The Expressiveness of the Body and the Divergence of Greek and Chinese Medicine* (New York: Zone Books, 1999), 258.

30. Zhu Danxi, *Jingui gouxuan*; as quoted in Simonis, "Mad Acts," 121.

31. Ma Peizhi, in *Menghe sijia yi'an yihua ji* [Medical case records from the four families of the Menghe lineage] (Shanxi: Shanxi kexue jishu chubanshe, 2009), 386–389.

32. Chao Weifang, in *Menghe sijia yi'an yihua ji*, 477.

33. Wang Mengying, *Wang Mengying yi'an yizhu* [Medical case records of Wang Mengying] (Beijing: Xueyuan chubanshe, 2009), 48.

34. The five *zang* organs, which produce and store vital fluids and *qi*, include the heart, lungs, liver, spleen, and kidneys. The six *fu* organs, which are involved in processes of digestion and transmission, include the stomach, small and large intestines, gall bladder, urinary bladder, and triple burner (*san jiao*).

35. *Nan Jing*, issue 34. These associations varied in different texts. Compare, for instance, to Hsiu-fen Chen's discussion of *Huangdi neijing* in "Emotional Therapy and Talking Cures in Late Imperial China," in Chiang, *Psychiatry and Chinese History*, 37–54.

36. Ning Yu, *The Chinese HEART in a Cognitive Perspective: Culture, Body, and Language* (Berlin: Mouton de Gruyter, 2009), 44–61. Despite the heart's role as "ruler," Shigehisa Kuriyama has pointed out that "power circulated" within the Chinese medical body, and thus no single organ was hegemonic. *Expressiveness of the Body*, 161.

37. Although, as Volker Scheid points out, the Menghe lineage purposely crafted itself as a distinct medical tradition, it was also influenced by, and shared common assumptions with, other medical lineages of the time. Scheid, *Currents of Tradition*, 156–157, 277–278.

38. Ding Ganren, *Ding Ganren yi'an* [Medical cases of Ding Ganren] (Shanxi: Shanxi kexue jishu chubanshe, 2013), 65–69.

39. In the Western world, Greek physicians like Hippocrates (c. 460–357 BC) were the first to advance naturalistic accounts of madness. See Andrew Scull, *Madness in Civilization: A Cultural History of Insanity from the Bible to Freud, from the Madhouse to Modern Medicine* (London: Thames & Hudson, 2015), 26–36.

40. Humoral explanations for madness remained surprisingly influential among physicians well into the 1800s. See Lynn Gamwell and Nancy Tomes, *Madness in America: Cultural and Medical Perceptions of Mental Illness before 1914* (Ithaca, NY: Cornell University Press, 1995), 70–71.

41. Selden, "Work among the Chinese," 7.

42. Selden, "Treatment of the Insane II," 228.

43. Sivin, *Traditional Medicine in Contemporary China*, 3.

44. Ning, *Chinese HEART*, 138; Keh-Ming Lin, "Traditional Chinese Medical Beliefs and Their Relevance for Mental Illness and Psychiatry," in *Normal and Abnormal Behavior in Chinese Culture*, ed. Arthur Kleinman and Tsung-Yi Lin (Boston: D. Reidel Publishing, 1981), 95–111.

45. Ma Peizhi, in *Menghe sijia yi'an yihua ji*, 387.

46. Zhou Xiaonong, *Zhou Xiaonong yi'an, di'er ban* [Medical case records of Zhou Xiaonong, vol. 2] (Shanghai: Shanghai kexue jishu chubanshe, 2008), 13. This was a reference to the belief that anger injures the liver and overthinking injures the spleen. See Ning, *Chinese HEART*, 127–129.

47. Ding Ganren, *Ding Ganren yi'an*, 65–69.

48. *Lengyu yihua* [Medical discussions of the cold shack]; as cited in Zheng Zhong and Liu Jingyu, eds., *Minzhong chuantong zhibing xiao juezhao* [Unique tricks to cure illness in popular tradition] (Beijing: Zhongguo zhongyiyao chubanshe, 2012), 216.

49. Much work, particularly in the field of medical anthropology, has focused on the somatization of mental illness in contemporary Chinese culture. For example, Keh-Ming Lin, Arthur Kleinman, and Tsung-Yi Lin, "Overview of Mental Disorders in Chinese Cultures: Review of Epidemiological and Clinical Studies," in Kleinman and Lin, *Normal and Abnormal Behavior in Chinese Culture*, 237–272; Arthur Kleinman and David Mechanic, "Mental Illness and Psychosocial Aspects of Medical Problems in China," in Kleinman and Lin, *Normal and Abnormal Behavior in Chinese Culture*, 331–356; Arthur Kleinman, *Patients and Healers in the Context of Culture* (Berkeley: University of California Press, 1980), 133–145.

50. Ma Peizhi, in *Menghe sijia yi'an yihua ji*, 388.

51. Zhou, *Zhou Xiaonong yi'an*, 41.

52. Kuriyama, *Expressiveness of the Body*, 168.

53. Wang, *Wang Mengying yi'an*, 222.

54. Ibid., 153.

55. Charlotte Furth, *A Flourishing Yin: Gender in China's Medical History, 960–1665* (Berkeley: University of California Press, 1999), 52.

56. For a longer discussion, see Simonis, "Mad Acts," 367–406.

57. Chen, "Making of Madness," 171–178.

58. More broadly, many scholars have differentiated Chinese from Western medicine on the basis that the latter tends to focus on disease entities while the former emphasizes disease patterns. For the specific case of *shenzhi* (mental faculty) disease patterns, see Yanhua Zhang, *Transforming Emotions with Chinese Medicine: An Ethnographic Account from Contemporary China* (Albany: State University of New York Press, 2007), 85.

59. Simonis, "Medicaments and Persuasion," 59.

60. Lin, "Traditional Chinese Medical Beliefs," 95.

61. Richard von Glahn, *The Sinister Way: The Divine and the Demonic in Chinese Religious Culture* (Berkeley: University of California Press, 2004).

62. John Dudgeon, "Medical Mission Work in Peking," *North China Herald*, October 21, 1885.

63. For example, "Yusui chengfeng" [Meeting an evil spirit and becoming mad], *Shen bao*, August 27, 1882.

64. As Richard von Glahn writes, "Chinese attributed illness, like misfortune in general, either to adventitious affliction by some malefic entity or to just punishment inflicted on the victim for his or her own moral transgressions." *Sinister Way*, 98. Paul Cohen's groundbreaking work on experiences of drought in north China also underscores the role that supernatural forces played in communal interpretations of poor weather and bodily possession. Paul Cohen, *History in Three Keys: The Boxers as Event, Experience, and Myth* (New York: Columbia University Press, 1997), especially 96–118.

65. Huang Junbo, ed., *Zui zhong zui: Qingmo minchu qi'an jishi* [Crimes within crimes: A collection of strange cases from the end of the Qing dynasty] (Beijing: Huaxia chubanshe, 2012), 294.

66. Ingram, "Pitiable Condition of the Insane," 153.

67. (No title), *Shen bao*, August 13, 1893.

68. "Xiaoci guangji" [Filial, loving, and extensive aid], *Shen bao*, October 20, 1891.

69. Dudgeon, "Medical Mission Work."

70. John Nevius, *Demon Possession* (Grand Rapids, MI: Kregel Publications, 1968), 44–48. It is well known that acupuncture did not become an elite medical practice until the mid-twentieth century. There is little textual evidence, however, to show precisely how and why illiterate healers employed acupuncture prior to this time. For more on the history of acupuncture, see Andrews, *Making of Modern Chinese Medicine*, 185–205.

71. Andrew H. Woods, "The Nervous Diseases of the Chinese," *Archives of Neurology and Psychiatry* 21 (March 1929): 27.

72. Dudgeon, "Medical Mission Work."

73. Hugh White, *Demonism Verified and Analyzed* (Shanghai: Presbyterian Mission Press, 1922), 18.

74. Zhou, *Zhou Xiaonong yi'an*, 45–46.

75. Wang, *Wang Mengying yi'an*, 262.

76. Selden, "Work among the Chinese," 7.

77. White, *Demonism*, 33, 56–57.

78. Timothy Richard, "The Spiritual Benefits of Christianity," *Chinese Recorder and Missionary Journal*, April 1, 1891.

79. Cohen, *History in Three Keys*, 84, 96–118.

80. White, *Demonism*, 74.

81. Dudgeon, "Medical Mission Work."

82. According to Ichisada Miyasaki, boys typically finished their classical education at the age of fifteen, which was the same age as Shuqin when he went mad. Ichisada Miyasaki, *China's Examination Hell: The Civil Service Examinations of Imperial China* (New Haven, CT: Yale University Press, 1976), 16.

83. Benjamin Elman, *A Cultural History of Civil Examinations in Late Imperial China* (Berkeley: University of California Press, 2000), 368; P. M. Yap, "The Mental Illness of Hung Hsiuch'uan, Leader of the Taiping Rebellion," *Far Eastern Quarterly* 13, no. 3 (May 1954): 287–304.

84. "Kaotong fafeng" [Examinee goes mad], *Shen bao*, November 18, 1881.

85. "Xiangguan chengbing" [Thinking of becoming an official and getting sick], *Shen bao*, December 6, 1883.

86. Zheng and Liu, *Minzhong chuantong zhibing*, 216.

87. Benjamin Hobson, "General Report on the Hospital at Kam-li-fau in Canton," *Chinese Repository*, June 1, 1850.

88. Robert Ross, "The Insane in China: Examination Hints," *China Medical Journal* 24 (1920): 517.

89. Ibid., 515–517. See also Charles Selden, "Conditions in South China in Relation to Insanity," *American Journal of Insanity* 70, nos. 2–4 (1913): 411–426.

90. For a discussion of the patriarchal politics involved in hysteria, see Showalter, *Female Malady*.

91. On "public sympathy" and the rise of a Chinese public sphere, see Eugenia Lean, *Public Passions: The Trial of Shi Jianqiao and the Rise of Popular Sympathy in Republican China* (Berkeley: University of California Press, 2007).

92. "Yinjing chengbing."

93. "Jiyuan chengji" [Storing up bitterness leads to illness], *Wushen quannian huabao*, no. 24 (spring 1908).

94. "Youfu wei yuzhou feng" [Woman goes mad from the universe], *Qianshuo riri huabao*, September 15, 1913.

95. Ross, "Insane in China," 514–518.

96. Chen, *Guilty of Indigence*, 5–6.

Chapter Two

1. BMA J181-018-04774.

2. For intellectual discussions on the deficiencies of the imperial state and the requirements of a strong modern nation, see Peter Zarrow, *After Empire: The Conceptual Transformation of the Chinese State, 1885–1924* (Stanford, CA: Stanford University Press, 2012), chapter 3, and Edmund Fung, *The Intellectual Foundations of Chinese Modernity: Cultural and Political Thought in the Republican Era* (Cambridge: Cambridge University Press, 2010), chapter 5. On the modern state and hygiene more specifically, see Rogaski, *Hygienic Modernity*, chapters 5–8, and Lei, *Neither Donkey nor Horse*, chapter 1.

3. This idea was most famously articulated through Michel Foucault's concept of "bio-power." Bio-power, which refers to the modern nation-state's ability to regulate its people by controlling, monitoring, and optimizing biological acts and life processes, was first discussed in Foucault's *History of Sexuality*, vol. 1 (New York: Vintage Books, 1990 [1978]), 140–144.

4. Although the Qing legal code specified, from 1762 onward, that people found guilty of "killing because of madness" be permanently confined, the same mandate did not apply to the insane who had not committed homicide.

5. Stephen MacKinnon, *Power and Politics in Late Imperial China* (Berkeley: University of California Press, 1980), chapter 5; Julia Strauss, "Creating 'Virtuous and Talented Officials' for the Twentieth Century: Discourse and Practice in *Xinzheng* China," *Modern Asian Studies* 37, no. 4 (October 2003): 831–850.

6. The usual date given for the opening of the institution is 1898. The refuge was actually founded in 1897, but did not receive its first patient until one year later. Charles Selden, "The Life of John G. Kerr," *Chinese Medical Journal* 49 (1935): 374.

7. Kerr, "Refuge for the Insane," 177.

8. Charles Selden, "Work among the Chinese," 5.

9. As Zhiying Ma has shown in regard to the John Kerr Refuge, Western missionaries often replicated the form of restraint used by Chinese families but labeled it therapeutic rather than carceral. Zhiying Ma, "An 'Iron Cage' of Civilization? Missionary Psychiatry, the Chinese Family, and a Colonial Dialectic of Enlightenment," in Chiang, *Psychiatry and Chinese History*, 91–110.

10. In the Kerr Refuge Annual Report for 1907–1908, the rate of cure is listed at 31 to 32 percent of those admitted; nevertheless, it is also noted that "this *somewhat high percentage of cures* is probably due to a larger proportion of manic-depressive cases and to the fewer of paresis than is found at home" (emphasis mine), 7–8. In the United States, the typical rate of improvement also hovered around 30 percent. Herbert Day Lamson, *Social Pathology in China: A Source Book for the Study of Problems of Livelihood, Health, and the Family* (Shanghai: Commercial Press, 1935), 429.

11. On medicine, religion, and cultural and national reform, see Jonathan Spence, *To Change China: Western Advisers in China, 1620–1960* (New York: Penguin, 1969), chapter 2; Heinrich, *Afterlife of Images*, chapter 2.

12. Bryn Mawr College Archives (hereafter, BMCA), Andrew Woods Papers, Box 1, diary entry, April 20, 1903.

13. Kerr, "Refuge for the Insane," 177–178. See also Peter Szto, "Psychiatric Space and Design Antecedents: The John G. Kerr Refuge for the Insane," in Chiang, *Psychiatry and Chinese History*, 71–90.

14. Kerr Refuge Annual Report, 1907–1908, 4.

15. Kerr Refuge Annual Report, 1909, 1–2.

16. Huang Pandong, "Shili jingshen bing liaoyang yuan zhi shilüe ji jinkuang" [Brief history and current situation of the municipal psychopathic hospital], *Guangzhou weisheng* 2 (1936): 105–106. For a discussion of the practical benefits of institutionalization from the perspective of the municipal police, see also Neil Diamant, "China's 'Great Confinement'? Missionaries, Municipal Elites, and Police in the Establishment of Chinese Mental Hospitals," *Republican China* 19, no. 1 (November 1994): 11, and Ma, "Iron Cage," 99.

17. AS 02-12-010-01-062.

18. Akira Hashimoto, "The Invention of a 'Japanese Gheel': Psychiatric Family Care from a Historical and Transnational Perspective," in *Transnational Psychiatries*, ed. Waltraud Ernst and Thomas Mueller (Newcastle upon Tyne: Cambridge Scholars Publishing, 2010), 152–153.

19. AS 02-20-009-01-050; 02-20-009-01-051.

20. AS 02-20-009-10-074; 02-20-013-10-002; 02-20-009-01-076.

21. "Berlin International Congress," *British Journal of Psychiatry* 56, no. 233 (April 1910): 385.

22. AS 02-12-010-01-062; Conolly Norman, "The Family Care of the Insane," *Medical Press and Circular* 131 (November 29, 1905): 557–560.

23. AS 02-12-010-01-062.

24. Susan Burns, "Contemplating Places: The Hospital as Modern Experience in Meiji Japan," in *New Directions in the Study of Meiji Japan*, ed. Helen Hardacre and Adam L. Kern (Leiden: Brill, 1997), 704. See also Rogaski, *Hygienic Modernity*, chapter 5; Susan Burns, "Constructing the National Body: Public Health and the Nation in Nineteenth-Century Japan," in *Nation Work: Asian Elites and National Identities*, ed. Timothy Brook and Andre Schmid (Ann Arbor: University of Michigan Press, 2000), 17–50. On the rehabilitation of deviant bodies, see Daniel Botsman, *Punishment and Power in the Making of Modern Japan* (Princeton, NJ: Princeton University Press, 2005), chapter 6.

25. Burns, "Constructing the National Body," 41.

26. Unlike the Qing bureaucracy, which used the term "person with a mad illness" in official documents, Japan had officially adopted the term "mental illness" (*seishinbyō*) in medical and legislative matters. See Karen Nakamura, *A Disability of the Soul: An Ethnography of Schizophrenia and Mental Illness in Contemporary Japan* (Ithaca, NY: Cornell University Press, 2013), 43.

27. Formal regulations mandating the institutionalization of the insane within an asylum would not be written into law until 1919. Akihito Suzuki, "State, Family, and the Insane in Japan, 1900–1945," in *The Confinement of the Insane: International Perspectives, 1800–1965*, ed. Roy Porter and David Wright (Cambridge: Cambridge University Press, 2003), 193–225; Akihito Suzuki, "Global Theory, Local Practice: Shock Therapies in Japanese Psychiatry, 1920–1945," in Ernst and Mueller, *Transnational Psychiatries*, 116–141; Junko Kitanaka, *Depression in Japan: Psychiatric Cures for a Society in Distress* (Princeton, NJ: Princeton University Press, 2012), 42–44.

28. Liu Yuzhen and Sun Xuemei, eds., *Riben zhengfa kaocha ji* [Records on observations of Japanese politics and law] (Shanghai: Shanghai guji, 2002), 171, 313, 319.

29. Rogaski, *Hygienic Modernity*, 303.

30. "Da Yingguo: Shouyang fengdian" [Great Britain: Care of the insane], *Wanguo gongbao*, no. 611 (1880): 17; Hua Zhi'an, "Youdai diankuang" [Giving preferential treatment to the insane], *Wanguo gongbao*, no. 640 (1881): 5–8.

31. "Fengren yifang" [Madmen should be guarded against], *Qianshuo riri huabao*, September 17, 1908.

32. Jacques Gernet, for example, has referred to Qing rule as a form of "authoritarian paternalism." Jacques Gernet, *A History of Chinese Civilization* (Cambridge: Cambridge University Press, 1982), part 8.

33. Keller, *Colonial Madness*, 80, 78.

34. As Andrew Scull has rightly remarked, "therapy and social control" were not necessarily considered mutually exclusive aims. Andrew Scull, *The Insanity of Place/The Place of Insanity* (London: Routledge, 2006), 108.

35. AS 02-20-009-01-051.

36. Shen Jiaben, *Da Qing xianxing xinglü anyu* [Commentary on the great Qing penal code currently in use] (Beijing: Falü guan, 1909), 87.

37. William Rowe, *China's Last Empire: The Great Qing* (Cambridge, MA: Harvard University Press, 2009), 286.

38. Strand, *Rickshaw Beijing*, 66–69.

39. Chen, *Guilty of Indigence*, 27.

40. It has long been a matter of confusion when the asylum was erected. Sidney Gamble, who visited the facility in 1918, mistakenly believed that it had been established in 1912. K. C. Wong, in "A Short History of Psychiatry and Mental Hygiene in China," *Chinese Medical Journal* 68 (1950): 44–48, gives the incorrect date of 1906, which has been repeated in later sources.

41. *Zhengzhi guanbao* [Political report], no. 369 (1908): 196–197. The first announcement about the facility that I have seen is "Ni tianshe fengren yuan" [Drafting plans to establish an asylum], *Shen bao*, March 17, 1907.

42. Asylum regulations referred to the facility as "an attached asylum" (*fushe fengren yuan*) to the municipal poorhouse. "Fushe fengren yuan jianzhang" [Regulations for the attached asylum], in *Qingmo Beijing chengshi guanli fagui* [Statutes on the administration of Beijing at the end of the Qing dynasty], ed. Tian Tao and Guo Chengwei (Beijing: Beijing yanshan chubanshe, 1996), 269–271. See also BMA J181-018-06205, J181-019-01896.

43. Police records from 1916, in particular BMA J181-018-06205, discuss the problem of overcrowding at the earlier facility. For an overview of the renovated facility, see Yuan Xi, *Beijing chengshi fazhan shi, jindai juan* [History of Beijing's development, modern edition] (Beijing: Beijing yanshan chubanshe, 2008), 65, and Ding Rui, *Guanli Beijing: Beiyang zhengfu shiqi jingshi jingcha ting yanjiu* [Governing Beijing: Research into the municipal police during the era of the Beiyang government] (Shanxi: Shanxi jingli chubanshe, 2013), 347–349.

44. "Fushe fengren yuan jianzhang," 269. For examples, see BMA J181-019-05591, J181-019-05607, J181-018-06464.

45. Sidney Gamble, *Peking: A Social Survey* (New York: George H. Doran Company, 1921), 125. Police files such as BMA J181-019-21289 also note that lunatics "passed through the police station [before being] sent to the asylum."

46. "Fushe fengren yuan jianzhang," 269–271. In practice, however, it was not uncommon for the individual to remain within the asylum regardless of how well he or she had been rehabilitated. In the case of Wang Weifang (BMA J181-018-12813), for example, the inmate's family

refused to come to the capital to collect him after he had been treated and cured. Wang became ill and died at the asylum soon thereafter.

47. In the original facility, men were housed in sixteen outer rooms, while women were placed in ten inner rooms. In the expanded facility, men and women occupied separate courtyards. See BMA J181-019-01866; Diamant, "China's 'Great Confinement'?," 24.

48. Gamble, *Peking*, 125.

49. BMA J181-019-01866.

50. Gamble, *Peking*, 125–126; Beiping Ministry of Health, ed., *Beiping shi zhengfu weisheng chu yewu baogao* [Report on tasks administered by the Beiping municipal department of health] (Beiping: Beiping shi zhengfu weisheng ju, 1934), 125–128.

51. For example, BMA J181-019-41640, J181-019-29027.

52. BMCA, Andrew Woods diary, February 7, 1921.

53. Although physicians were responsible for separating the insane by the severity of their condition, they were not responsible for determining the existence of madness in the first place. "Fushe fengren yuan jianzhang," 269.

54. For examples of rhetoric in Qing legal cases, see Simonis, "Mad Acts," chapter 13.

55. Zhang was provisionally replaced by Wang Baohua in 1921, who was soon thereafter replaced by Chen Zizhen. However, because Chen misplaced a casket containing the corpse of an inmate, he was quickly relieved of his position and replaced by yet a new manager, Wang Chengxun, in 1922. All of these men were simultaneously employed at separate municipal institutions and received no payment for their work at the asylum. The issue of payment would not be resolved until 1929. BMA J181-018-12553, J181-018-14374, J002-001-00010.

56. Chen, *Guilty of Indigence*, 47, 2.

57. Zwia Lipkin, *Useless to the State: Social Problems and Social Engineering in Nationalist Nanjing, 1927–1937* (Cambridge, MA: Harvard University Asia Center, 2006), 8.

58. Dong, *Republican Beijing*, 239. The ratio of police to civilians was estimated at twelve per thousand residents, more than any other country in the world at the time. Li, Dray-Novey, and Kong, *Beijing*, 138.

59. Yamin Xu, "Policing Civility on the Streets: Encounters with Litterbugs, 'Nightsoil Lords,' and Street Corner Urinators in Republican Beijing," *Twentieth-Century China* 30, no. 2 (2005): 28–71.

60. Strand, *Rickshaw Beijing*, 91.

61. Ibid., 76.

62. Diamant, "China's 'Great Confinement'?," 29. According to Frank Ki Chun Yee, the law "abstractly [gave] the police authority the right to enforcement without stating the exact circumstances under which the police must act." Frank Ki Chun Yee, "Police in Modern China" (PhD diss., University of California, Berkeley, 1942), 77.

63. BMA J181-019-01890.

64. BMA J181-019-05591.

65. BMA J181-019-09923.

66. Although the Qing had passed an "anti-vagrancy" law in 1907, the stipulation had lapsed following the overthrow of the dynasty and the Republican government did not renew the provision until 1916. See Chen, *Guilty of Indigence*, 34.

67. Pierre-Etienne Will, *Bureaucracy and Famine in Eighteenth-Century China* (Stanford, CA: Stanford University Press, 1990), chapter 2; Philip Kuhn, *Soulstealers: The Chinese Sorcery Scare of 1768* (Cambridge, MA: Harvard University Press, 1990), 111–118; on the "rootless rascal"

(*guanggun*), see Matthew Sommer, *Sex, Law, and Society in Late Imperial China* (Stanford, CA: Stanford University Press, 2002), 14.

68. BMA J181-019-09923.

69. Michael Dutton, *Policing and Punishment in China* (Cambridge: Cambridge University Press, 1992), 163.

70. Michel Foucault has made a similar observation about the history of madness in classical France. "Unreason," he argues, was often affiliated with an individual's unwillingness to labor and propensity for idleness. Michel Foucault, *Madness and Civilization* (New York: Random House, 1965), 72.

71. BMA J181-019-05578.

72. BMA J181-019-01875.

73. Jan Kiely, *The Compelling Ideal: Thought Reform and the Prison in China, 1901–1956* (New Haven, CT: Yale University Press, 2014), 30–32; Frank Dikötter, *Crime, Punishment, and the Prison in Modern China* (New York: Columbia University Press, 2002), 162–164; Klaus Mülhahn, *Criminal Justice in China: A History* (Cambridge, MA: Harvard University Press, 2007), 101–104.

74. These are the rationales given, for example, in Kiely, *Compelling Ideal*, 10; Dikötter, *Crime, Punishment, and the Prison*, 162.

75. Simonis, "Mad Acts," chapter 15.

76. BMA J181-019-10080.

77. BMA J181-019-01840.

78. BMA J181-019-01875.

79. BMA J181-019-09923.

80. BMA J181-019-01892.

81. S. A. Smith, "Talking Toads and Chinless Ghosts: The Politics of 'Superstitious Rumor' in the People's Republic of China, 1961–65," *American Historical Review* 111, no. 2 (April 2006): 405–427.

82. Rebecca Nedostup, *Superstitious Regimes: Religion and the Politics of Chinese Modernity* (Cambridge, MA: Harvard University Asia Center, 2009), 194–195.

83. BMA J181-019-21301.

84. BMA J181-019-50743.

85. Elizabeth Packard, *Modern Persecution, or Insane Asylums Unveiled* (New York: Pelletreau and Raynor, 1873), 95.

86. One need think only of the Taiping Rebellion. It is instructive, moreover, to compare the police response to Yin and Yang with earlier historical precedents. In Philip Kuhn's *Soulstealers*, for instance, the Qianlong emperor (1711–1799) was confronted with a movement of mass superstition that also threatened the power of the dynasty. He called for the culprits of the movement to be "arrested forthwith and punished severely," but there was no effort to link their activities to madness (76).

87. For example, BMA J191-002-11357, J181-019-01880, J181-019-13502, J181-019-41632.

88. The treatment of madness in England in the eighteenth and early nineteenth centuries consisted to a large degree of physical restraint. Restraint was not just employed to prevent the insane from injuring themselves and others; it was also "considered as a remedy." Parry-Jones, *Trade in Lunacy*, 171.

89. Ingram, "Pitiable Condition of the Insane," 153–154.

90. Gamble, *Peking*, 125.

91. "Fushe fengren yuan jianzhang," 271.

92. The new Qing code represented an effort to align Chinese laws with those of the international community. See *Da Qing fagui daquan, falü bu* [Comprehensive collection of the laws and regulations of the Great Qing, section on laws] (Taibei: Kaozheng chubanshe, 1972). On the similarities and differences between the revised Qing code and the temporary Republican code, see Zhou Shaoyuan, *Zhongguo jindai xingfa de zhaoduan* [The beginnings of modern Chinese criminal law] (Beijing: Shangwu yinshu guan, 2012), 218–223.

93. Beijing Ministry of Justice, "Xingfa cao'an" [Penal code draft], in *Zhengfu gongbao* (Beijing: n.p., 1912), article twelve. This article was likely a response to foreign precedents such as the British M'Naghten rules, which stipulated that a convict could be judged "not guilty by reason of insanity" and spared a punitive sentence.

94. Earlier Qing substatutes pertaining to the punishment of homicidal lunatics also mandated that they be imprisoned. However, because no such institution as an asylum existed, these individuals were typically sent to a local jail. See Simonis, "Mad Acts," 781.

95. For example, BMA J181-019-25208, J181-018-16111, J181-019-35272, J181-019-35273.

96. BMA J181-018-13183.

97. Bruce J. Ennis and Thomas R. Litwack, "Psychiatry and the Presumption of Expertise: Flipping Coins in the Courtroom," *California Law Review* 62, no. 3 (May 1974): 693–752.

98. Xu Xiaoqun, "The Fate of Judicial Independence in Republican China, 1912–1937," *China Quarterly* 149 (March 1997): 3.

99. BMA J181-018-07345; also J181-019-35361.

100. Kiely, *Compelling Ideal*, 93–94.

101. Discretionary rules in Republican penal codes granted judges a certain degree of leeway when it came to criminal sentencing, thereby allowing them to "mediate between legal ideals and social reality." Jennifer Neighbors, "The Long Arm of Qing Law? Qing Dynasty Homicide Rulings in Republican Courts," *Modern China* 35, no. 1 (2009): 3–37.

102. BMA J1810-019-13506.

103. Gamble, *Peking*, 126.

104. Strand, *Rickshaw Beijing*, 71.

Chapter Three

1. Gamble, *Peking*, 126.

2. "The Climate of China and Insanity," *North China Herald*, June 15, 1906. See also S. R. H., "China as a Field for Research in Nervous Diseases," *China Medical Missionary Journal* 3, no. 4 (December 1889): 167–168; Ilza Veith, "Psychiatric Thought in Chinese Medicine," *Journal of the History of Medicine and Allied Sciences* 10 (1955): 261–268. Foreigners in China also noted— incorrectly—that the Chinese were immune from the physical diseases to which Westerners succumbed, such as blood poisoning and smallpox. For example, Edward Alsworth Ross, *The Changing Chinese: The Conflict of Oriental and Western Cultures in China* (London: T. Fisher Unwin, 1911), chapter two.

3. The discourse linking modernity to madness was widespread in Western Europe and the United States during the late nineteenth and early twentieth centuries. Isaac Ray (1807–1881), an American psychiatrist, hypothesized that insanity would continue to increase "at a rate unparalleled in any former period" as a result of the excessive demands put on the brain by the exigencies of modern life. As quoted in Rothman, *Discovery of the Asylum*, 115. For a longer discussion, see Scull, *Madness in Civilization*, 168–170, 224–229.

4. Gamble, *Peking*, 126.

5. Rockefeller Archive Center (hereafter, RAC), China Medical Board (hereafter, CMB), Inc., Record Group (hereafter, RG) IV2B9, Box 96, Folder 689, Andrew Woods, "The Peking Union Medical College and the Problem of Insanity in China," December 27, 1920; CMB, Inc., RG IV2B9, Box 96, Folder 689, Richard Pearce to George Vincent, January 6, 1921.

6. "Editorial," *China Medical Journal* 34 (1920): 50.

7. J. A. Hofmann, "A Report of the Patients Discharged from the John G. Kerr Hospital for Insane During 1912," *China Medical Journal* 27 (1913): 369.

8. Woods, "Nervous Diseases of the Chinese," 524.

9. It is very likely that the municipality had strategically arranged Gamble's visit to correspond to the opening of the new facility. When Gamble asked how the municipality was caring for the insane who were not institutionalized, the interpreter "refused to translate the question," and the manager pleaded ignorance. After pushing for a response, Gamble received the following reply: "Why do you ask that? Here is room for 80 patients and there are only 32 inmates. There can't be any more insane in the city." *Peking*, 126.

10. Historians of England, who have attempted to determine why the incidence of madness appeared to increase so sharply in tandem with the introduction of the asylum, have observed similar phenomena. See Scull, *Most Solitary of Afflictions*, 352–363; Andrew Scull, "Was Insanity Increasing?" in *Social Order/Mental Disorder* (Berkeley: University of California Press, 1989), 239–249.

11. For a discussion of political factionalism in China following Yuan's death, see Andrew Nathan, *Peking Politics, 1918–1923: Factionalism and the Failure of Constitutionalism* (Berkeley: University of California Press, 1976).

12. Li, Dray-Novey, and Kong, *Beijing*, 137; Shi, "Beijing Transforms," 25–87.

13. By 1920, Beijing offered the following institutions: two reformatories (*jiaoyang yuan*), one almshouse (*jiuji yuan*), one poorhouse in the outer city and one in the inner city (*shouyang pinmin suo*), a handicraft workshop (*xiyi gongchang*), a reformatory for prostitutes (*funü ganhua suo*), a vagrant workshop, an asylum, and an orphanage. See Li Xiaowei, ed., *Xin Zhongguo jianli chuqi de shehui jiuzhu yanjiu* [Research into charitable works in the early years of new China] (Beijing: Shehui kexue wenxian chubanshe, 2012), 47.

14. Strand, *Rickshaw Beijing*, 65. See also William Ker Muir Jr., *Police: Streetcorner Politicians* (Chicago: University of Chicago Press, 1977).

15. "Fengren keju" [Madmen are frightening], *Wushen quannian huabao*, September 5, 1909; "Fengren yiguan" [Madmen should be controlled], *Qianshuo riri xinwen huabao*, September 21, 1909.

16. Barbara Mittler, *A Newspaper for China? Power, Identity, and Change in Shanghai's News Media, 1872–1912* (Cambridge, MA: Harvard East Asian Monographs, 2004), 37–39.

17. "Fengfu shuo fenghua, jingcha gai huiqi" [A madwoman speaks mad words, the police must be unlucky], *Shishi gongbao*, March 8, 1913.

18. "Xuesheng yuzhe fengzi" [A student comes across a madman], *Shengjing shibao*, October 17, 1917; "Fengfu naojie" [A madwoman makes a ruckus in the street], *Shengjing shibao*, September 7, 1912.

19. "Fengren yiguan."

20. "The Insane in China," *North China Herald*, May 17, 1924.

21. "Fengren yijin" [Madmen should be detained], *Shengjing shibao*, March 28, 1928.

22. BMA J181-019-05591.

23. BMA J181-018-04704.

24. BMA J181-019-50762.

25. BMA J181-018-16487 and J181-033-01851.

26. Michel Foucault raises a similar point about the suppression of sex and sexuality in *History of Sexuality*, part 1.

27. Lao She, *Luotuo Xiangzi* [Camel Xiangzi], first published in serial format in *Yuzhou feng* [Cosmic wind], vols. 25–48 (1936–1937).

28. Lu Xun, "Yijian xiaoshi" [An incident], first published in July 1920, compiled in *Nahan* [A call to arms] (Shanghai: Xin chaoshe chubanshe, 1923).

29. On warlordism and refugees, see Lillian Li, *Fighting Famine in North China: State, Market, and Environmental Decline, 1690s–1990s* (Stanford, CA: Stanford University Press, 2007), chapters 10 and 11.

30. Li Jinghan, "Beiping zuidi xiandu di shenghuo chengdu di taolun" [Discussion of the lowest standard of living in Beiping], *Shehui xue jie*, no. 3 (September 1929): 1–16; Sidney Gamble, *How Chinese Families Live in Peiping* (New York: Funk & Wagnalls, 1933), 3–4.

31. "Jingji pinmin zhi siwang lü: suinian zengjia" [Death rates of the poor in the capital: Increasing every year], *Liming bao*, March 3, 1923.

32. "Daobi qigai heduo" [Why are there so many dead beggars?], *Shishi baihua bao*, December 3, 1924.

33. "Qigai yinbing siwang" [Beggar dies of illness], *Shengjing shibao*, August 4, 1912.

34. "Pinmin xiezhen" [Portrait of poor people], *Shishi baihua bao*, October 23, 1922, and "Jieshao cishan" [Introducing philanthropists], *Shishi baihua bao*, December 13, 1922.

35. "Beijing de pinmin rijian zengduo" [The poor in Beijing are increasing by the day], *Beijing baihua bao*, January 31, 1921.

36. Families who earned between five and nine yuan per month averaged only 3.0 members, while those who earned above two hundred yuan per month averaged 8.5 members, including servants. Gamble, *How Chinese Families Live in Peiping*, 315.

37. In families making less than ten yuan per month, over 90 percent of household income was spent on food, rent, and heat. Gamble, *How Chinese Families Live in Peiping*, 320–321.

38. BMA J181-018-13082.

39. A similar list was produced in 1925. See BMA J181-018-18207.

40. *Jingshi jingcha gongbao* [Capital police bulletin], December 31, 1927 and March 2, 1927.

41. Kerr Refuge Annual Report, 1909, 4. In the 1916 edition of the report, 20.0 percent of admitted patients had died at the facility; by the time the 1923 report was compiled, this number had increased to 27.7 percent.

42. RAC CMB, Inc., Box 96, Folder 690, "Insane Asylum," Richard Lyman to Roger Greene, May 14, 1934.

43. As two examples, BMA J181-019-38439, J181-019-35310.

44. Jian Hu, "Pinglun: Guomin zhi jingshen bing" [Critique: The people's mental illness], *Dongfang zazhi* 18, no. 4 (1921): 1–3; Chen Wanli, "Jingshen bing shi shenme?" [What is mental illness?], *Tongsu yishi yuekan* 2 (1919): 16–20.

45. Weng Zhilong, "Jingshen bingyuan yingyou de shebei" [The equipment that insane asylums should have], *Minzhong yibao* 6 (1931): 35–41.

46. BMA J181-019-32402.

47. BMA J181-019-38420.

48. BMA J181-018-19237.

49. For example, BMA J181-019-38420, J1810-019-38398, among others.

50. BMA J181-019-21289.

51. BMA J181-019-46448. It might perhaps seem strange that both Guan Yanchang and Fang Yujing were able to so lucidly describe their mad disorder. The police, however, recognized that madness was often a sporadic condition (the illness "comes and goes" [*shifa shiyu*] was a common refrain in police documents), and they therefore took the men's testimonies into consideration alongside the corroborating testimonies provided by their relatives.

52. BMA J181-019-25183.

53. Tang Erhe, "Jingshen bing yu qi zhiliao" [Mental illness and its treatment], *Dongfang zazhi* 21, no. 8 (1924): 92–94. For more on Tang, see David Luesink, "State Power, Governmentality, and the (Mis)remembrance of Chinese Medicine," in *Historical Epistemology and the Making of Modern Chinese Medicine*, ed. Howard Chiang (Manchester: Manchester University Press, 2015), 160–187.

54. Weng, "Jingshen bingyuan yingyou de shebei," 35.

55. Since the police-managed asylum did not keep statistics on its inmates, it is difficult to say how many admittances were brought by either their families or the police. It was not until the 1930s that statistical data were compiled. Francis L. K. Hsü, "A Brief Report on the Police Cooperation in Connection with Mental Cases in Peiping," in *Social and Psychological Studies in Neuropsychiatry in China*, ed. R. Lyman, V. Maeker, and P. Liang (Peking: Henri Vetch, 1939), 203.

56. Eric Hobsbawm, "Peasants and Politics," *Journal of Peasant Studies* 1, no. 1 (1973): 13.

57. In this sense, I provide an alternative viewpoint to studies of peasant politics that mainly focus on covert, "Brechtian" forms of resistance to the state. Most notably, James Scott, *Weapons of the Weak: Everyday Forms of Peasant Resistance* (New Haven, CT: Yale University Press, 1985).

58. BMA J181-019-32372.

59. BMA J181-019-13484.

60. Their complicity with new municipal norms does not suggest, however, that either woman was acting out of a concern for broader modernization projects; as Hanchao Lu has shown, ordinary people were more often moved by pragmatism than ideology, and this was undoubtedly the case in both incidents described here. Hanchao Lu, *Beyond the Neon Lights: Everyday Shanghai in the Early Twentieth Century* (Berkeley: University of California Press, 1999), 295.

61. In a way, these examples recall Erving Goffman's argument that mental patients enter the asylum not because they "distinctively suffer . . . from mental illness" but because of various "contingencies" that combine to justify their institutionalization. Erving Goffman, *Asylums: Essays on the Social Situation of Mental Patients and Other Inmates* (Chicago: Aldine, 1961), 135.

62. BMA J181-018-12813.

63. BMA J181-019-35373.

64. BMA J181-019-41735 and J181-019-38508.

65. Xu Ke, *Shiyong Beijing zhinan* [Practical guide to Beijing] (Shanghai: Shangwu yinshuguan, 1920).

66. Although this is the first time I have seen a parallel being drawn between madness and animality in the Republican context, the relationship was much more salient in the West. Roy Porter, citing Foucault, argues that the cause of the English madman's social alienation was his idleness and "animality." Roy Porter, "Foucault's Great Confinement," *History of the Human Sciences* 3, no. 1 (February 1990): 49.

67. BMA J181-018-12813.

68. BMA J181-019-41632.

69. On Britain, see Peter Bartlett, *The Poor Law of Lunacy: The Administration of Pauper Lunatics in Mid-Nineteenth Century England* (London: Leicester University Press, 1999), 100–102. For an overview of Japan's modern history of mental illness, see Sachiko Horiguchi, "Mental Health and Therapy in Japan," in *Critical Issues in Contemporary Japan*, ed. Jeff Kingston (London: Routledge, 2014), 223–234.

70. Foucault, *Madness and Civilization*, chapter 2. See also Diamant, "China's 'Great Confinement'?"

71. Foucault speaks of the "undifferentiated mass" of people who were institutionalized within the Hôpital Général. Foucault, *Madness and Civilization*, 48. Others have challenged the historical veracity of this assertion. Roy Porter, for instance, argues that Foucault's claims "[do] not fit the facts" and are "hyperbolic," especially considering that the number of insane confined in the Hôtel Dieu throughout the eighteenth century remained relatively small. Roy Porter, *Madmen: A Social History of Madhouses, Mad-Doctors, and Lunatics* (Stroud, UK: Tempus, 2004), 20–22.

72. BMA J181-019-47038.

73. Ibid.

74. Often, such letters were written by a hired intermediary who was familiar with bureaucratic language. Indeed, the phrases the letter-writer uses to describe Mrs. Zhang's madness were entirely in keeping with the tropes of madness discussed in chapter 2. See Chen, *Guilty of Indigence*, 105.

75. A *mu* is equivalent to 0.165 acres.

76. BMA J184-002-15920.

77. Throughout the republic, the number of women confined within the asylum was significantly lower than that of men. According to the *Jingshi jingcha gongbao*, the ratio of men to women in the asylum was typically around 3:2 (usually 60 men to 40 women, though these figures fluctuated). Although these numbers could partially be attributed to the gender disparity in the general population, later survey data from the Peking Union Medical College suggest that the police were far less willing to detain women than men; consequently, a greater percentage of women were brought to the asylum by their families than by the police. Of the individuals brought to the asylum by the police, 66.6 percent were men and 33.3 percent were women; of the individuals brought by their families, 56.7 percent were men and 43.3 percent were women. Hsü, "Report on the Police Cooperation in Peiping," 204.

78. Hsü, "Report on the Police Cooperation in Peiping," 204.

79. Foucault, *Madness and Civilization*, 41.

80. Although the Republican period witnessed an unprecedented rise in discourses related to women's rights and gender equality, the lived experiences of women were slow to keep pace with feminist ideologies. With certain exceptions, many women continued to be viewed as interlopers into the patrilineal household; and the woman's perceived role as caregiver, rather than economic provider, similarly served to undermine her standing and power both within the home and in the workplace. See, for instance, Christina Gilmartin, *Engendering the Chinese Revolution: Radical Women, Communist Politics, and Mass Movements in the 1920s* (Berkeley: University of California Press, 1995), 109–112.

81. Showalter, *Female Malady*, 73; Akihito Suzuki, *Madness at Home: The Psychiatrist, the Patient, and the Family in England 1820–1860* (Berkeley: University of California Press, 2006), 146–150; Andrew Scull, *Hysteria: The Disturbing History* (Oxford: Oxford University Press, 2011), 71–73.

82. "Shanghai fengdian yiyuan feifa jingu yi jianfu" [Shanghai asylum illegally detains a healthy woman], *Funü yuebao* 2, no. 3 (1936): 44–47; "Patient of Local Asylum Files Charge," *China Press*, March 24, 1936.

83. For an account of the various types of "mad doctors" who profited from the trade in lunacy, see Parry-Jones, *Trade in Lunacy*, chapter 4.

84. Compare, for instance, with the British Lunacy Act of 1845, which made county asylums mandatory; or the French law of June 30, 1838, which mandated the establishment of asylums in every département, to be staffed by full-time physicians. On the significance of the latter, see Goldstein, *Console and Classify*, chapter 8.

85. Hsü, "Report on the Police Cooperation in Peiping," 222–223.

86. "Yin shenghuo jiannan dafa fengkuang" [Going insane from everyday hardships], *Shehui ribao*, June 14, 1924.

Chapter Four

1. For example, BMA J181-019-32402, J1810-019-29027, J181-019-41640, among others.

2. Woods, "Nervous Diseases of the Chinese," 542.

3. For example, Zhou, *Zhou Xiaonong yi'an*, 41–46.

4. James W. Bennett, "Pills of Ten Thousand Efficacies," *Asia: Journal of the American Asiatic Association* 30 (September 1930): 620.

5. "Li Guishan de shenjing bing" [The madness of Li Guishan], *Liming bao*, June 11, 1924, 3.

6. Bennett, "Pills of Ten Thousand Efficacies," 618.

7. Stephen R. MacKinnon, "Toward a History of the Chinese Press in the Republican Period," *Modern China* 23, no. 1 (January 1997): 3–32.

8. Psychiatric entrepreneurs did not refer to themselves as such, of course. Medical advertisements did not even mention the word "psychiatry" (*jingshen bingxue* or *jingshen yixue*), which was still a relatively recent neologism.

9. Sherman Cochran, *Chinese Medicine Men: Consumer Culture in China and Southeast Asia* (Cambridge, MA: Harvard University Press, 2006), 3.

10. In his discussion of Shanghai, Hanchao Lu distinguishes between the "elites" (literati, Western-educated professionals like doctors and lawyers, merchants, and struggling writers who "lived among the populace while maintaining the mentality of an elite"), the petty urbanites, and the urban poor (former peasants who were mostly unskilled and illiterate). Although intellectuals were not always financially well-off (in fact, many were quite poor), they still considered themselves part of the "elite" classes because of their educational status. Lu, *Beyond the Neon Lights*, 55–66. On the rise of a middle class, see Wen-hsin Yeh, *Shanghai Splendor: Economic Sentiments and the Making of Modern China, 1843–1949* (Berkeley: University of California Press, 2007).

11. The rise of "nervous illnesses" was certainly not unique to China. For one of the first tracts on the subject in the Western world, see George Cheyne, *The English Malady* (London: Strahan, 1733).

12. Leslie E. Gill, *Advertising and Psychology* (London: Routledge, 2013 [1954]), 11.

13. James Flath, "Temple Fairs and the Republican State in North China," *Twentieth-Century China* 30, no. 1 (November 2004): 39–63; Susan Naquin, *Peking: Temples and City Life, 1400–1900* (Berkeley: University of California Press, 2000), 622–637.

14. Dong, *Republican Beijing*, 164.

15. Ibid., 163–169; Madeleine Yue Dong, "Juggling Bits: Tianqiao as Republican Beijing's Recycling Center," *Modern China* 25, no. 3 (July 1999): 303–342.

16. Mittler, *Newspaper for China*, 315–322; Huaiting Wu, "The Construction of a Consumer Population in Advertising in 1920s China," *Discourse & Society* 20, no. 1 (January 2009): 147–171.

17. Rogaski, *Hygienic Modernity*, 226–233; Barbara Mittler, "Gendered Advertising in China: What History Do Images Tell?" *European Journal of East Asian Studies* 6, no. 1 (2007): 13–41; Sherman Cochran, "Marketing Medicine and Advertising Dreams in Shanghai, 1900–1940," in *Becoming Chinese: Passages to Modernity and Beyond*, ed. Wen-hsin Yeh (Berkeley: University of California Press, 2000), 62–97; Karl Gerth, *China Made: Consumer Culture and the Creation of the Nation* (Cambridge, MA: Harvard University Press, 2003).

18. And vice versa. Western products also adopted a Chinese vocabulary in order to appeal to native consumers. Emily Baum, "Health by the Bottle: The Dr. Williams' Medicine Company and the Commodification of Well-Being in the *Liangyou* Pictorial," in *Liangyou: Kaleidoscopic Modernity and the Shanghai Global Metropolis*, ed. Paul Pickowicz, Shen Kuiyi, and Zhang Yingjin (Leiden: Brill, 2013), 71–93.

19. Eugenia Lean, "The Modern Elixir: Medicine as Consumer Item in the Early Twentieth-Century Chinese Press," *UCLA Historical Journal* 15 (1995): 65–92.

20. Beiping Hongren Tang, "Beiping Hongren Tang lejia lao yaopu wansan gaodan jiamu" [Beiping Hongren Tang happy family apothecary medication price guide] (Beiping: Hongren Tang, 1935).

21. For example, Hinrichs and Barnes, *Chinese Medicine and Healing*, 97–128.

22. Peter Buck, *American Science and Modern China, 1876–1936* (Cambridge: Cambridge University Press, 1980), 24–27.

23. Yang Nianqun, *Zaizao bingren: Zhongxi yi chongtu xia de kongjian zhengzhi, 1832–1985* [Remaking patients: Politics of space in the conflicts between traditional Chinese medicine and Western medicine] (Beijing: Renmin daxue chubanshe, 2006).

24. Buck, *American Science and Modern China*, 23–24.

25. By the early 1920s, many hospitals were reporting debts due to lack of patient fees. In 1922, one Shanghai hospital reported a deficit of over $31,000, while another hospital in Guangzhou reported a deficit of close to $36,000. "Hospital Reports," *China Medical Missionary Journal* 37, no. 11 (November 1923): 953–955.

26. Rogaski, *Hygienic Modernity*, chapter 8; Croizier, *Traditional Medicine in Modern China*, 72–74.

27. Lei, *Neither Donkey nor Horse*, 1–2.

28. "President Li Yuan-Hung on Medical Work in China," *China Medical Missionary Journal* 37, no. 7 (July 1923): 588–589.

29. Peiyao Zhang et al., "An Exploratory Spatial Analysis of Western Medical Services in Republican Beijing," *Applied Geography* 32, no. 2 (March 2012): 556–565.

30. "Xu Fu'an fengke zhuanjia tonggao bingjia" [Xu Fu'an, specialist in madness medicine, makes an announcement to those who are ill], *Shishi gongbao*, July 26, 1936.

31. According to Sidney Gamble, average household expenditures for health-related items ranged between 1.1 and 2.0 percent of a family's annual budget. For families making less than $100 per year, inpatient hospital costs would have been out of the question. *How Chinese Families Live in Peiping*, 171–173.

32. "Ziran zhiliao yiguan" [Natural healing hospital], *Chen bao*, November 19, 1924.

33. "Shi Sunzhi jingshen zhiliao" [Shi Sunzhi spirit healing], Chen bao, October 1, 1924. Related advertisements in Chen bao include "Guomin jingshen yangcheng hui: jingshen zhiliao yuan" [People's spirit cultivation society: Mental healing hospital], Chen bao, September 10, 1926; "Jingshen liaoyang yuan" [Mental rehabilitation hospital], Chen bao, October 23, 1927.

34. "Jingshen xue zhuanjia Shi Sunzhi" [Psychiatric specialist Shi Sunzhi], Chen bao, May 22, 1928.

35. Hypnotism, which had gained a following in the Western world in the last two decades of the nineteenth century, was introduced to China around the turn of the Republican period. The Chinese Institute of Mentalism (Zhongguo xinling yanjiu hui), one of the first and most successful study societies for the art of hypnotism, was established in Tokyo in 1911 and moved to Shanghai about one decade later. By 1931, membership in the institute had surpassed eighty thousand people. Yu Pingke, Cuimian shu hanshou jiangyi [Correspondence teaching materials on hypnotism] (Shanghai: Zhongguo xinling yanjiu hui, 1931), 48–50.

36. "Fengdian yiyuan" [Madness hospital], Shishi huabao, February 1, 1932. For a discussion of zangzao, see chapter 7.

37. "Baikui yiyuan" [Baikui Hospital], in Beiping lüxing zhinan [Beiping travel guide] (Beiping: Shibao yingye bu faxing, 1935).

38. "Xu Fu'an fengke zhuanjia."

39. Wei Hongsheng, "Zongzhi" [Preface], in Jingshen jiankang shiyan lu [Records of healthy spirit practice] (Beiping: Jingshen xue yanjiu hui faxing, 1937).

40. Bao Fangzhou advertised his research society widely and over many years. Advertisements appeared most prominently in the Shanghai newspaper Shen bao (as one example, September 25, 1935) but were also featured in newspapers from northeast China, in particular Shengjing shibao. For example, see "Zhongguo jingshen yanjiu hui: jingshen liaobing yuan" [Chinese Spirit Research Association: Mental therapeutics hospital], Shengjing shibao, January 14, 1920.

41. Bao referenced a well-known expression: "Illnesses of mind require mind medicines" (xinbing haixu xin yaoyi). The motto of his research society similarly expressed an emphasis on mind over body: "Treatment of the mind is most important; treatment of the body is secondary; treatment of the illness is of least importance" (yixin weishang, yishen cizhi, yibing weixia).

42. Zhongguo jingshen yanjiu hui, ed., Zhongguo jingshen yanjiu hui jingshen tekan [Chinese Spirit Research Association special issue] (Shanghai: Zhongguo jingshen yanjiu hui chubanshe, 1936), 51.

43. Ibid., 7.

44. Wei Hongsheng, "Huan bingzhe wenda" [Questions and answers for those who are ill], in Jingshen duanlian zhiliao shiyan wenda [Questions and answers on experiments related to the exercise and treatment of the spirit] (Beiping: n.p., 1936), 36–37.

45. Ibid., 39–40.

46. Ma uses the term "six doors" (liumen). The "six doors" refers to the six pathogenic influences of wind, summer heat, dampness, fire, dryness, and cold. Chinese medicine believes that these influences comprise the major external causes of illness.

47. Wei, Jingshen duanlian zhiliao shiyan wenda, 25–27.

48. Lee J. Vance, "Evolution of Patent Medicine," Popular Science Monthly, May 1891, 76.

49. Samuel Hopkins Adams, "The Great American Fraud," Collier's Weekly, October 7, 1905, 4.

50. James Harvey Young, The Toadstool Millionaires: A Social History of Patent Medicines in America before Federal Regulation (Princeton, NJ: Princeton University Press, 1972); James

Harvey Young, *American Health Quackery* (Princeton, NJ: Princeton University Press, 1992). See also Roy Porter, *Health for Sale: Quackery in England, 1660–1850* (Manchester: Manchester University Press, 1989).

51. Bridie Andrews has argued that patent medicines existed in China since at least the Ming dynasty. Although Chinese pharmacies did produce similar types of cure-alls, they were not nationally mass-produced or sold on a scale equivalent to that of twentieth-century proprietary medicines. Andrews, *Making of Modern Chinese Medicine*, 46.

52. Thomas Sammons, *Proprietary Medicine and Ointment Trade in China* (Washington, DC: Government Printing Office, 1917), 3.

53. Bridie Andrews, "Blood in the History of Modern Chinese Medicine," in *Historical Epistemology and the Making of Modern Chinese Medicine*, 130.

54. Hugh Shapiro, "The Puzzle of Spermatorrhea in Republican China," *positions* 6, no. 3 (1998): 571.

55. "Yangjiao feng banshen busui diankuang miaoyao" [Miraculous medicine for epilepsy, semiparalysis, and madness], *Chen bao*, December 23, 1922. Costs at the municipal hospital were priced on a sliding scale. According to BMA J181-019-32317, the Beijing Outer City Hospital charged third-class patients three jiao (thirty cents) per day.

56. "Fengdian zhenjing wan" [Madness suppressing pill], *Jingshi jingcha gongbao*, March 2, 1927.

57. "Quanqiu diyi tanmi fengdian wan" [World's number-one mucous confusion and madness pill], *Chen bao*, October 2, 1924. The advertisement, in various iterations, continued to run through 1926. See also "Wenwu fengdian" [Civil and martial madness], *Shehui ribao*, March 8, 1923.

58. Cochran, "Marketing Medicine and Advertising Dreams in Shanghai," 67.

59. Although these advertisements did not specifically reveal how the medications worked, the "Mucous Confusion and Madness Pill" provides a hint. Unlike other drugs, it claimed, this product "did not cause vomiting or diarrhea" and was "perfectly safe."

60. As just a few examples, "Fengfu zixing zhashang boxiang" [Mad woman slits open her own throat], *Shishi baihua bao*, March 21, 1923; "Fengsun si zumu" [Mad grandson kills grandmother], *Beijing baihua bao*, June 8, 1922; "Fenghan huodu canwen" [The tragic tale of the madman disemboweling himself], *Beijing baihua bao*, July 1, 1922.

61. Samuel Hopkins Adams argued that many such testimonials featured men and women who had never actually used the proprietary medicine, but who nonetheless agreed to attach their names to the advertisement "for the joy of appearing in print." Adams, "Great American Fraud," 6.

62. Thomas Sammons noted, "Testimonial advertising has met with success in China" and "many spontaneous letters of gratitude are received daily by patent medicine firms here." Sammons, *Proprietary Medicine and Ointment Trade in China*, 7.

63. "Jieshao tanmi fengdian wan" [Introducing the Mucous Confusion and Madness Pill], *Baihua guoqiang bao*, March 13, 1924.

64. "Wuxie zhiyu fengkuang shuchuang" [Sincerely expressing gratitude for healing madness and scrofula], *Shengjing shibao*, October 3, 1934.

65. Recent research has also tackled the question of how direct-to-consumer medical advertising has reduced the stigma of certain mental health conditions, such as depression. For example, Andrew Payton and Peggy Thoits, "Medicalization, Direct-to-Consumer Advertising, and Mental Illness Stigma," *Society and Mental Health* 1, no. 1 (March 2011): 55–70; Patrick Corrigan

et al., "How Does Direct to Consumer Advertising Affect the Stigma of Mental Illness?" *Community Mental Health Journal* 50, no. 7 (2014): 792–799.

66. Well into the 1980s, neurasthenia remained "the most common psychiatric outpatient diagnosis for neurotic disorders in China." Arthur Kleinman, *Social Origins of Distress and Disease: Depression, Neurasthenia, and Pain in Modern China* (New Haven, CT: Yale University Press, 1988), 3.

67. George Beard, "Neurasthenia, or Nervous Exhaustion," *Boston Medical and Surgical Journal* 3, no. 18 (April 29, 1869): 217–221; also George Beard, *American Nervousness: Its Causes and Consequences* (New York: Putnam, 1881), vii.

68. Beard, *American Nervousness*, vi.

69. Tom Lutz has argued that the disorder was "not suffered so much as 'enjoyed.'" Tom Lutz, "Varieties of Medical Experience: Doctors and Patients, Psyche and Soma in America," in *Cultures of Neurasthenia from Beard to the First World War*, ed. Marijke Gijswijt-Hofstra and Roy Porter (Amsterdam: Rodopi, 2001), 51.

70. John Harvey Kellogg, *Neurasthenia, or Nervous Exhaustion* (Battle Creek, MI: Good Health Publishing, 1915), 15–16.

71. Thomas Dixon Savill, *Clinical Lectures on Neurasthenia* (London: Henry J. Glaisher, 1908), 23.

72. Janet Oppenheim, *Shattered Nerves: Doctors, Patients, and Depression in Victorian England* (Oxford: Oxford University Press, 1991), 97.

73. Yu-chuan Wu, "A Disorder of Ki: Alternative Treatments for Neurasthenia in Japan, 1890–1945" (PhD diss., University College London, 2012), 9–10. On a brief history of neurasthenia in Japan, see Kenji Kitanishi and Kyoichi Kondo, "The Rise and Fall of Neurasthenia in Japanese Psychiatry," *Transcultural Psychiatric Research Review* 31, no. 2 (1994): 137–152.

74. Ishikawa Hanzan, *Shinkei suijaku oyobi sono kaifuku* [Neurasthenia and its recovery] (Tokyo: Kōgakukai, 1909), 1.

75. Furukawa Hisashi, *Sōseki no shokan* [Sōseki's letters] (Tokyo: Tōkyōdō shuppan, 1970).

76. Wu, "Disorder of Ki," 28–29.

77. Song Jiaoren, *Song Jiaoren riji* [The diary of Song Jiaoren] (Changsha: Hunan renmin chubanshe, 1980), 187, 191; Zhang Yaojie, *Xuanàn bainian: Song Jiaoren an yu Guomindang* [An unsettled case of the century: The case of Song Jiaoren and the Guomindang] (Taibei: Guojia tushuguan chuban, 2010), 12.

78. Peng Hsiao-yen, *Dandyism and Transcultural Modernity: The Dandy, the Flaneur, and the Translator in 1930s Shanghai, Tokyo, and Paris* (London: Routledge, 2010), 176–177.

79. Between 1918 and 1919, the Peking Union Medical College saw only 11 cases of neurasthenia but 728 cases of syphilis. Peking Union Medical College Eleventh Annual Report, 1918–1919 (Peking: Bureau of Engraving and Printing, 1919), 43, 45. Likewise, the first mention of psychoneuroses in annual reports for the Kerr Refuge did not appear until 1922–1923. In this report, only 3 patients out of 464 were diagnosed with psychoneuroses. Kerr Refuge Annual Report, 1922–1923, 12.

80. W. M. Royds, "Japanese Patent Medicines," *Transactions of the Asiatic Society of Japan* 35–36 (1907): 5.

81. "Patent Medicines in Japan," *British Medical Journal* 1, no. 2455 (January 18, 1908): 161–163.

82. Sammons, *Proprietary Medicine and Ointment Trade in China*, 4.

83. These statistics come from a 1907 report; by the 1910s, there were likely far more licensed dealers operating in China. See Royds, "Japanese Patent Medicines," 7–11.

84. Zheng Shibin, *Riben jiating yao* [Japanese home medicine] (Taiwan: Pasidun Publishing, 2015), 94; Wu Yongmei and Li Peide [Pui-tak Lee], *Tuxiang yu shangye wenhua: fenxi Zhongguo jindai guanggao* [Graphic images and consumer culture: Analysis of modern advertising culture in China] (Hong Kong: Hong Kong University Press, 2014), 183.

85. For example, "Jiannao wan" [Brain-strengthening pill], *Shengjing shibao*, August 13, 1912; "You zenme yang de nao shenjing bing liangyao" [Miraculous medicine for whatever kind of brain and nervous illnesses], *Shengjing shibao*, March 22, 1916; "Nao shenjing bing texiao wan" [Particularly effective medicine for brain and nervous illnesses], *Shengjing shibao*, November 21, 1917.

86. "Naozheng liangyao lingpian" [Efficacious pills for brain ailments], *Shengjing shibao*, February 1, 1921.

87. "Bunao mishen lingyao" [Efficacious brain-bolstering potion], *Shengjing shibao*, August 2, 1912.

88. "Shenjing shuairuo zhi liangyao" [Wonderful medicine for neurasthenia], *Shen bao*, April 18, 1925.

89. "Shenjing shuairuo texiao nao yixin" [Particularly effective for neurasthenia and revitalizing the brain], in *Beiping lüxing zhinan*.

90. "Bunao zhuangjin wan" [Brain-bolstering and muscle-strengthening pill], *Chen bao*, September 8, 1926; "Luo Wei shi tingzhuang wan" [Mr. Luo Wei strengthening pill], *Beijing baihua bao*, July 12, 1929. On the relationship between seminal emission (spermatorrhea) and "mental" illness, see Shapiro, "Puzzle of Spermatorrhea."

91. The first reference to neurasthenia in an advertisement for Ailuo Brain Tonic that I have found is "Zhiliao shenjing shuairuozheng de texiao yao: Ailuo bunaozhi" [Particularly effective medicine for treating neurasthenia: Ailuo brain tonic], *Shen bao*, April 13, 1926.

92. "Wuxie Yuantian yishi" [Greatly thank doctor Harada], *Liming bao*, January 20, 1924.

93. Max K. W. Huang, "Medical Advertising and Cultural Translation: The Case of *Shenbao* in Early Twentieth-Century China," in *Print, Profit, and Perception: Ideas, Information, and Knowledge in Chinese Societies, 1895–1949*, ed. Pei-yin Lin and Weipin Tsai (Leiden: Brill, 2014), 135.

94. BMA J005-003-00063 and J181-020-31062.

95. Zhang Ning, "Nao wei yishen zhi zhu: cong 'Ailuo Bunaozhi' kan jindai Zhongguo shenti guan de bianhua" [From heart to brain: Ailuo brain tonic and the new concept of the body in modern China], *Zhongyang yanjiuyuan jindaishi yanjiusuo jikan* 74 (December 2011): 1–40.

96. Stuart Ewen, *Captains of Consciousness: Advertising and the Social Roots of the Consumer Culture* (New York: McGraw Hill, 2001 [1976]), 35.

97. William Leiss, Stephen Kline, and Sut Jhally, *Social Communication in Advertising: Persons, Products, and Images of Well-Being* (London: Routledge, 1997), 23.

98. I have borrowed the term "illness narrative" from Arthur Kleinman. Kleinman defines an illness narrative as "a story the patient tells, and significant others retell, to give coherence to the distinctive events and long-term course of suffering." Kleinman, *Illness Narratives*, 49.

99. Zhou Zuoren, "Shanzhong zaxin" [Assorted letters from the mountain], in *Jingdian zuopin xuan* [Anthology of classic works] (Beijing: Dangdai shijie chubanshe, 2002), 63–64. The letter quoted is dated June 29, 1921.

100. Zhou Zuoren, "Guanyu sanyue shiba ri de sizhe" [On those who died on March 18], in *Jingdian zuopin xuan*, 18. The quotation is from a 1926 diary entry.

101. Zhou, "Shanzhong zaxin," 64. The letter quoted is dated July 14, 1921.

102. On a detailed look at Gu's experience with neurasthenia, see Wang Wenji, "Zhixing weibi heyi: Gu Jiegang yu shenjing shuairuo de ziwo guanli" [Gu Jiegang and the management

of neurasthenia in Republican China], in *Weisheng yu yiliao* (Taibei: Zhongyang yanjiu yuan, 2013), 65–99.

103. For example, "Wenda" [Q & A], *Huabei yibao*, no. 16 (February 1, 1930): 3. On *Dongfang zazhi*, see Wang, "Zhixing weibi heyi," 66.

104. Liao Qichong, "Wode shenjing shuairuo bing yuhou de shuohua" [My testimony on having recovered from neurasthenia], *Dazhong yikan*, no. 13 (1931): 54.

105. Wu Jiangleng, "Shenjing bing de shiren" [The nervous poet], *Shaonian shehui* 2 (1919): 15–16.

106. Ding X, "Yige jingshen bing huanzhe de laiyuan yu shigao" [A letter and draft of a poem from a mentally ill person], *Tianfeng*. Accessed at Shanghai Municipal Archives (hereafter, SMA) D2-0-923.

107. Peng, *Dandyism and Transcultural Modernity*, 178–181.

108. Hugh Shapiro has argued that the appeal of neurasthenia had to do with its "anatomic resonance" to traditional Chinese disorders of depletion and lassitude. This explanation is no doubt true, but it does not necessarily explain the willingness of intellectuals to adopt a neurasthenic identity. Hugh Shapiro, "Neurasthenia and the Assimilation of Nerves into China" (paper presented at the Symposium on the History of Disease, Academia Sinica, Taiwan, June 16–18, 2000); Hugh Shapiro, "How Different Are Chinese and Western Medicine? The Case of Nerves," in *Medicine across Cultures: History and Practice of Medicine in Non-Western Cultures*, ed. Helaine Selin (New York: Kluwer, 2003), 351–372.

109. Richard Elliott, "Making Up People: Consumption as a Symbolic Vocabulary for the Construction of Identity," in *Elusive Consumption*, ed. Karin Ekstrom and Helene Brembeck (Oxford: Berg, 2004), 129–144.

110. Lu Xun, "Kuangren riji."

111. Peng Hsiao-yen, "A Traveling Disease: The 'Malady of the Heart,' Scientific Jargon, and Neo-Sensation," in *China and Its Others: Knowledge Transfer through Translation, 1829–2010*, ed. James St. André and Peng Hsiao-yen (Amsterdam: Rodopi, 2012), 116.

112. Lei, *Neither Donkey nor Horse*, 1–2.

Chapter Five

1. The Peking Union Medical College, for instance, treated only a small number of patients suffering from "diseases of the mind" and disorders of the nervous system. Peking Union Medical College Eleventh Annual Report, 1918–1919, 44–46.

2. For example, Ju Zhongzhou, *Biantai xinli xue jiangyi lu* [Teaching materials on abnormal psychology] (Beijing: Zhonghua biantai xinli xue hui, 1923); Pang Jing, *Shiyong cuimian shu* [Applied hypnotism] (Shanghai: Zhonghua shuju, 1923); Lu Shoujian, *Shenjing shuairuo liaoyang fa* [Treatment for neurasthenia] (Shanghai: Zhonghua shuju, 1917).

3. Richard Lyman, "Psychiatry in China," *Archives of Neurology and Psychiatry* 37, no. 4 (April 1937): 768.

4. Ibid., 766.

5. RAC CMB, Inc., RG IV2B9, Box 22, Folder 155, "Survey of Psychiatric Hospitals," 1933.

6. RAC RG 1, Series 601, Box 12, Folder 129, "Report on Visit to China, June 9–July 3, 1931."

7. Lyman, "Psychiatry in China," 769.

8. RAC CMB, Inc., RG IV2B9, Box 22, Folder 155, Roger Greene to Max Mason, January 1, 1931.

9. Diamant, "China's 'Great Confinement'?," 27.

10. For a discussion of the role of the state in the advancement of biomedicine more broadly, see Lei, *Neither Donkey nor Horse*, chapter 3.

11. As quoted in Dong, *Republican Beijing*, 85–87.

12. For reasons of ease and consistency, I will continue to refer to the city as Beijing. On the transformation of the city during the Nanjing Decade, see Madeleine Yue Dong, "Defining Beiping: Urban Reconstruction and National Identity, 1928–1936," in Esherick, *Remaking the Chinese City*, 121–138.

13. "Jieban jingshen bing liaoyang yuan" [Taking over the psychopathic hospital], *Shizheng pinglun*, nos. 1–2 (1935): 19.

14. BMA J002-001-00010.

15. BMA J181-020-02578.

16. BMA J002-001-00010.

17. Egon Erwin Kisch, *Secret China* (originally published in German as *China Geheim*) (London: Butler & Tanner, 1935 [1933]), 173.

18. "Beiping tebie shi shehui ju jiuji shiye xiaoshi" [Brief history of the charitable undertakings of the Beiping Municipal Social Affairs Bureau], in *Minguo shiliao congkan*, vol. 734, ed. Zhang Yan and Sun Yanjing (Zhengzhou: Daxiang chubanshe, 2009), 46.

19. Hsü, "Report on the Police Cooperation in Peiping," 227. See also, for instance, BMA J181-021-11691, J181-021-08633, J181-021-11625.

20. Kisch, *Secret China*, 170.

21. *Zhonghua minguo xingfa* [Penal code of the Republic of China] (Nanjing: Sifa bu, 1928). The earlier draft version of the penal code, promulgated in 1927, copied the language of the 1912 code verbatim. In contrast, the 1928 code replaced the term "mentally ill" (*jingshen bingren*) with the vaguer term "those who have lost their minds" (*xinshen sangshi*) and the clause "not considered a crime" (*buwei zui*) with the clause "not [legally] punishable" (*bufa*). See section 2, article 12 of *Zhonghua minguo zanxing xin xinglü* [Temporary new penal code of the Republic of China] (Shanghai: Commercial Press, 1927).

22. Hsü, "Report on the Police Cooperation in Peiping," 222.

23. The Republican judicial system was based on the German model. A panel of judges, rather than a jury of peers, decided verdicts. In contrast to the deviant behaviors discussed in chapter 2, which were handled internally by the police, criminal behavior like murder was tried in court. See Lean, *Public Passions*, 112–115.

24. BMA J181-031-03253.

25. In government memoranda, such as the ones mentioned below, the task of "treating" (*zhiliao*) the insane was always listed as secondary to the task of "taking them in [off the streets]" (*shourong* or *shouyang*).

26. "Benshi jiangshe fengren yuan" [This city will establish an asylum], *Shoudu shizheng gongbao*, no. 58 (1930): 13; see also "Choushe fengren yuan" [Planning to build an asylum], *Shoudu shizheng gongbao*, no. 82 (1931): 1. In the end, the asylum would not be completed until 1947.

27. "Shoudu fengren yuan" [Capital asylum], *Huabei yibao*, no. 56 (March 21, 1931): 3.

28. Kisch, *Secret China*, 171.

29. For example, BMA J181-021-05225, J181-021-11625.

30. Kisch, *Secret China*, 172.

31. RAC CMB, Inc., RG IV2B9, Box 96, Folder 690, Roger Greene to Margery Eggleston, June 9, 1933; Diamant, "China's 'Great Confinement'?," 27.

32. The original grounds of the PUMC, which had been established in 1906 as the "Union Medical College," were purchased from the London Missionary Society by the Rockefeller Foundation's China Medical Board in 1915. Peking Union Medical College, *Dedication Ceremonies and Medical Conference, September 15–22, 1921* (Peking: n.p., 1922); Mary Brown Bullock, *An American Transplant: The Rockefeller Foundation and Peking Union Medical College* (Berkeley: University of California Press, 1980), 3.

33. See, for instance, Clifford Beers, *A Mind That Found Itself* (New York: Longmans, Green, 1908).

34. Rockefeller Foundation Annual Report, 1913–1914 (New York: Rockefeller Foundation, 1914), 21–23.

35. RAC RG 1 Projects, Box 26, Series 601, Folder 240, "Preliminary Report of the China Medical Commission to the Rockefeller Foundation," September 24, 1914.

36. RAC CMB, Inc., RG IV2B9, Box 96, Folder 689, Thomas Salmon to Wallace Buttrick, September 5, 1919.

37. "Andrew H. Woods, M.D. Obituary," *AMA Archives of Psychology and Neurology* 79, no. 2 (1958): 175–176; BMCA, Andrew Woods diary, September 24, 1919.

38. BMCA, Andrew Woods diary, April 20 and November 13, 1903.

39. Woods, "Peking Union Medical College and the Problem of Insanity in China."

40. Andrew Woods, "The Menace of Insanity to Popular Government," *National Medical Journal of China* 7, no. 1 (March 1921): 204.

41. Woods, "Peking Union Medical College and the Problem of Insanity in China."

42. BMCA, Andrew Woods diary, July 4, 1919.

43. "Psychological diseases are diseases of the brain" was the slogan adopted by Wilhelm Griesinger (1817–1868) upon his assumption of the chair of psychiatry and neurology at Berlin in 1865. For a brief history of the development of neuropsychiatry as a single field, see Edward Brown, "Neurology's Influence on American Psychiatry, 1865–1915," in *History of Psychiatry and Medical Psychology*, ed. Edwin Wallace and John Gach (New York: Springer, 2008), 519–532; John Gach, "Biological Psychiatry in the Nineteenth and Twentieth Centuries," in Wallace and Gach, *History of Psychiatry and Medical Psychology*, 380–412; George Makari, *Soul Machine: The Invention of the Modern Mind* (New York: W. W. Norton, 2015), chapter 19.

44. Wenjing Li and Heinz-Peter Schmiedebach, "German Wine in an American Bottle: The Spread of Modern Psychiatry in China, 1898–1949," *History of Psychiatry* 26, no. 3 (2015): 348–358.

45. For an example of the PUMC's evolving classification of nervous system disorders, see Peking Union Medical College Eleventh Annual Report, 1918–1919, and Peking Union Medical College Twentieth Annual Report, 1928 (Peking: PUMC Press, 1928).

46. RAC CMB, Inc., RG IV2B9, Box 96, Folder 689, Roger Greene to Edwin Wayte, September 12, 1922; BMCA Andrew Woods diary, April 17, 1921. In 1921, Woods's title was changed from "Professor of Neurology and Psychiatry" to "Professor of Neurology."

47. RAC CMB, Inc., RG IV2B9, Box 96, Folder 689, Roger Greene to Margery Eggleston, June 14, 1928, and January 20, 1932.

48. RAC CMB, Inc., RG IV2B9, Box 96, Folder 689, Roger Greene, interview with Ludwik Rajchman, December 21, 1930.

49. RAC CMB, Inc., RG IV2B9, Box 96, Folder 689, Roger Greene, "China Medical Education," January 1, 1931.

50. Bullock, *American Transplant*, 152. See also Lei, *Neither Donkey nor Horse*, 59–60; RAC RG 1, Series 601, Box 12, Folder 129, Selskar Gunn to Max Mason, January 23, 1934.

51. RAC CMB, Inc., RG IV2B9, Box 96, Folder 689, Roger Greene to Margery Eggleston, January 20, 1932, and May 15, 1933. In a memorandum to the China Medical Board, Greene wrote that "our decision to [hire] Dr. Lyman was due to our conviction . . . that we ought to give proper instruction in psychiatry. Thus the appointment followed the realization of a need rather than vice versa."

52. RAC RG 1, Series 601, Box 11, Folder 117, Roger Greene to Alan Gregg, October 26, 1932; RAC RG 1, Series 601, Box 11, Folder 118, Roger Greene to Alan Gregg, February 23, 1933.

53. RAC CMB, Inc., RG IV2B9, Box 96, Folder 690, Roger Greene to Margery Eggleston, April 8, 1933.

54. RAC RG 1, Series 601, Box 11, Folder 118, Roger Greene to Max Mason, January 28, 1933.

55. RAC RG 1, Series 601, Box 11, Folder 118, Alan Gregg to Roger Greene, April 10, 1933, and Max Mason diary excerpt, April 5, 1933.

56. BMA J002-001-00010.

57. RAC CMB, Inc., RG IV2B9, Box 96, Folder 690, Board of Trustees, "Executive Committee Report," June 8, 1933.

58. RAC RG 1, Series 601, Box 11, Folder 118, Roger Greene to Alan Gregg, February 23, 1933; CMB, Inc., RG IV2B9, Box 22, Folder 155, Roger Greene to Max Mason, January 1, 1931.

59. Board of Trustees, "Executive Committee Report"; RAC CMB, Inc., RG IV2B9, Box 96, Folder 690, Roger Greene to Margery Eggleston, June 9, 1933, and Francis Dieuaide to Roger Greene, October 17, 1933. It was estimated that the monthly expenditure for the facility would total 1,141 yuan. While the municipality agreed to pay for the grounds of the facility and the expenses associated with each patient, the PUMC provided the salaries for doctors and staff, purchased necessary supplies and equipment, and undertook costs associated with the general improvement of the institution. In total, the municipality contributed 600 yuan per month toward the arrangement, leaving 541 yuan to be provided by the PUMC.

60. Francis Dieuaide to Roger Greene, October 17, 1933.

61. Henry Houghton, introduction to Lyman, Maeker, and Liang, Social and Psychological Studies in Neuropsychiatry in China, 1.

62. Joel Braslow, Mental Ills and Bodily Cures: Psychiatric Treatment in the First Half of the Twentieth Century (Berkeley: University of California Press, 1997), 51.

63. For one particularly frightening example, see Andrew Scull, Madhouse: A Tragic Tale of Megalomania and Modern Medicine (New Haven, CT: Yale University Press, 2007), chapter 3.

64. BMA J002-001-00108; RAC CMB, Inc., RG IV2B9, Box 96, File 690, Roger Greene to Margery Eggleston, February 12, 1934.

65. Zhang Kan and Zhao Chengjie, Zhongguo dangdai yixue jia huicui [Compilation of modern Chinese doctors] (Jilin: Jilin kexue jishu chubanshe, 1991), 296; BMA J002-001-00117.

66. Beiping Ministry of Health, Beiping shi zhengfu weisheng chu yewu baogao, 125–128.

67. RAC CMB, Inc., RG 4, Series 4, An Eight-Month Experiment, 1933–1934.

68. "Beiping shi weisheng ju jingshen bing liaoyang yuan zhuyuan guize" [Regulations on being admitted to the Beiping municipal psychopathic hospital], Beiping shi shizheng gongbao, no. 264 (August 24, 1934): 9–11.

69. BMA J001-003-00071, J001-003-00069. Psychiatric nurses were first made to complete a specialized training program at the PUMC.

70. "Beiping shi zhengfu jingshen bing liaoyang yuan tanshi guize" [Visiting regulations for the municipal psychopathic hospital], July 5, 1934, in Beijing weisheng dashi ji [Important events in Beijing hygiene], ed. Wang Kangjiu (Beijing: Beijing kexue jishu chubanshe, 1994).

71. "Beiping shi weisheng ju ershisi nian er yuefen jingshen bing liaoyang yuan zhencha bing-ren cishu yuebao biao" [Monthly report on patient examinations at the Beiping Psychopathic Hospital for February 1935], *Beiping shi shizheng gongbao*, no. 299 (1935): 1; L. C. Chou and Y. C. Lu, "A Sociological Study of Chinese Mental Patients," in Lyman, Maeker, and Liang, *Social and Psychological Studies in Neuropsychiatry in China*, 64.

72. First-class patients paid three yuan per day. Patients in the lower-class wards paid either one jiao (ten cents) per day or had their fees waived. "Beiping shi zhengfu weisheng ju jingshen bing liaoyang yuan shoufei guize" [Regulations for collecting fees at the municipal psychopathic hospital], July 28, 1934, in *Beijing weisheng dashi ji*.

73. Chou and Lu, "Sociological Study of Chinese Mental Patients," 42–48.

74. Between January and June 1935, medicinal treatments were employed a total of 4,308 times. "Gexiang zhiliao renshu tongji biao" [Statistics on the types of treatments administered], in Beiping Ministry of Health, *Beiping shi zhengfu weisheng chu yewu baogao*, chart 97.

75. Francisco López-Muñoz et al., "The History of Barbiturates a Century after Their Clini-cal Introduction," *Neuropsychiatric Disease and Treatment* 1, no. 4 (December 2005): 329–343. On a longer history of drug use and psychiatry, see David Healy, *The Antidepressant Era* (Cam-bridge, MA: Harvard University Press, 1997).

76. W. H. Chao, Y. K. Hsu, and R. S. Lyman, "Comments on the Treatment of Drug Ad-diction with Protracted Narcosis," *Journal of Nervous and Mental Disease* 87, no. 4 (April 1938): 454–463.

77. Lyman, "Psychiatry in China," 768. Fever therapy never underwent clinical trials before being replaced by penicillin.

78. Braslow, *Mental Ills and Bodily Cures*, 40.

79. Lyman, "Psychiatry in China," 768. In Chinese, this form of therapy was referred to as "social therapy" (*shehui zhiliao*) and was used sparingly in contrast to other medicinal cures (a total of 271 times over a six-month period). Beiping Ministry of Health, *Beiping shi zhengfu weisheng chu yewu baogao*, 130. The 1935 report listed an additional form of "psychotherapy" (*jingshen zhiliao*), but this had no relation to talk therapy; instead, it simply referred to an activ-ity room where patients could play ping-pong, read newspapers, and practice musical instru-ments. Beiping Ministry of Health, ed., *Beiping shi zhengfu weisheng ju yewu baogao* [Report on tasks administered by the Beiping municipal ministry of health] (Beiping: Beiping shi zhengfu weisheng ju, 1935), 233.

80. Beiping Ministry of Health, *Beiping shi zhengfu weisheng chu yewu baogao*, 129; Beiping Ministry of Health, *Beiping shi zhengfu weisheng ju yewu baogao*, 232.

81. Yolanda Eraso, "A Burden to the State: The Reception of the German 'Active Therapy' in an Argentinean 'Colony-Asylum' in the 1920s and 1930s," in Ernst and Mueller, *Transnational Psychiatries*, 51–79.

82. "Zhuyuan shouyuan chuyuan siwang gexiang renshu tongji bijiao tubiao" [Statistics on those admitted, remaining, discharged, and deceased at the hospital], in Beiping Ministry of Health, *Beiping shi zhengfu weisheng chu yewu baogao*, chart 98.

83. Hsü, "Report on the Police Cooperation in Peiping," 212.

84. "Weisheng yaowen" [Important health news], *Weisheng yuekan* 3, nos. 5–6 (1936): 92–93.

85. As quoted in Anne Rose, "Racial Experiments in Psychiatry's Provinces: Richard S. Ly-man and His Colleagues in China and the American South, 1932–51," *History of Psychiatry* 23, no. 419 (2012): 420.

86. Lyman, "Psychiatry in China," 768.

87. Beiping Ministry of Health, *Beiping shi zhengfu weisheng chu yewu baogao*, 130.

88. Ibid., 127–129.

89. Ibid., 129, and Beiping Ministry of Health, *Beiping shi zhengfu weisheng ju yewu baogao*, 232.

90. "Bianyan" [Preface], in Beiping Ministry of Health, *Beiping shi zhengfu weisheng chu yewu baogao*, 1–2.

91. RAC RG 1, Series 601, Box 12, Folder 129, "China and the Rockefeller Foundation," January 23, 1934.

92. Between 1934 and 1935, the police were responsible for 63.5 percent of admittances to the psychopathic hospital, either by detaining the individual directly or by facilitating the family's request for institutionalization. Moreover, despite the fact that the police were technically no longer allowed to make final determinations about the psychological state of men and women in their custody, an unofficial police "judge" frequently adjudicated the mental competency of potentially insane criminals. Hsü, "Report on the Police Cooperation in Peiping," 203.

93. Ibid., 225.

94. Ibid., 222–227.

95. BMA J181-020-23460.

96. BMA J181-020-23466.

97. Hsü, "Report on the Police Cooperation in Peiping," 224.

98. "Xin Zhonghua minguo xingfa" [New penal code for the Republic of China], *Zhonghua minguo xingfa xinjiu quanwen duizhao biao* [Comparison chart of the old and new Republican penal codes] (Beiping: n.p., 1935).

99. Hsü, "Report on the Police Cooperation in Peiping," 228–230.

100. M. Marjorie King, "The Social Service Department Archives: Peking Union Medical College, 1928–1951," *American Archivist* 59 (Summer 1996): 341. See also Ida Pruitt, "Hospital Social Service in Diagnosis and Treatment," *Chinese Medical Journal*, no. 28 (1928): 432–443.

101. S. D. Lamb, *Pathologist of the Mind: Adolf Meyer and the Origins of American Psychiatry* (Baltimore: Johns Hopkins University Press, 2014), 162; Jerome Schneck, *A History of Psychiatry* (Springfield, IL: Charles C. Thomas, 1960), 152.

102. Lyman, "Psychiatry in China," 768–769.

103. Beiping Ministry of Health, *Beiping shi zhengfu weisheng chu yewu baogao*, 130; Chou and Lu, "Sociological Study of Chinese Mental Patients," 31–116.

104. Song Siming, *Jingshen bing zhi shehui de yinsu yu fangzhi* [The social causes and prevention of mental illness] (Shanghai: Zhonghua shuju, 1944), 22.

105. As one example, Ida Pruitt describes the case of a man in the early stages of neurosyphilis who refused to accept a lumbar puncture as treatment. Pruitt explained to him the deadly effects of neurosyphilis and eventually persuaded him to undergo the procedure. Pruitt, "Hospital Social Service," 435.

106. Pruitt, "Hospital Social Service," 439–440; King, "Social Service Department Archives," 342–344. Unfortunately, patient records and sociological data from the PUMC are currently inaccessible to researchers. The only information I have been able to obtain about these files has come from published articles and related primary sources.

107. An interesting case that demonstrates the disjuncture between old and new psychiatric vocabularies can be found in BMA J181-025-07786. This case, from 1936, includes the record of a police interrogation with a mentally ill woman. The woman, who was twenty-five, was brought to the police by her husband after he claimed that she had tried to stab him in the head.

Her husband referred to her as "crazy" (*feng*), and the woman also described herself as a "mad person" (*fengzi*). The police, however, referred to the woman as "mentally ill" (*jingshen bing*).

108. Houghton, introduction to Lyman, Maeker, and Liang, *Social and Psychological Studies in Neuropsychiatry in China*, 1.

109. BMA J181-020-19112.

Chapter Six

1. Woods, "Menace of Insanity," 201–206.

2. Gerald Grob, *Mental Illness and American Society, 1875–1940* (Princeton, NJ: Princeton University Press, 1983), 144–178; Theresa Richardson, *The Century of the Child: The Mental Hygiene Movement and Social Policy in the United States and Canada* (Albany: State University of New York Press, 1989), 3–4.

3. Woods, "Menace of Insanity," 202.

4. Rockefeller Foundation Annual Report, 1936, 22–23.

5. Lloyd Eastman, *The Abortive Revolution: China under Nationalist Rule, 1927–1937* (Cambridge, MA: Harvard University Press, 1990), xii.

6. Julia Strauss, *Strong Institutions in Weak Polities: State Building in Republican China, 1927–1940* (Oxford: Oxford University Press, 1998), 59.

7. As quoted in Marie-Claire Bergère, *Sun Yat-sen*, trans. Janet Lloyd (Stanford, CA: Stanford University Press, 1998), 372.

8. Beers, *Mind That Found Itself*, 12–15.

9. Ibid., 52.

10. Clifford W. Beers, *The Mental Hygiene Movement: Origin and Growth* (Norwood, MA: Plimpton Press, 1917), part 5.

11. Grob, *Mental Illness*, 144; Johannes Pols, "Managing the Mind: The Culture of American Mental Hygiene, 1910–1950" (PhD diss., University of Pennsylvania, 1997).

12. Martin Stone, "Shellshock and the Psychologists," in *The Anatomy of Madness: Essays in the History of Psychiatry*, vol. 2, ed. William Bynum, Roy Porter, and Michael Shepherd (London: Routledge, 1985), 242–271.

13. William White, "The Origin, Growth, and Significance of the Mental Hygiene Movement," *Science* 72, no. 1856 (July 25, 1930): 79.

14. Adolf Meyer, "Organization of Community Facilities for Prevention, Care, and Treatment of Nervous and Mental Diseases," in *Proceedings of the First International Congress on Mental Hygiene* (New York: International Committee for Mental Hygiene, 1932), 248.

15. Daniel Wolford La Rue, *Mental Hygiene* (New York: Macmillan Company, 1932), 9–11.

16. Edwin Kirkpatrick, *Mental Hygiene for Effective Living* (New York: D. Appleton-Century, 1934), 326.

17. Frankwood Williams, *Mental Hygiene* (Chicago: American Library Association, 1929), 15.

18. White, "Mental Hygiene Movement," 79. On homosexuality and mental pathology, see Margot Canaday, *The Straight State: Sexuality and Citizenship in Twentieth-Century America* (Princeton, NJ: Princeton University Press, 2009), 66–69.

19. Ian Dowbiggin, *The Sterilization Movement and Global Fertility in the Twentieth Century* (Oxford: Oxford University Press, 2008), 26–30; also, Harry Bruinius, *Better for All the World: The Secret History of Forced Sterilization and America's Quest for Racial Purity* (New York: Random House, 2006).

20. Beers, *Mental Hygiene Movement*, 311-312.

21. As Mathew Thomson has pointed out, the mental hygiene movement unfolded differently in different locations, but its underlying impulse arose from a similar source. Mathew Thomson, "Mental Hygiene as an International Movement," in *International Health Organizations and Movements, 1918-1939*, ed. Paul Weindling (Cambridge: Cambridge University Press, 1995), 283-304.

22. Liang Qichao, "Fojiao xinli xue ceyan" [Putting Buddhist psychology to the test], *Xinli zazhi xuancun*, July 3, 1923; Gao Juefu, *Zhongguo xinli xue shi* [History of Chinese psychology] (Beijing: Renmin jiaoyu chubanshe, 1985), 27-28.

23. The school of behaviorism best exemplified this goal. See John Mills, *Control: A History of Behavioral Psychology* (New York: New York University Press, 1998), 6-7; John B. Watson, *Behaviorism* (Chicago: University of Chicago Press, 1924); John B. Watson, "Psychology as the Behaviorist Views It," *Psychological Review* 20 (1913): 158-177.

24. Geoffrey Blowers, "The Origins of Scientific Psychology in China, 1898-1949," in *Internationalizing the History of Psychology*, ed. Adrian Brock (New York: New York University Press, 2006), 97.

25. Yan Guocai, ed., *Zhongguo xinli xue shi ziliao xuanbian, di si juan* [Collection of materials on the history of Chinese psychology, vol. 4] (Beijing: Renmin jiaoyu chubanshe, 1990), 15.

26. Louise Higgins and Mo Zheng, "An Introduction to Chinese Psychology: Its Historical Roots until the Present Day," *Journal of Psychology* 136, no. 2 (2002): 225-239.

27. Huang Weirong, *Biantai xinli xue ABC* [The ABCs of abnormal psychology] (Shanghai: Shijie shuju, 1929), 103. On Huang Weirong, behaviorism, and his aversion to psychoanalysis, see Geoffrey Blowers, "La psychoanalyse en Chine avant 1949: le rejet ou la distortion" [Psychoanalysis in China before 1949: Rejection or distortion], *Perspectives chinoises* 39 (1997): 33-39.

28. Guo Renyuan, *Xinli xue ABC* [The ABCs of psychology] (Shanghai: Shijie shuju, 1928), 51.

29. Wang Zucheng, "Ji Zhongguo diyi wei nüxing jingshen bing xue jia: Gui Zhiliang jiaoshou" [Remembering China's first female psychiatrist: Professor Gui Zhiliang] *Jingshen yixue lishi* 23, no. 3 (2011): 191-192.

30. Gui Zhiliang, *Xiandai jingshen bingxue* [Modern psychiatry] (Shanghai: Xinyue shudian, 1932), 11, 81.

31. Sun Xiong, *Biantai xingwei* [Abnormal behavior] (Shanghai: Shijie shuju, 1939), 1.

32. Si Yi, "Jingshen bing yu xiandai shehui" [Mental illness and modern society], *Qinghua zhoukan* 43, no. 4 (1935): 6-17.

33. Zhang Kecheng, *Nannü shengzhi qixing shenjing shuairuo de yufang ji zhiliao* [Prevention and treatment of sexual neurasthenia in men and women] (Shanghai: Shenghuo yiyuan, 1934); Zhao Han'en, *Jingshen bingxue* [Psychiatry] (Shanghai: Shangwu yinshu guan, 1929), 13.

34. The belief that mental illness was on the rise was a universal phenomenon. For a discussion of the subject in England, see Scull, *Social Order/Mental Disorder*, 310-311.

35. Si, "Jingshen bing," 6.

36. Sun, *Biantai xingwei*, 2-3. Also, Liu Xiong, *Nao shenjing bing* [Brain and nervous diseases] (Shanghai: Shangwu yinshu guan, 1931), 13, 48.

37. "Ni you shenjing bing ma?" [Are you crazy?], *Liangyou huabao*, no. 124 (1937): 36-37.

38. Wu Nanxuan, "Shehui kongzhi dineng de zhongyao he fangfa" [The importance and methods of the social control of the feebleminded], *Guoli zhongyang daxue jiaoyu congkan* 1, no. 1 (1933): 86.

39. Song, *Jingshen bing*, 15.

40. Sun, *Biantai xingwei*, 1.

41. Song, *Jingshen bing*, 20.

42. Wu "Shehui kongzhi dineng de zhongyao he fangfa," 88. Wu provides this translation.

43. *Proceedings of the First International Congress on Mental Hygiene*, ix, 23.

44. Ibid., 94–95.

45. The John Kerr Refuge for the Insane in Guangzhou had also attempted to spread knowledge about the subject through two mental hygiene campaigns in 1921 and 1922. Robert Ross,
"Mental Hygiene," *China Medical Journal* 40 (1926): 8–13.

46. RAC CMB, Inc., RG IV2B9, Box 96, Folder 689, Thomas Salmon to Wallace Buttrick,
September 5, 1919; Rockefeller Foundation Annual Report, 1915, 26–29.

47. RAC CMB, Inc., RG IV2B9, Box 97, Folder 697, Dai Bingham to Margery Eggleston,
December 3, 1934.

48. RAC CMB, Inc., RG IV2B9, Box 97, Folder 697, Richard Lyman to Dai Bingham, January 15, 1935.

49. Shu Yueyu, "Zhang Yinian: Zhongguo xinli weisheng de kaituo zhe" [Zhang Yinian:
Progenitor of Chinese mental hygiene], *Ziran bianzheng fa tongxun*, no. 6 (2015): 138–146.

50. Zhang Yinian, *Xinli weisheng gailun* [Introduction to mental hygiene] (Shanghai:
Shangwu yinshu guan, 1936), 1–11.

51. Zhang Yinian, "Xinli weisheng yu ertong xundao" [Mental hygiene and the guidance of
children], in *Xinli weisheng*, ed. Tai Shuangqiu (Shanghai: Jiaoyu bianyi guan chuban, 1935), 16.

52. Zhang Yinian, "Xinli weisheng zai xuexiao ji jiating zhong de yingyong" [The utility of
mental hygiene in the school and at home], *Xinli jikan* 2, no. 2 (1937): 1–11.

53. Zhang, "Xinli weisheng yu ertong xundao," 25.

54. Other psychologists also shared this position. See, for instance, Xiao Xiaorong, "Xinli
weisheng zhi jiben yuanze" [Basic principles of mental hygiene], *Guoli zhongyang daxue jiaoyu
congkan* 2, no. 1 (1934): 1–13.

55. Wu Nanxuan, "Guoji xinli weisheng yundong" [The international mental hygiene move-
ment], *Guoli zhongyang daxue jiaoyu congkan* 2, no. 1 (1934): 38–39; also, Wu Nanxuan, "Xinli
weisheng yiyi fanwei yu zhongyao xing" [The meaning and importance of mental hygiene],
Guoli zhongyang daxue jiaoyu congkan 2, no. 1 (1934): 1–11.

56. Wu, "Guoji xinli weisheng yundong," 20–21.

57. Wu, "Shehui kongzhi dineng de zhongyao he fangfa," 63–97.

58. Ernst Rüdin, "The Significance of Eugenics and Genetics for Mental Hygiene," *Proceedings of the First International Congress on Mental Hygiene*, 472.

59. Norman Dain, *Clifford W. Beers: Advocate for the Insane* (Pittsburgh, PA: University of
Pittsburgh Press, 1980), 164.

60. Wu, "Shehui kongzhi dineng de zhongyao he fangfa," 91–93.

61. It is worth noting that by the time the Chinese mental hygiene movement had gotten
under way, Frankwood Williams, medical director of the NCMH from 1922 to 1931, had resigned
his position and turned his attention to the Soviet Union as a better structural and political
model for the achievement of mental health. His new position on mental hygiene, which was
widely propagated in China, involved the idea that self-abnegation and the pursuit of communal welfare could act as the basis of psychological strength. As he was quoted in a 1935 Chinese
article, "In the modern Soviet Union, the individual is important [only] because he is part of
society. . . . In this nation, there is only one loyalty: and that is to the society. Outside of society
there is no self; being loyal to oneself is the same as being loyal to society!" As quoted in Si,

"Jingshen bing," 17; see also Frankwood E. Williams, *Russia, Youth, and the Present-Day World: Further Studies in Mental Hygiene* (New York: Farrar & Reinhart, 1934).

62. Zhang Yinian, "Zhongguo xinli weisheng xiehui yuanqi" [Genesis of the Chinese Mental Hygiene Association], in Zhang, *Xinli weisheng gailun*, 225.

63. Out of the eleven guiding principles of the Chinese Mental Hygiene Association, only one—number eight—mentions improvement in care given to the individual patient. The other principles stress the "public utility" (*gonggong shiye*) of mental hygiene research and education.

64. Zhang and Wu were two of seven leading committee members of the association. "Jiaoyu wenhua xiaoxi: Zhongguo xinli weisheng xiehui chengli" [News on education and culture: Establishment of the Chinese Mental Hygiene Association], *Jiao yu xue* 1, no. 12 (1936): 286.

65. "Zhongguo xinli weisheng xiehui yuanqi" and "Zhongguo xinli weisheng xiehui jianzhang" [Regulations of the Chinese Mental Hygiene Association], in Zhang, *Xinli weisheng gailun*, 225–229. On the accomplishments of the association, see "Zhongguo xinli weisheng xiehui gongzuo baogao" [Work report for the Chinese Association of Mental Hygiene], *Jianguo jiaoyu*, no. 1 (1938): 39–41. A brief summary of the organization and its members can be found at Zhu Ziqiang and Gao Zhanxiang, *Zhongguo wenhua da baike quanshu, jiaoyu juan* [Encyclopedia of Chinese culture, education edition] (Changchun: Changchun chubanshe, 1994), 787, and Zhang Xianwen and Fang Qingqiu, *Zhonghua minguo shi da cidian* [Dictionary of Republican history] (Jiangsu: Jiangsu guji chubanshe, 2001), 330.

66. "Zhongguo xinli weisheng xiehui gongzuo baogao," 41.

67. Lyman, "Psychiatry in China," 771.

68. Chiang, *Social Engineering*, 1.

69. Wen-hsin Yeh, *The Alienated Academy: Culture and Politics in Republican China, 1919–1937* (Cambridge, MA: Harvard University Press, 1990), 169.

70. General information about the academic careers of Chinese psychologists can be found in several sources, including Li Shengping, *Zhongguo jinxiandai renming da cidian* [Biographical dictionary of modern China] (Beijing: Zhongguo guoji guangbo chubanshe, 1989); Zhou Chuan, *Zhongguo jinxiandai gaodeng jiaoyu renwu cidian* [Dictionary of figures in higher education in modern China] (Fujian: Fujian jiaoyu chubanshe, 2012).

71. Sun Zhongshan (Sun Yat-sen), *Xinli jianshe* [Psychological reconstruction] (Chongqing: Hangkong weiyuan hui, 1940), 2, originally published as part of Sun Zhongshan, *Sunwen xueshuo* [Doctrines of Sun Wen] (Shanghai: Minzhi shuzhu, 1925).

72. H. H. Chang, *Chiang Kai-shek: Asia's Man of Destiny* (New York: Doran and Company, 1944), 189–190. See also Jiang Jieshi (Chiang Kai-shek), "Guomin xinli de jianshe" [The psychological reconstruction of the people], in *Jiang Zongtong dui guofu sixiang shijian duxing yu ronghui guantong* [President Chiang's conscientious implementation and comprehensive mastery of Sun Yat-sen thought], ed. Qin Xiaoyi (Taibei: Zhonghua minguo gejie jinian guofu bainian danchen choubei weiyuan hui, 1965), 660–662.

73. Chen Lifu, "Xinli jianshe yu jinhou zhi zhengzhi jianshe" [Psychological reconstruction and future political reconstruction], *Ziqiu* 19 (1930): 35–36.

74. Zhang Shoutao, "Minguo zhongyang daxue danghua jiaoyu yanjiu" [Research into the partification of education at National Central University during the Republican period], *Dang'an yu jianshe* 3 (2015): 56–58; Yeh, *Alienated Academy*, 167–182.

75. *Guoli Zhejiang daxue yaolan* [Guidebook to Zhejiang University] (Hangzhou, 1935), 6.

76. *Guoli Zhejiang daxue bugao* [Zhejiang University bulletin], no. 37 (June 29, 1934): 1953–1954; "Qu Guo xuanyan" [Expel Guo manifesto], *Guoli Zhejiang daxue xiaokan* 24, no. 203

(December 23, 1935). In his unpublished autobiography, Guo confesses that he wanted to "demonstrate to Chiang Kai-shek and his men what should and could be done in higher education." American Philosophical Society Archives (hereafter, APSA), *Confessions of a Chinese Scientist* (1953), chapter 6.

77. Guo Renyuan, *Shehui kexue gailun* [Outline of the social sciences] (Shanghai: Shangwu yinshu guan, 1928), 21–22. I expand on this argument in Emily Baum, "Controlling Minds: Guo Renyuan, Behavioral Psychology, and Fascism in Republican China," *Chinese Historical Review* 22, no. 2 (2015): 141–159.

78. An Kun, *Wei lishi* [Microhistory] (Beijing: Tuanjie chubanshe, 2012), 144.

79. Guo Renyuan, *Xingwei zhuyi xinli xue jiangyi* [Teaching materials on behavioral psychology] (Shanghai: Shangwu yinshu guan, 1928), 128.

80. Li Yuan, *Biantai xinli yu gaizao Zhongguo* [Abnormal psychology and the reformation of China] (Shanghai: Xinsheng shuju, 1932), 3.

81. Ibid., 31.

82. Ibid., 49–57.

83. Pichon P. Y. Loh, "The Ideological Persuasion of Chiang Kai-shek," *Modern Asian Studies* 4, no. 3 (1970): 212–213. This formulation comes from the classical Confucian text *Daxue* (Great learning).

84. Jiang Jieshi (Chiang Kai-shek), "Xin shenghuo yundong gangyao" [Essentials of the New Life Movement], as translated by William Theodore de Bary, *Sources of Chinese Tradition*, vol. 2 (New York: Columbia University Press, 2000), 341–344.

85. Jiang Jieshi, "Guomin xinli de jianshe."

86. Arif Dirlik, "The Ideological Foundations of the New Life Movement," *Journal of Asian Studies* 34, no. 4 (August 1975): 945–980; Lloyd Eastman et al., *The Nationalist Era in China, 1927–1949* (Cambridge: Cambridge University Press, 1991), 31–32.

87. Wei Yulin, "Cong yanjiu jingshen bing tandao jingshen weisheng" [Speaking of mental hygiene from the perspective of psychiatric research], *Weisheng yuekan* 2, nos. 7–8 (1936): 28–31.

88. RAC CMB, Inc., RG IV2B9, Box 97, Folder 697, Richard Lyman to Dai Bingham, January 15, 1935.

89. Wang Wenji, "Yufang, shiying yu gaizao: Minguo shiqi de xinli weisheng" [Prevent, conform, and transform: Republican-era mental hygiene], in *Jiankang yu shehui* [Health and society], ed. Zhu Pingyi (Taibei: Lianjing, 2013), 246–247; Fan Tingwei and Huang Jian, "Ding Zan yu xinli fenxi de yingyong" [Ding Zan and the application of psychoanalysis], *Zhonghua yishi zazhi* 40, no. 5 (2010): 306–310.

90. "Shehui weisheng jiaoyu: Shiji gongzuo" [Social hygiene education: Practical work], *Beiping shi weisheng ju di'er weisheng qu shiwu suo nianbao*, no. 2 (1935): 115–118.

91. Wang Ziming, "Guangbo jiangyan: Jingshen bing yu shehui" [Broadcast speech: Mental illness and society], *Weisheng yuekan* 1, nos. 8–9 (1935): 71–74.

92. On public health and politics, see Rogaski, *Hygienic Modernity*; Lei, *Neither Donkey nor Horse*; Ka-che Yip, *Health and National Reconstruction in Nationalist China: The Development of Modern Health Services, 1929–1937* (Ann Arbor, MI: Association of Asian Studies, 1995).

93. As a point of comparison, Ernst Rüdin (1874–1952), who spoke at the International Congress on Mental Hygiene on the benefits of eugenics, became a loyal advisor to Adolf Hitler prior to the Second World War.

94. Foucault, *History of Sexuality*, 136–142.

95. Baum, "Controlling Minds," 150–151; "Qinghua daxue qu Wu zhenxiang" [Facts of the Expel Wu (Movement) at Qinghua University], *Zhongguo sheying xuehui huabao* 6, no. 297 (1931): 1.

Chapter Seven

1. Lyman, "Psychiatry in China," 770.

2. Wei Yulin, "Duiyu jingshen bingren ying zhuyi de shixiang" [Matters to which attention should be paid regarding the mentally ill], *Weisheng yuekan* 2, no. 1 (1936): 8–10.

3. On the modernist divide between nature and culture, see Bruno Latour, *We Have Never Been Modern* (Cambridge, MA: Harvard University Press, 1993).

4. Andrews, *Making of Modern Chinese Medicine*, 1–2.

5. Lei, *Neither Donkey nor Horse*, 289n2. The prescriptions were published in *Chen bao*, February 21, 1925, 3.

6. Xiaoqun Xu, "National Essence vs. Science: Chinese Native Physicians' Fight for Legitimacy, 1912–1937," *Modern Asian Studies* 31, no. 4 (October 1997): 847–877.

7. Scheid, *Currents of Tradition*, chapter 8; Lei, *Neither Donkey nor Horse*, chapter 4; Andrews, *Making of Modern Chinese Medicine*, 122–133.

8. Yi-Li Wu, "Bodily Knowledge and Western Learning in Late Imperial China: The Case of Wang Shixiong (1808–68)," in *Historical Epistemology and the Making of Modern Chinese Medicine*, 80–112; Andrews, *Making of Modern Chinese Medicine*, 133–136.

9. Zong Zihe, "Shuo nao" [Speaking of the brain], *Dazhong yixue yuekan* 1, no. 7 (1933): 22.

10. Li Jianyi, "Diankuang bing" [Madness], *Zhongyi shijie* 4, no. 24 (1932): 25.

11. In a way, the takeaway of the debate had surprising resonances to Aristotelian beliefs on the heart-brain nexus. Aristotle likewise believed that the heart functioned as the center of cognition, sensation, and movement, yet he also recognized that the brain played an essential, if secondary, role in these processes. See Charles Gross, "Aristotle on the Brain," *Neuroscientist* 1, no. 4 (July 1995): 245–250.

12. Yu Shenchu, "Diankuang bing zhi yanjiu" [Research on madness], *Dazhong yixue yuekan* 1, no. 2 (1933): 14–16.

13. Zong, "Shuo nao," 22–23.

14. Li, "Diankuang bing," 26–27.

15. Ibid.

16. Wang Qiuyuan, "Nao zhi shengli: Xin yu nao zhi yanjiu" [Physiology of the brain: Research on the heart and brain], *Dazhong yixue yuekan* 1, nos. 9–10 (1934): 4–5.

17. Yu, "Diankuang bing zhi yanjiu," 16.

18. Li, "Diankuang bing," 27.

19. Zong, "Shuo nao," 23.

20. Despite his use of this neologism, Wang was arguably envisioning the Chinese medical body rather than the biomedical one. Although he states that thoughts and movements run through the *shenjing*, he also claims that the *shenjing* are "lubricated" by blood, which enables thoughts to move smoothly and not become coagulated or stuck.

21. Wang, "Nao zhi shengli," 5.

22. In her essay on psychiatric translation in the Republican period, Angelika Messner gives other examples of the effort to render the brain and heart "complementary" to one another. Angelika C. Messner, "On 'Translating' Western Psychiatry into the Chinese Context in Republican

China," in *Mapping Meanings: The Field of New Learning in Late Qing China*, ed. Michael Lackner and Natascha Vittinghoff (Leiden: Brill, 2004), 639–658.

23. For a discussion, see Michael Lackner, Iwo Amelung, and Joachim Kurtz, eds., *New Terms for New Ideas: Western Knowledge and Lexical Change in Late Imperial China* (Leiden: Brill, 2001).

24. As Lydia Liu has previously argued, "One does not translate between equivalents; rather, one creates tropes of equivalence in the middle zone of interlinear translation between the host and the guest languages." Lydia Liu, *Translingual Practice: Literature, National Culture, and Translated Modernity* (Stanford, CA: Stanford University Press, 1995), 40.

25. The term would later be revised to *xinli xue* (the study of the principles of the heart-mind). Peng, "Traveling Disease," 102–107.

26. Sean Lei gives a similar description of this phenomenon using the example of *weisheng* (hygiene). Rather than interpreting *weisheng* as "hygienic modernity," as Ruth Rogaski does, Lei argues that it was instead interpreted in the far more mundane way of "maintaining health" or "nurturing life." Sean Hsiang-lin Lei, "Moral Community of *Weisheng*: Contesting Hygiene in Republican China," *East Asian Science, Technology, and Society* 3, no. 4 (2009): 475–504, and "Weisheng weihe bushi baowei shengming? Minguo shiqi de linglei de weisheng, ziwo yu jianbing" [Why weisheng is not about guarding life: Alternative conceptions of hygiene, self, and illness in Republican China], *Taiwan shehui yanjiu jikan* 54 (2004): 17–59.

27. For a deeper synopsis of these terms, see Zhang, *Transforming Emotions with Chinese Medicine*, 36–38.

28. Robert Hans van Gulik, *Sexual Life in Ancient China: A Preliminary Survey of Chinese Sex and Society* (Leiden: Brill, 1961), 145–146.

29. For example, the Confucian philosopher Mencius (372–289 BC) once remarked that *shen* was the "sacred thing that cannot be known." Mengzi, *Jinxin xia* [Exhaust one's heart, part two].

30. For a contemporary definition, see Xie Guan, *Zhongguo yixue da cidian* [Dictionary of Chinese medicine] (Shanghai: Shangwu yinshu guan, 1927).

31. In the doctrine of Five Phases (*wu xing*), which the historian Paul Unschuld describes as a theory of "systematic correspondence" linking material and abstract phenomena, the phase of water is affiliated with the kidneys, while the phase of fire is affiliated with the heart. Paul Unschuld, *Medicine in China: A History of Ideas* (Berkeley: University of California Press, 2010 [1985]), 6.

32. Wei Hongsheng, "Lun jingshen zhi yuan ji gongyong" [On the origins and uses of the *jingshen*], in *Jingshen duanlian zhiliao shiyan wenda*, 1–2.

33. Ibid., 2.

34. Liu, *Translingual Practice*, 40.

35. For another example of the misreading of *jingshen bing*, see Zhou Lichuan, *Jingshen bing guangyi* [The broad meaning of mental illness] (Shanghai: Siming yiyi shuwu, 1931), 2.

36. Yang Huanwen, "Kuangdianxian zhi yanjiu" [Research on kuang, dian, and xian], *Dazhong yixue yuekan* 1, no. 9 (1933): 64–69.

37. "Quanqiu diyi tanmi fengdian wan" [World's number-one mucous confusion and madness pill], *Baihua guoqiang bao*, March 13, 1924.

38. "Zepu renqun mingyi wei rendao jin zhonggao" [Famous doctor of Zepu gives the people advice], *Liangyou huabao*, no. 18 (1927): 15.

39. As quoted in Scull, *Hysteria*, 7.

40. One of the earliest mentions of hysteria that I have seen is in Ju, *Biantai xinli xue jiangyi lu*, 88.

41. The standard term for hysteria, at least according to the 1935 *Psychiatric Terminology Dictionary*, was *yibing*. However, few scholars employed this term in their writings. Most, like Wang, used *xiesideli* or a variant, like *xiesidiya*. Others, like the hypnotist Pang Jing, employed the term *xinfeng* (heart wind), while the aesthetician Zhu Guangqian (1897–1986) used the term *mikuang zheng* (an illness of confused mania). See *Jingshen bing lixue mingci* [Psychiatric terminology dictionary] (Shanghai: Shangwu yinshu guan, 1935), 71; Pang, *Shiyong cuimian shu*, 51; Zhu Guangqian, *Biantai xinli xue* [Abnormal psychology] (Shanghai: Shangwu yinshu guan, 1933), chapter 3.

42. "Furen zabing" [Miscellaneous women's diseases], in *Jingui yaolüe* [Essential prescriptions of the golden cabinet].

43. Wang Runmin, "Zangzao—Xiesideli zhi yanjiu" [Research on zangzao—hysteria], in Zhou, *Jingshen bing guangyi*, 15.

44. Richard Hutchings, *A Psychiatric Word Book* (New York: State Hospitals Press, 1930), 70–71.

45. Scull, *Hysteria*, 30. Andrew Woods discusses cases of male hysteria in "Nervous Diseases of the Chinese," 27; Ida Pruitt also gives an example of male hysteria in "Hospital Social Service," 434.

46. *Yizong jinlan* [Golden mirror of medicine], 1742.

47. Furth, *Flourishing Yin*, 44.

48. Shapiro, "View from a Chinese Asylum," 131.

49. Ibid., 141. The writer Zhao Han'en also observed that most people fall ill with mental illness in the summer due to heat. Zhao, *Jingshen bingxue*, 9.

50. Gu Wenjun, *Shanghai fengdian zhuanmen yiyuan* [Shanghai specialized hospital for the insane] (Shanghai: Fengdian zhuanmen yiyuan faxing, 1934), cases 75, 78, 84, and 87, among others; BMA J181-019-41632.

51. King, "Social Service Department Archives," 345.

52. Wei, *Jingshen duanlian zhiliao shiyan wenda*, 25.

53. Gu, *Zhuanmen yiyuan*, case 48.

54. On "mental overwork," see Pang, *Shiyong cuimian shu*, 51; Ju, *Biantai xinli xue jiangyi lu*, section 23; Liu, *Nao shenjing bing*, 48. On "morbid introspection," see Andrew Woods, "The Incidence of Nervous Diseases in China," *China Medical Journal* 40 (1926): 1070–1082.

55. Woods, "Nervous Diseases of the Chinese," 26–27.

56. Shapiro, "View from a Chinese Asylum," 139.

57. McCartney, "Neuropsychiatry in China," 94.

58. C. C. Kao, T. Ting, and E. H. Hsü, "Content of Thought: A Review of the Mental Status with Special Reference to the Parergastic Reaction-Type," in Lyman, Maeker, and Liang, *Social and Psychological Studies in Neuropsychiatry in China*, 349.

59. Gu, *Zhuanmen yiyuan*, cases 23 and 26.

60. Kleinman, *Patients and Healers in the Context of Culture*, chapter 5; see also Lin, Kleinman, and Lin, "Overview of Mental Disorders in Chinese Cultures," 237–272; Kleinman and Mechanic, "Mental Illness and Psychosocial Aspects of Medical Problems in China," 331–356.

61. Ida Pruitt, "Medical Social Workers: Their Work and Training," *Chinese Medical Journal* 49 (1935): 909–916. See also Pruitt, "Hospital Social Service," 432–443.

62. BMA J181-019-17247, J181-019-38420, J181-019-32378, among others.

63. McCartney, "Neuropsychiatry in China," 89. Charles Selden made a similar observation approximately two decades earlier.

64. BMA J181-019-50667.

65. For example, BMA J183-002-05704, J181-019-35373, J181-019-50667.

66. P. Liang, "Verbal Expressions of Emotion in Chinese," in Lyman, Maeker, and Liang, *Social and Psychological Studies in Neuropsychiatry in China*, 252.

67. Ibid., 254.

68. As another example, the terms for depression in Chinese—*youyu* and *yiyu*—literally translate to "sorrow and stagnation" and "repression and stagnation." As Zhiying Ma has shown, these terms often influence the "symptom phenomenology" of psychiatric patients. Zhiying Ma, "Psychiatric Subjectivity and Cultural Resistance: Experience and Explanations of Schizophrenia in Contemporary China," in *Chinese Modernity and the Individual Psyche*, ed. Andrew Kipnis (New York: Palgrave Macmillan, 2012), 213.

69. Shapiro, "View from a Chinese Asylum," 124–126.

70. For examples of the role that social workers played in this mediating process, see Toh Woo, "An Analysis of 2,330 Case Work Records of the Social Service Department, Peiping Union Medical College," in *Bulletins of the Social Research Department, 1928–1933* (New York: Garland, 1982 [1931]).

71. RAC CMB, Inc., RG IV2B9, Box 96, File 690, Richard Lyman to Roger Greene, May 14, 1934.

72. Ibid. According to Lyman, "No bid is made for patients with psychogenic disorders."

73. Dai Bingham, "The Patient as Person," in Lyman, Maeker, and Liang, *Social and Psychological Studies in Neuropsychiatry in China*, 3–4.

74. RAC CMB, Inc., RG IV2B9, Box 96, Folder 689, Andrew Woods to Franklin McLean, March 24, 1920.

75. Dai, "Patient as Person," 3.

76. Dai Bingham, "Personality Problems in Chinese Culture," *American Sociological Review* 6, no. 5 (October 1941): 688.

77. Ibid., 692. Dai points out that economic pressures were relevant in 26.5 percent of cases for men but only 6.3 percent of cases for women; problems with one's family constituted 32.9 percent of cases for women but only 10.2 percent of cases for men.

78. Lamson, *Social Pathology in China*, 425.

79. Woods, "Nervous Diseases of the Chinese," 26.

80. Song, *Jingshen bing*, 13, 17.

81. Gu, *Zhuanmen yiyuan*, cases 18 and 79.

82. Shapiro, "View from a Chinese Asylum," 143.

83. Hugh Shapiro, "Pathologizing Marriage: Neuropsychiatry and the Escape of Women in Early Twentieth-Century China," in Chiang, *Psychiatry and Chinese History*, 129–142. See also Hugh Shapiro, "Operatic Escapes: Performing Madness in Neuropsychiatric Beijing," in *Science and Technology in Modern China, 1880s–1940s*, ed. Jing Tsu and Benjamin Elman (Leiden: Brill, 2014), 297–326.

84. Song Siming pointed out that some patients so enjoyed their regimented lifestyle within the psychopathic hospital that when it came time for their discharge, they refused to leave. Song, *Jingshen bing*, 44.

85. See chapter 5.

86. Appalachian State University Special Collections (hereafter, ASUSC), George Kriegman, "Bingham Dai and 'Wu-Wei,'" *Academy Forum (American Academy of Psychoanalysis)* 23, no. 3 (Autumn 1979): 12–13.

87. Dai, "Patient as Person," 4–5.

88. Ibid., 5–7.

89. Ibid., 7–18; also ASUSC, Dai Bingham, "Chinese Philosophy of Life," unpublished paper.

90. Kriegman, "Bingham Dai," 13.

91. ASUSC, Dai Bingham, "Zen as a Form of Psychotherapy," unpublished paper.

92. For instance, Peking Union Medical College Nineteenth Annual Report (Peking: Bureau of Engraving and Printing, 1927), 95.

93. ASUSC, Dai Bingham, "*Ren*: A Chinese Ideal of Mental Health," unpublished paper; Dai Bingham, "Being Fully Human: A Chinese Ideal of Mental Health," *Highland Highlights* (1981), 14.

94. Kriegman, "Bingham Dai," 12.

95. Dai, "Patient as Person," 25–26; Dai, "Being Fully Human," 9.

96. Dai, "Being Fully Human," 14.

97. Dai, "Patient as Person," 28.

98. By the 1950s and 1960s, American psychologists like Abraham Maslow (1908–1970), Carl Rogers (1902–1987), and Erich Fromm (1900–1980) were also beginning to integrate Chinese philosophy into their clinical practices. Though perhaps not directly influenced by Dai himself, they appropriated concepts like *wu wei*, *ren*, and *Dao* to create a more "client-centered" approach. Maslow believed that Daoism could enable the patient to "break through the defenses against his own self-knowledge," and Rogers, who traveled through China for a period of six months in 1922, also became inspired by the psychotherapeutic capabilities of meditation and Daoism. See Edmund Hermsen, "Person-Centered Psychology and Taoism: The Reception of Lao-tzu by Carl R. Rogers," *International Journal for the Psychology of Religion* 6, no. 2 (1996): 107–125; Abraham Maslow, *The Farther Reaches of Human Nature* (New York: Viking Press, 1971), 52.

99. RAC CMB, Inc., RG IV2B9, Box 22, Folder 155, W. W. Yen, "Western Medicine in China."

Conclusion

1. RAC CMB, Inc., RG IV2B9, Box 96, File 690, Henry Houghton to Edwin Lobenstine, January 25, 1938, February 10, 1938, and August 9, 1939.

2. BMA J005-001-00530.

3. For a discussion of PUMC physicians during wartime, see Bullock, *American Transplant*, chapter 8.

4. BMA J005-002-00373, J002-006-00247.

5. Fan Tingwei, "Cong shourong dao kexue zhiliao: Wei Yulin yu Beiping jingshen bing liaoyang yuan de chuangjian" [From custody to scientific therapy: Wei Yulin's contribution to the founding of the Peiping Municipal Psychopathic Hospital], *Zhonghua yishi zazhi* 43, no. 6 (November 2013): 345–350.

6. Robin Munro, *Dangerous Minds: Political Psychiatry in China Today and Its Origins in the Mao Era* (New York: Human Rights Watch, 2002), 52.

7. Kriegman, "Bingham Dai," 13. The Francis L. K. Hsü papers are held at the Northwestern University library.

8. Robert Chin and Ai-li Chin, *Psychological Research in Communist China, 1949–1966* (Cambridge, MA: MIT Press, 1969), 21–23; Matthias Petzold, "The Social History of Chinese Psychology," in *Psychology in Twentieth-Century Thought and Society*, ed. Mitchell Ash and William Woodward (Cambridge: Cambridge University Press, 1987), 213–232; Hsuan-Ying Huang, "From Psychotherapy to Psycho-Boom: A Historical Overview of Psychotherapy in China," *Psychoanalysis and Psychotherapy in China* 1 (2015): 1–30.

9. Ruth Sidel, "The Role of Revolutionary Optimism in the Treatment of Mental Illness in the People's Republic of China," *American Journal of Orthopsychiatry* 43, no. 5 (1973): 732–736; Victor Sidel and Ruth Sidel, *Serve the People: Observations on Medicine in the People's Republic of China* (Boston: Beacon Press, 1973), 156–174.

10. Munro, *Dangerous Minds*, 69.

11. An anthropological inquiry into neurasthenia in China can be found in Kleinman, *Social Origins of Distress and Disease*; Sing Lee and Arthur Kleinman, "Are Somatoform Disorders Changing with Time? The Case of Neurasthenia in China," *Psychosomatic Medicine* 69, no. 9 (December 2007): 846–849.

12. In the United States, homosexuality was excised from the Diagnostic and Statistical Manual of Mental Disorders (DSM) in 1973. In China, homosexuality was still considered a mental illness until 2001, when it was removed from the Chinese Psychiatric Association's official list of mental disorders.

13. For a discussion, see Veronica Pearson, "The Development of Psychiatric Services in China: Christianity, Communism, and Community," in *Medical Transitions in Twentieth-Century China*, ed. Bridie Andrews and Mary Bullock (Bloomington: Indiana University Press, 2014), 146–172.

14. Benjamin Schwartz, "Culture, Modernity, and Nationalism: Further Reflections," *Daedalus* 122, no. 3 (Summer 1993): 208.

15. It is difficult to assess the state of mental illness in rural China during this time due to an absence of historical sources. However, judging from anthropological research conducted in the later People's Republic, it is likely that urban psychiatric discourses had not fully infiltrated remote rural areas during the Republican period.

16. Recent work has just begun to explore this theme in colonized regions throughout Asia. For example, Claire Edington, "Going In and Getting Out of the Colonial Asylum: Families and Psychiatric Care in French Indochina," *Comparative Studies in Society and History* 55, no. 3 (2013): 725–755.

17. One such facility was the Mercy Hospital, which opened to the public in 1935. See "Insane in China to Be Aided Soon: Effort to Revolutionize Hospitalization, Civil Code Is Planned," *China Press*, October 20, 1935; "Mental Hospice to Be Opened End of June," *China Press*, June 1, 1935; SMA U1-16-590.

18. Gu Wenjun, "Yuanwu gaiyao shuhou" [Postscript on the essentials of asylum duties], in *Shanghai fengdian zhuanmen yiyuan*, 1–2.

19. For example, one woman whose only child had recently died arrived at the refuge wishing to learn how to pray, while another woman who had gone mad (or perhaps feigned it) prior to being sold into "slavery" remained at the refuge on a long-term basis doing industrial work rather than being returned to her family. Kerr Refuge Annual Report, 1922–1923, 4–5.

20. Selden, "Treatment of the Insane II," 228; Selden, "Work among the Chinese," 8.

21. For an extended treatment of this subject, see Emily Baum, "Choosing Cures for Mental Ills: Psychiatry and Chinese Medicine in Early Twentieth-Century China," *Asian Review of World Histories* 6, no. 1 (January 2018): 8–32.

22. Linda Poon, "They're Invisible in China: Portraits of the Mentally Ill," *NPR*, August 22, 2015.

23. Sharon LaFraniere, "Life in Shadows for Mentally Ill in China," *New York Times*, November 10, 2010.

24. Lotus Yuen, "Unable to Cope: China's Inadequate Care of the Mentally Ill," *Atlantic*, July 29, 2013.

25. Cesar Chelala, "How China Leaves Mental Health Problems Unaddressed," *Globalist*, August 24, 2014.

26. Johan Nylander, "China's Mental Health Care System Is Lacking," *CNN*, May 6, 2014.

27. LaFraniere, "Life in Shadows."

28. Jin Liu et al., "Mental Health System in China: History, Recent Service Reform, and Future Challenges," *World Psychiatry* 10, no. 3 (October 2011): 210–216.

29. For a discussion, see Michael Phillips et al., "China's New Mental Health Law: Reframing Involuntary Treatment," *American Journal of Psychiatry* 170, no. 6 (June 2013): 588–591.

30. "Xinli hexie: shehui hexie de zhongyao neirong" [Psychological harmony: The important substance of social harmony], *Guangming ribao*, October 31, 2005.

31. Doris F. Chang and Arthur Kleinman, "Growing Pains: Mental Health Care in a Developing China," *Yale-China Health Journal* 1, no. 1 (2002): 85–98.

32. Michael Phillips et al., "Prevalence, Treatment, and Associated Disability of Mental Disorders in Four Provinces in China during 2001–05," *Lancet* 373, no. 9680 (2009): 2041–2053.

33. Mao-Sheng Ran et al., *Family-Based Mental Health Care in Rural China* (Hong Kong: Hong Kong University Press, 2005), 27.

34. Ma, "Psychiatric Subjectivity and Cultural Resistance," 203–228.

35. Hsuan-Ying Huang, "The Emergence of the Psycho-Boom in Contemporary Urban China," in Chiang, *Psychiatry and Chinese History*, 183–205.

36. Ian Hacking, *Mad Travelers: Reflections on the Reality of Transient Mental Illnesses* (Charlottesville: University Press of Virginia, 1998), 1.

Bibliography

Archives

Academia Sinica Institute of Modern History Archives (AS)
American Philosophical Society Archives (APSA)
Appalachian State University Special Collections (ASUSC)
Beijing Municipal Archives (BMA)
Bryn Mawr College Archives (BMCA)
Columbia Theological Seminary
National Library of China
Rockefeller Archive Center (RAC)
Shanghai Municipal Archives (SMA)
Shanghai Municipal Library
Yale Divinity School Library

Periodicals

The Atlantic
Baihua guoqiang bao
Beijing baihua bao
Chen bao
China Press
Chinese Repository
The Globalist
Guangming ribao
Huabei yibao
Jingshi jingcha gongbao
Liangyou huabao
Liming bao
The New York Times
North China Herald
Qianshuo riri huabao
Qianshuo riri xinwen huabao

Shehui ribao
Shen bao
Shengjing shibao
Shishi baihua bao
Shishi gongbao
Shishi huabao
Shoudu shizheng gongbao
Wanguo gongbao
Wushen quannian huabao
Zhengfu gongbao
Zhengzhi guanbao

Books and Articles

Abbott, Andrew. *The System of Professions: An Essay on the Division of Expert Labor.* Chicago: University of Chicago Press, 1988.

Adams, Samuel Hopkins. "The Great American Fraud." *Collier's Weekly,* October 7, 1905.

Anderson, Warwick. *Colonial Pathologies: American Tropical Medicine, Race, and Hygiene in the Philippines.* Durham, NC: Duke University Press, 2006.

"Andrew H. Woods, M.D. Obituary." *AMA Archives of Psychology and Neurology* 79, no. 2 (1958): 175–176.

Andrews, Bridie. "Blood in the History of Modern Chinese Medicine." In *Historical Epistemology and the Making of Modern Chinese Medicine,* edited by Howard Chiang, 113–136. Manchester: Manchester University Press, 2015.

———. *The Making of Modern Chinese Medicine, 1850–1960.* Honolulu: University of Hawaii Press, 2014.

Andrews, Jonathan, and Andrew Scull. *Customers and Patrons of the Mad Trade: The Management of Lunacy in Eighteenth-Century London.* Berkeley: University of California Press, 2003.

An Kun. *Wei lishi* [Microhistory]. Beijing: Tuanjie chubanshe, 2012.

Arnold, David. *Colonizing the Body: State Medicine and Epidemic Disease in Nineteenth-Century India.* Berkeley: University of California Press, 1993.

Bartlett, Peter. *The Poor Law of Lunacy: The Administration of Pauper Lunatics in Mid-Nineteenth Century England.* London: Leicester University Press, 1999.

Baum, Emily. "Choosing Cures for Mental Ills: Psychiatry and Chinese Medicine in Early Twentieth-Century China." *Asian Review of World Histories* 6, no. 1 (January 2018): 8–32.

———. "Controlling Minds: Guo Renyuan, Behavioral Psychology, and Fascism in Republican China." *Chinese Historical Review* 22, no. 2 (2015): 141–159.

———. "Health by the Bottle: The Dr. Williams' Medicine Company and the Commodification of Well-Being in the *Liangyou* Pictorial." In *Liangyou: Kaleidoscopic Modernity and the Shanghai Global Metropolis,* edited by Paul Pickowicz, Shen Kuiyi, and Zhang Yingjin, 71–93. Leiden: Brill, 2013.

Beard, George. *American Nervousness: Its Causes and Consequences.* New York: Putnam, 1881.

———. "Neurasthenia, or Nervous Exhaustion." *Boston Medical and Surgical Journal* 3, no. 18 (April 29, 1869): 217–221.

Beers, Clifford. *The Mental Hygiene Movement: Origin and Growth.* Norwood, MA: Plimpton Press, 1917.

———. *A Mind That Found Itself.* New York: Longmans, Green, 1908.

Beijing Ministry of Justice. "Sifa bu ling faguan duiyu jingshen bingren zhi fanzui wuyi diaocha queshi zhengju wen" [Ministry of Justice orders the courts that the crimes of the mentally ill should be investigated with reliable evidence]. *Zhengfu gongbao fenlei hui*, no. 15 (1915): 49.

———. "Sifa bu ling xuangao sixing fan ru li jingshen bing huo yunfu jun ying tingzhi zhixing wen" [Ministry of Justice orders that if a criminal suffers from mental illness or pregnancy they should not be executed]. *Zhengfu gongbao fenlei hui*, no. 15 (1915): 48–49.

———. "Xingfa cao'an" [Penal code draft]. *Zhengfu gongbao.* Beijing: n.p., 1912.

Beiping Hongren Tang. "Beiping Hongren Tang lejia lao yaopu wansan gaodan jiamu" [Beiping Hongren Tang happy family apothecary medication price guide]. Beiping: Hongren Tang, 1935.

Beiping lüxing zhinan [Beiping travel guide]. Beiping: Shibao yingye bu faxing, 1935.

Beiping Ministry of Health, ed. *Beiping shi zhengfu weisheng chu yewu baogao* [Report on tasks administered by the Beiping municipal department of health]. Beiping: Beiping shi zhengfu weisheng ju, 1934.

———. *Beiping shi zhengfu weisheng ju yewu baogao* [Report on tasks administered by the Beiping municipal ministry of health]. Beiping: Beiping shi zhengfu weisheng ju, 1935.

"Beiping shi weisheng ju ershisi nian er yuefen jingshen bing liaoyang yuan zhencha bingren cishu yuebao biao" [Monthly report on patient examinations at the Beiping Psychopathic Hospital for February 1935]. *Beiping shi shizheng gongbao*, no. 299 (1935): 1.

"Beiping shi weisheng ju jingshen bing liaoyang yuan zhuyuan guize" [Regulations on being admitted to the Beiping municipal psychopathic hospital]. *Beiping shi shizheng gongbao*, no. 264 (August 24, 1934): 9–11.

Benedict, Carol. *Bubonic Plague in Nineteenth-Century China.* Stanford, CA: Stanford University Press, 1996.

Bennett, James W. "Pills of Ten Thousand Efficacies." *Asia: Journal of the American Asiatic Association* 30 (September 1930): 616–621.

Bergère, Marie-Claire. *Sun Yat-sen.* Translated by Janet Lloyd. Stanford, CA: Stanford University Press, 1998.

"Berlin International Congress." *British Journal of Psychiatry* 56, no. 233 (April 1910): 385.

Blowers, Geoffrey. "La psychoanalyse en Chine avant 1949: le rejet ou la distortion" [Psychoanalysis in China before 1949: Rejection or distortion]. *Perspectives chinoises* 39 (1997): 33–39.

———. "The Origins of Scientific Psychology in China, 1898–1949." In *Internationalizing the History of Psychology*, edited by Adrian Brock, 94–111. New York: New York University Press, 2006.

Blowers, Geoffrey, and Shelley Wang Xuelai. "Gone with the West Wind: The Emergence and Disappearance of Psychotherapeutic Culture in China, 1936–68." In Chiang, *Psychiatry and Chinese History*, 143–160.

Botsman, Daniel. *Punishment and Power in the Making of Modern Japan.* Princeton, NJ: Princeton University Press, 2005.

Braslow, Joel. *Mental Ills and Bodily Cures: Psychiatric Treatment in the First Half of the Twentieth Century.* Berkeley: University of California Press, 1997.

Brown, Edward. "Neurology's Influence on American Psychiatry, 1865–1915." In Wallace and Gach, *History of Psychiatry and Medical Psychology*, 519–532.

Bruinius, Harry. *Better for All the World: The Secret History of Forced Sterilization and America's Quest for Racial Purity.* New York: Random House, 2006.

Bu, Liping. "Social Darwinism, Public Health, and Modernization in China, 1895–1925." In *Uneasy Encounters: The Politics of Medicine and Health in China, 1900–1937*, edited by Iris Borowy, 93–124. New York: Peter Lang, 2009.

Buck, Peter. *American Science and Modern China, 1876–1936*. Cambridge: Cambridge University Press, 1980.

Bullock, Mary Brown. *An American Transplant: The Rockefeller Foundation and Peking Union Medical College*. Berkeley: University of California Press, 1980.

Burns, Susan. "Constructing the National Body: Public Health and the Nation in Nineteenth-Century Japan." In *Nation Work: Asian Elites and National Identities*, edited by Timothy Brook and Andre Schmid, 17–50. Ann Arbor: University of Michigan Press, 2000.

———. "Contemplating Places: The Hospital as Modern Experience in Meiji Japan." In *New Directions in the Study of Meiji Japan*, edited by Helen Hardacre and Adam L. Kern, 702–718. Leiden: Brill, 1997.

Canaday, Margot. *The Straight State: Sexuality and Citizenship in Twentieth-Century America*. Princeton, NJ: Princeton University Press, 2009.

Cassell, Eric. "Illness and Disease." *Hastings Center Report* 6, no. 2 (April 1976): 27–37.

Certeau, Michel de. *The Practice of Everyday Life*. Vol. 1. Berkeley: University of California Press, 1984.

Chang, Doris F., and Arthur Kleinman. "Growing Pains: Mental Health Care in a Developing China." *Yale-China Health Journal* 1, no. 1 (2002): 85–98.

Chang, H. H. *Chiang Kai-shek: Asia's Man of Destiny*. New York: Doran and Company, 1944.

Chao, W. H., Y. K. Hsu, and R. S. Lyman. "Comments on the Treatment of Drug Addiction with Protracted Narcosis." *Journal of Nervous and Mental Disease* 87, no. 4 (April 1938): 454–463.

Chen Daqi. *Xinli xue dagang* [Outline of psychology]. Beijing: Beijing daxue, 1918.

Chen, Hsiu-fen. "Articulating 'Chinese Madness.'" Paper presented at the first annual Asian Society for the History of Medicine meeting, 2003.

———. "Dang bingren jiandao gui: shilun Ming-Qing yizhe duiyu 'xiesui' de taidu" [The patient sees a ghost: The attitude of Ming-Qing physicians on evil spirits]. In *Zongjiao yu yiliao* [Religion and medicine], edited by Lin Fushi, 329–364. Taibei: Lianjing, 2011.

———. "Emotional Therapy and Talking Cures in Late Imperial China." In Chiang, *Psychiatry and Chinese History*, 37–54.

———. "Medicine, Society, and the Making of Madness in Imperial China." PhD diss., University of London, 2003.

Chen, Janet. *Guilty of Indigence: The Urban Poor in China, 1900–1953*. Princeton, NJ: Princeton University Press, 2012.

Chen Lifu. "Xinli jianshe yu jinhou zhi zhengzhi jianshe" [Psychological reconstruction and future political reconstruction]. *Ziqiu*, no. 19 (1930): 35–36.

Chen Wanli. "Jingshen bing shi shenme?" [What is mental illness?]. *Tongsu yishi yuekan*, no. 2 (1919): 16–20.

Chen Zhongquan. "Diankuang zhi fenxi yanjiu" [Research into the difference between dian and kuang]. *Zhongyi shijie* 2, no. 11 (1931): 34–35.

Cheyne, George. *The English Malady*. London: Strahan, 1733.

Chiang, Howard, ed. *Psychiatry and Chinese History*. London: Pickering & Chatto, 2014.

Chiang, Yung-chen. *Social Engineering and the Social Sciences in China, 1919–1949*. Cambridge: Cambridge University Press, 2001.

Chin, Robert, and Ai-li Chin. *Psychological Research in Communist China, 1949–1966*. Cambridge, MA: MIT Press, 1969.

"China as a Field for Research in Nervous Diseases." *China Medical Missionary Journal* 3, no. 4 (December 1889): 167–168.

Chiu, Martha Li. "Mind, Body, and Illness in a Chinese Medical Tradition." PhD diss., Harvard University, 1986.

Chou, L. C. and Y. C. Lu, "A Sociological Study of Chinese Mental Patients." In Lyman, Maeker, and Liang, *Social and Psychological Studies in Neuropsychiatry in China*, 31–116.

Chow, Tse-tung. *The May Fourth Movement: Intellectual Revolution in Modern China*. Cambridge, MA: Harvard University Press, 1960.

Cochran, Sherman. *Chinese Medicine Men: Consumer Culture in China and Southeast Asia*. Cambridge, MA: Harvard University Press, 2006.

———. "Marketing Medicine and Advertising Dreams in Shanghai, 1900–1940." In Yeh, *Becoming Chinese: Passages to Modernity and Beyond*, 62–97.

Cohen, Paul. *History in Three Keys: The Boxers as Event, Experience, and Myth*. New York: Columbia University Press, 1997.

Corrigan, Patrick, Kristin Kosyluk, J. Konadu Fokuo, and Jin Hee Park. "How Does Direct to Consumer Advertising Affect the Stigma of Mental Illness?" *Community Mental Health Journal* 50, no. 7 (2014): 792–799.

Croizier, Ralph. *Traditional Medicine in Modern China: Science, Nationalism, and the Tensions of Cultural Change*. Cambridge, MA: Harvard University Press, 1968.

Dai Bingham. "Being Fully Human: A Chinese Ideal of Mental Health." *Highland Highlights*, 1981.

———. "The Patient as Person." In Lyman, Maeker, and Liang, *Social and Psychological Studies in Neuropsychiatry in China*, 1–30.

———. "Personality Problems in Chinese Culture." *American Sociological Review* 6, no. 5 (October 1941): 688–696.

Dain, Norman. *Clifford W. Beers: Advocate for the Insane*. Pittsburgh, PA: University of Pittsburgh Press, 1980.

Da Qing fagui daquan, falü bu [Comprehensive collection of the laws and regulations of the Great Qing, section on laws]. Taibei: Kaozheng chubanshe, 1972.

"Da Yingguo: Shouyang fengdian" [Great Britain: Care of the insane]. *Wanguo gongbao*, no. 611 (1880): 17.

De Bary, William Theodore. *Sources of Chinese Tradition*. Vol. 2. New York: Columbia University Press, 2000.

Deutsch, Albert. *The Mentally Ill in America: A History of Their Care and Treatment from Colonial Times*. New York: Doubleday, 1937.

Diamant, Neil. "China's 'Great Confinement'? Missionaries, Municipal Elites, and Police in the Establishment of Chinese Mental Hospitals." *Republican China* 19, no. 1 (November 1994): 3–50.

Digby, Anne. *Madness, Morality, and Medicine: A Study of the York Retreat, 1796–1914*. Cambridge: Cambridge University Press, 1985.

Dikötter, Frank. *Crime, Punishment, and the Prison in Modern China*. New York: Columbia University Press, 2002.

Ding Ganren. *Ding Ganren yi'an* [Medical cases of Ding Ganren]. Shanxi: Shanxi kexue jishu chubanshe, 2013.

Ding Rui. *Guanli Beijing: Beiyang zhengfu shiqi jingshi jingcha ting yanjiu* [Governing Beijing: Research into the municipal police during the era of the Beiyang government]. Shanxi: Shanxi jingli chubanshe, 2013.

Dirlik, Arif. "The Ideological Foundations of the New Life Movement." *Journal of Asian Studies* 34, no. 4 (August 1975): 945–980.

Dong, Madeleine Yue. "Defining Beiping: Urban Reconstruction and National Identity, 1928–1936." In Esherick, *Remaking the Chinese City*, 121–138.

———. "Juggling Bits: Tianqiao as Republican Beijing's Recycling Center." *Modern China* 25, no. 3 (July 1999): 303–342.

———. *Republican Beijing: The City and Its Histories*. Berkeley: University of California Press, 2003.

Dong, Madeleine Yue, and Joshua Goldstein, eds. *Everyday Modernity in China*. Seattle: University of Washington Press, 2006.

Dowbiggin, Ian. *Keeping America Sane: Psychiatry and Eugenics in the United States and Canada, 1880–1940*. Ithaca, NY: Cornell University Press, 1997.

———. *The Sterilization Movement and Global Fertility in the Twentieth Century*. Oxford: Oxford University Press, 2008.

Dutton, Michael. *Policing and Punishment in China*. Cambridge: Cambridge University Press, 1992.

Eastman, Lloyd. *The Abortive Revolution: China under Nationalist Rule, 1927–1937*. Cambridge, MA: Harvard University Press, 1990.

Eastman, Lloyd, Jerome Ch'en, Suzanne Pepper, and Lyman Van Slyke. *The Nationalist Era in China, 1927–1949*. Cambridge: Cambridge University Press, 1991.

Edington, Claire. "Going In and Getting Out of the Colonial Asylum: Families and Psychiatric Care in French Indochina." *Comparative Studies in Society and History* 55, no. 3 (2013): 725–755.

"Editorial." *China Medical Journal* 34 (1920): 50.

Elliott, Richard. "Making Up People: Consumption as a Symbolic Vocabulary for the Construction of Identity." In *Elusive Consumption*, edited by Karin Ekstrom and Helene Brembeck, 129–144. Oxford: Berg, 2004.

Elman, Benjamin. *A Cultural History of Civil Examinations in Late Imperial China*. Berkeley: University of California Press, 2000.

Ennis, Bruce J., and Thomas R. Litwack. "Psychiatry and the Presumption of Expertise: Flipping Coins in the Courtroom." *California Law Review* 62, no. 3 (May 1974): 693–752.

Eraso, Yolanda. "A Burden to the State: The Reception of the German 'Active Therapy' in an Argentinean 'Colony-Asylum' in the 1920s and 1930s." In Ernst and Mueller, *Transnational Psychiatries*, 51–79.

Ernst, Waltraud. *Mad Tales from the Raj: Colonial Psychiatry in South Asia, 1800–1858*. New York: Anthem, 2010.

Ernst, Waltraud, and Thomas Mueller, eds. *Transnational Psychiatries: Social and Cultural Histories of Psychiatry in Comparative Perspective, 1800–2000*. Newcastle upon Tyne: Cambridge Scholars Publishing, 2010.

Esherick, Joseph, ed. *Remaking the Chinese City: Modernity and National Identity, 1900–1950*. Honolulu: University of Hawaii Press, 1999.

Ewen, Stuart. *Captains of Consciousness: Advertising and the Social Roots of the Consumer Culture*. New York: McGraw Hill, 2001 [1976].

Fanon, Frantz. *The Wretched of the Earth.* New York: Grove Press, 1963 [1961].

Fan Tingwei. "Cong shourong dao kexue zhiliao: Wei Yulin yu Beiping jingshen bing liaoyang yuan de chuangjian" [From custody to scientific therapy: Wei Yulin's contribution to the founding of the Peiping Municipal Psychopathic Hospital]. *Zhonghua yishi zazhi* 43, no. 6 (November 2013): 345–350.

Fan Tingwei and Huang Jian. "Ding Zan yu xinli fenxi de yingyong" [Ding Zan and the application of psychoanalysis]. *Zhonghua yishi zazhi* 40, no. 5 (2010): 306–310.

Feder, Lillian. *Madness in Literature.* Princeton, NJ: Princeton University Press, 1980.

Fitzgerald, John. *Awakening China: Politics, Culture, and Class in the National Revolution.* Stanford, CA: Stanford University Press, 1996.

Flath, James. "Temple Fairs and the Republican State in North China." *Twentieth-Century China* 30, no. 1 (November 2004): 39–63.

Fortune, Robert. *Yedo and Peking.* London: J. Murray, 1863.

Foucault, Michel. *The History of Sexuality.* Vol. 1. New York: Vintage Books, 1990 [1978].

———. *Madness and Civilization.* New York: Random House, 1965.

———. *Power/Knowledge.* New York: Pantheon Books, 1972.

Fung, Edmund. *The Intellectual Foundations of Chinese Modernity: Cultural and Political Thought in the Republican Era.* Cambridge: Cambridge University Press, 2010.

Furth, Charlotte. *A Flourishing Yin: Gender in China's Medical History, 960–1665.* Berkeley: University of California Press, 1999.

Furukawa Hisashi. *Sōseki no shokan* [Sōseki's letters]. Tokyo: Tōkyōdō shuppan, 1970.

Gach, John. "Biological Psychiatry in the Nineteenth and Twentieth Centuries." In Wallace and Gach, *History of Psychiatry and Medical Psychology,* 380–412.

Gamble, Sidney. *How Chinese Families Live in Peiping.* New York: Funk & Wagnalls, 1933.

———. *Peking: A Social Survey.* New York: George H. Doran Company, 1921.

Gamwell, Lynn, and Nancy Tomes. *Madness in America: Cultural and Medical Perceptions of Mental Illness before 1914.* Ithaca, NY: Cornell University Press, 1995.

Gao Juefu. *Zhongguo xinli xue shi* [History of Chinese psychology]. Beijing: Renmin jiaoyu chubanshe, 1985.

Gernet, Jacques. *A History of Chinese Civilization.* Cambridge: Cambridge University Press, 1982.

Gerth, Karl. *China Made: Consumer Culture and the Creation of the Nation.* Cambridge, MA: Harvard University Press, 2003.

Gill, Leslie. *Advertising and Psychology.* London: Routledge, 2013 [1954].

Gilmartin, Christina. *Engendering the Chinese Revolution: Radical Women, Communist Politics, and Mass Movements in the 1920s.* Berkeley: University of California Press, 1995.

Goffman, Erving. *Asylums: Essays on the Social Situation of Mental Patients and Other Inmates.* Chicago: Aldine, 1961.

Goldstein, Jan. *Console and Classify: The French Psychiatric Profession in the Nineteenth Century.* Cambridge: Cambridge University Press, 1987.

Good, Byron. *Medicine, Rationality, and Experience: An Anthropological Perspective.* Cambridge: Cambridge University Press, 1994.

Greenfield, Liah. *Mind, Modernity, Madness: The Impact of Culture on Human Experience.* Cambridge, MA: Harvard University Press, 2013.

Grob, Gerald. *Mental Illness and American Society, 1875–1940.* Princeton, NJ: Princeton University Press, 1983.

———. *Mental Institutions in America: Social Policy to 1875.* New York: Free Press, 1972.

Gross, Charles. "Aristotle on the Brain." *Neuroscientist* 1, no. 4 (July 1995): 245–250.

Gui Zhiliang. *Xiandai jingshen bingxue* [Modern psychiatry]. Shanghai: Xinyue shudian, 1932.

Guoli Zhejiang daxue bugao [Zhejiang University bulletin], no. 37 (June 29, 1934): 1953–54.

Guoli Zhejiang daxue yaolan [Guidebook to Zhejiang University]. Hangzhou, 1935.

Guo Renyuan. *Shehui kexue gailun* [Outline of the social sciences]. Shanghai: Shangwu yinshu guan, 1928.

———. *Xingwei zhuyi xinli xue jiangyi* [Teaching materials on behavioral psychology]. Shanghai: Shangwu yinshu guan, 1928.

———. *Xinli xue ABC* [The ABCs of psychology]. Shanghai: Shijie shuju, 1928.

Gu Wenjun. *Shanghai fengdian zhuanmen yiyuan* [Shanghai specialized hospital for the insane]. Shanghai: Fengdian zhuanmen yiyuan faxing, 1934.

Hacking, Ian. *Mad Travelers: Reflections on the Reality of Transient Mental Illnesses*. Charlottesville: University Press of Virginia, 1998.

Hashimoto, Akira. "The Invention of a 'Japanese Gheel': Psychiatric Family Care from a Historical and Transnational Perspective." In Ernst and Mueller, *Transnational Psychiatries*, 142–171.

Healy, David. *The Antidepressant Era*. Cambridge, MA: Harvard University Press, 1997.

Heinrich, Ari. *The Afterlife of Images: Translating the Pathological Body between China and the West*. Durham, NC: Duke University Press, 2008.

Helman, Cecil. "Disease versus Illness in General Practice." *Journal of the Royal College of Medical Practitioners* 31 (September 1981): 548–552.

Hermsen, Edmund. "Person-Centered Psychology and Taoism: The Reception of Lao-tzu by Carl R. Rogers." *International Journal for the Psychology of Religion* 6, no. 2 (1996): 107–125.

Hershatter, Gail. *Dangerous Pleasures: Prostitution and Modernity in Twentieth-Century Shanghai*. Berkeley: University of California Press, 1997.

Higgins, Louise, and Mo Zheng. "An Introduction to Chinese Psychology: Its Historical Roots until the Present Day." *Journal of Psychology* 136, no. 2 (2002): 225–239.

Hinrichs, T. J., and Linda Barnes. *Chinese Medicine and Healing*. Cambridge, MA: Harvard University Press, 2013.

Hobsbawm, Eric. "Peasants and Politics." *Journal of Peasant Studies* 1, no. 1 (1973): 3–22.

Hofmann, J. A. "A Report of the Patients Discharged from the John G. Kerr Hospital for Insane during 1912." *China Medical Journal* 27 (1913): 369–379.

Horiguchi, Sachiko. "Mental Health and Therapy in Japan." In *Critical Issues in Contemporary Japan*, edited by Jeff Kingston, 223–234. London: Routledge, 2014.

"Hospital Reports." *China Medical Missionary Journal* 37, no. 11 (November 1923): 953–955.

Hsu, Elisabeth. *The Transmission of Chinese Medicine*. Cambridge: Cambridge University Press, 1999.

Hsü, Francis L. K. "A Brief Report on the Police Cooperation in Connection with Mental Cases in Peiping." In Lyman, Maeker, and Liang, *Social and Psychological Studies in Neuropsychiatry in China*, 199–230.

Huang, Hsuan-Ying. "The Emergence of the Psycho-Boom in Contemporary Urban China." In Chiang, *Psychiatry and Chinese History*, 183–205.

———. "From Psychotherapy to Psycho-Boom: A Historical Overview of Psychotherapy in China." *Psychoanalysis and Psychotherapy in China* 1 (2015): 1–30.

Huang Junbo, ed. *Zui zhong zui: Qingmo minchu qi'an jishi* [Crimes within crimes: A collection of strange cases from the end of the Qing dynasty]. Beijing: Huaxia chubanshe, 2012.

Huang, Max K. W. "Medical Advertising and Cultural Translation: The Case of *Shenbao* in Early Twentieth-Century China." In *Print, Profit, and Perception: Ideas, Information, and Knowledge in Chinese Societies, 1895–1949*, edited by Pei-yin Lin and Weipin Tsai, 114–147. Leiden: Brill, 2014.

Huang Pandong. "Shili jingshen bing liaoyang yuan zhi shilüe ji jinkuang" [Brief history and current situation of the municipal psychopathic hospital]. *Guangzhou weisheng*, no. 2 (1936): 105–106.

Huang Weirong. *Biantai xinli xue ABC* [The ABCs of abnormal psychology]. Shanghai: Shijie shuju, 1929.

Hua Zhi'an. "Youdai diankuang" [Giving preferential treatment to the insane]. *Wanguo gongbao*, no. 640 (1881): 5–8.

Hutchings, Richard. *A Psychiatric Word Book*. New York: State Hospitals Press, 1930.

Ingram, J. H. "The Pitiable Condition of the Insane in North China." *China Medical Journal* 32, no. 2 (March 1918): 153–154.

Ishikawa Hanzan. *Shinkei suijaku oyobi sono kaifuku* [Neurasthenia and its recovery]. Tokyo: Kōgakukai, 1909.

Jenkins, Janis. *Extraordinary Conditions: Culture and Experience in Mental Illness*. Berkeley: University of California Press, 2015.

Jiang Jieshi (Chiang Kai-shek). "Guomin xinli de jianshe" [The psychological reconstruction of the people]. In *Jiang Zongtong dui guofu sixiang shijian duxing yu ronghui guantong* [President Chiang's conscientious implementation and comprehensive mastery of Sun Yat-sen thought], edited by Qin Xiaoyi, 660–662. Taibei: Zhonghua minguo gejie jinian guofu bainian danchen choubei weiyuan hui, 1965.

Jian Hu. "Pinglun: Guomin zhi jingshen bing" [Critique: The people's mental illness]. *Dongfang zazhi* 18, no. 4 (1921): 1–3.

"Jiaoyu wenhua xiaoxi: Zhongguo xinli weisheng xiehui chengli" [News on education and culture: Establishment of the Chinese Mental Hygiene Association]. *Jiao yu xue* 1, no. 12 (1936): 286.

"Jieban jingshen bing liaoyang yuan" [Taking over the psychopathic hospital]. *Shizheng pinglun*, no. 1–2 (1935).

Jingshen bing lixue mingci [Psychiatric terminology dictionary]. Shanghai: Shangwu yinshu guan, 1935.

John G. Kerr Refuge for the Insane. Annual Reports.

Ju Zhongzhou. *Biantai xinli xue jiangyi lu* [Teaching materials on abnormal psychology]. Beijing: Zhonghua biantai xinli xue hui, 1923.

Kao, C. C., T. Ting, and E. H. Hsu. "Content of Thought: A Review of the Mental Status with Special Reference to the Parergastic Reaction-Type." In Lyman, Maeker, and Liang, *Social and Psychological Studies in Neuropsychiatry in China*, 341–370.

Kao, John J. *Three Millennia of Chinese Psychiatry*. New York: Institute for Advanced Research in Asian Medicine, 1979.

Keller, Richard. *Colonial Madness: Psychiatry in French North Africa*. Chicago: University of Chicago Press, 2007.

Kellogg, John Harvey. *Neurasthenia, or Nervous Exhaustion*. Battle Creek, MI: Good Health Publishing, 1915.

Kerr, J. G. "The 'Refuge for the Insane,' Canton." *China Medical Missionary Journal* 12, no. 4 (December 1898): 176–179.

Kiely, Jan. *The Compelling Ideal: Thought Reform and the Prison in China, 1901–1956*. New Haven, CT: Yale University Press, 2014.

King, M. Marjorie. "The Social Service Department Archives: Peking Union Medical College, 1928–1951." *American Archivist* 59 (Summer 1996): 340–349.

Kirkpatrick, Edwin. *Mental Hygiene for Effective Living*. New York: D. Appleton-Century, 1934.

Kisch, Egon Erwin. *Secret China*. London: Butler & Tanner, 1935 [1933].

Kitanaka, Junko. *Depression in Japan: Psychiatric Cures for a Society in Distress*. Princeton, NJ: Princeton University Press, 2012.

Kitanishi, Kenji, and Kyoichi Kondo. "The Rise and Fall of Neurasthenia in Japanese Psychiatry." *Transcultural Psychiatric Research Review* 31, no. 2 (1994): 137–152.

Kleinman, Arthur. *The Illness Narratives: Suffering, Healing, and the Human Condition*. New York: Basic Books, 1988.

———. *Patients and Healers in the Context of Culture*. Berkeley: University of California Press, 1980.

———. *Rethinking Psychiatry: From Cultural Category to Personal Experience*. New York: Free Press, 1988.

———. *Social Origins of Distress and Disease: Depression, Neurasthenia, and Pain in Modern China*. New Haven, CT: Yale University Press, 1988.

Kleinman, Arthur, and Tsung-Yi Lin, eds. *Normal and Abnormal Behavior in Chinese Culture*. Boston: D. Reidel Publishing, 1981.

Kleinman, Arthur, and David Mechanic. "Mental Illness and Psychosocial Aspects of Medical Problems in China." In Kleinman and Lin, *Normal and Abnormal Behavior in Chinese Culture*, 331–356.

Kriegman, George. "Bingham Dai and 'Wu-Wei.'" *Academy Forum (American Academy of Psychoanalysis)* 23, no. 3 (Autumn 1979): 12–13.

Kuhn, Philip. *Soulstealers: The Chinese Sorcery Scare of 1768*. Cambridge, MA: Harvard University Press, 1990.

Kuriyama, Shigehisa. *The Expressiveness of the Body and the Divergence of Greek and Chinese Medicine*. New York: Zone Books, 1999.

Kwok, D. W. Y. *Scientism in Chinese Thought, 1900–1950*. New Haven, CT: Yale University Press, 1965.

Lackner, Michael, Iwo Amelung, and Joachim Kurtz, eds. *New Terms for New Ideas: Western Knowledge and Lexical Change in Late Imperial China*. Leiden: Brill, 2001.

Lamb, S. D. *Pathologist of the Mind: Adolf Meyer and the Origins of American Psychiatry*. Baltimore: Johns Hopkins University Press, 2014.

Lamson, Herbert Day. *Social Pathology in China: A Source Book for the Study of Problems of Livelihood, Health, and the Family*. Shanghai: Commercial Press, 1935.

Lao She. *Luotuo Xiangzi* [Camel Xiangzi]. In *Yuzhou feng* [Cosmic wind], vols. 25–48 (1936–1937).

———. "Xisheng" [Sacrifice]. In *Yinghai ji* [Cherries and the sea]. Shanghai: Renjian shuwu, 1935.

La Rue, Daniel Wolford. *Mental Hygiene*. New York: Macmillan Company, 1932.

Latour, Bruno. *We Have Never Been Modern*. Cambridge, MA: Harvard University Press, 1993.

Lean, Eugenia. "The Modern Elixir: Medicine as Consumer Item in the Early Twentieth-Century Chinese Press." *UCLA Historical Journal* 15 (1995): 65–92.

———. *Public Passions: The Trial of Shi Jianqiao and the Rise of Popular Sympathy in Republican China*. Berkeley: University of California Press, 2007.

Lee, Leo Ou-fan. *Shanghai Modern: The Flowering of a New Urban Culture in China, 1930–1945*. Cambridge, MA: Harvard University Press, 1999.

Lee, Sing, and Arthur Kleinman. "Are Somatoform Disorders Changing with Time? The Case of Neurasthenia in China." *Psychosomatic Medicine* 69, no. 9 (December 2007): 846–849.

Lei, Sean Hsiang-lin. "Moral Community of *Weisheng*: Contesting Hygiene in Republican China." *East Asian Science, Technology, and Society* 3, no. 4 (2009): 475–504.

———. *Neither Donkey nor Horse: Medicine in the Struggle over China's Modernity*. Chicago: University of Chicago Press, 2014.

———. "Weisheng weihe bushi baowei shengming? Minguo shiqi de linglei de weisheng, ziwo yu jianbing" [Why weisheng is not about guarding life: Alternative conceptions of hygiene, self, and illness in Republican China]. *Taiwan shehui yanjiu jikan* 54 (2004): 17–59.

Leiss, William, Stephen Kline, and Sut Jhally. *Social Communication in Advertising: Persons, Products, and Images of Well-Being*. London: Routledge, 1997.

Li Jianyi. "Diankuang bing" [Madness]. *Zhongyi shijie* 4, no. 24 (1932): 25–27.

Li Jinghan. "Beiping zuidi xiandu di shenghuo chengdu di taolun" [Discussion of the lowest standard of living in Beiping]. *Shehui xue jie*, no. 3 (September 1929): 1–16.

Li, Lillian. *Fighting Famine in North China: State, Market, and Environmental Decline, 1690s–1990s*. Stanford, CA: Stanford University Press, 2007.

Li, Lillian, Alison Dray-Novey, and Haili Kong. *Beijing: From Imperial Capital to Olympic City*. New York: Palgrave Macmillan, 2007.

Li Shengping. *Zhongguo jinxiandai renming da cidian* [Biographical dictionary of modern China]. Beijing: Zhongguo guoji guangbo chubanshe, 1989.

Li, Wenjing, and Heinz-Peter Schmiedebach. "German Wine in an American Bottle: The Spread of Modern Psychiatry in China, 1898–1949." *History of Psychiatry* 26, no. 3 (2015): 348–358.

Li Xiaowei, ed. *Xin Zhongguo jianli chuqi de shehui jiuzhu yanjiu* [Research into charitable works in the early years of new China]. Beijing: Shehui kexue wenxian chubanshe, 2012.

Li Yuan. *Biantai xinli yu gaizao Zhongguo* [Abnormal psychology and the reformation of China]. Shanghai: Xinsheng shuju, 1932.

Liang, P. "Verbal Expressions of Emotion in Chinese." In Lyman, Maeker, and Liang, *Social and Psychological Studies in Neuropsychiatry in China*, 249–258.

Liang Qichao. "Fojiao xinli xue ceyan" [Putting Buddhist psychology to the test]. *Xinli zazhi xuancun*, July 3, 1923.

Liao Qichong. "Wode shenjing shuairuo bing yuhou de shuohua" [My testimony on having recovered from neurasthenia]. *Dazhong yikan*, no. 13 (1931): 54.

Lin, Keh-Ming. "Traditional Chinese Medical Beliefs and Their Relevance for Mental Illness and Psychiatry." In Kleinman and Lin, *Normal and Abnormal Behavior in Chinese Culture*, 95–111.

Lin, Keh-Ming, Arthur Kleinman, and Tsung-Yi Lin. "Overview of Mental Disorders in Chinese Cultures: Review of Epidemiological and Clinical Studies." In Kleinman and Lin, *Normal and Abnormal Behavior in Chinese Culture*, 237–272.

Linder, Birgit. "Trauma and Truth: Representations of Madness in Chinese Literature." *Journal of Medical Humanities* 32, no. 4 (2011): 291–303.

Lipkin, Zwia. *Useless to the State: Social Problems and Social Engineering in Nationalist Nanjing, 1927–1937*. Cambridge, MA: Harvard University Press, 2006.

Liu, Jin, Hong Ma, Yan-Ling He, Bin Xie, Yi-Feng Xu, Hong-Yu Tang, and Ming Li, et al. "Mental Health System in China: History, Recent Service Reform, and Future Challenges." *World Psychiatry* 10, no. 3 (October 2011): 210–216.

Liu, Lydia. *Translingual Practice: Literature, National Culture, and Translated Modernity*. Stanford, CA: Stanford University Press, 1995.

Liu Xiong. *Nao shenjing bing* [Brain and nervous diseases]. Shanghai: Shangwu yinshu guan, 1931.

Liu Yuzhen and Sun Xuemei, eds. *Riben zhengfa kaocha ji* [Records on observations of Japanese politics and law]. Shanghai: Shanghai guji, 2002.

Loh, Pichon P. Y. "The Ideological Persuasion of Chiang Kai-shek." *Modern Asian Studies* 4, no. 3 (1970): 211–238.

López-Muñoz, Francisco, Ronaldo Ucha-Udabe, and Cecilio Alamo. "The History of Barbiturates a Century after Their Clinical Introduction." *Neuropsychiatric Disease and Treatment* 1, no. 4 (December 2005): 329–343.

Lu, Hanchao. *Beyond the Neon Lights: Everyday Shanghai in the Early Twentieth Century*. Berkeley: University of California Press, 1999.

———. *Street Criers: A Cultural History of Chinese Beggars*. Stanford, CA: Stanford University Press, 2005.

Lu Shoujian. *Shenjing shuairuo liaoyang fa* [Treatment for neurasthenia]. Shanghai: Zhonghua shuju, 1917.

Lu Xun. "Kuangren riji" [Diary of a madman]. In *Selected Stories of Lu Hsun*. Beijing: Foreign Languages Press, 1960 [1918].

———. "Yijian xiaoshi" [An incident]. In *Nahan* [A call to arms]. Shanghai: Xin chaoshe chubanshe, 1923.

Luesink, David. "State Power, Governmentality, and the (Mis)remembrance of Chinese Medicine." In *Historical Epistemology and the Making of Modern Chinese Medicine*, edited by Howard Chiang, 160–187. Manchester: Manchester University Press, 2015.

Luhrmann, T. M., R. Padmavati, H. Tharoor, and A. Osei. "Differences in Voice-Hearing Experiences of People with Psychosis in the USA, India and Ghana: Interview-Based Study." *British Journal of Psychiatry* 206, no. 1 (June 26, 2014): 41–44.

Lutz, Tom. "Varieties of Medical Experience: Doctors and Patients, Psyche and Soma in America." In *Cultures of Neurasthenia from Beard to the First World War*, edited by Marijke Gijswijt-Hofstra and Roy Porter, 51–76. Amsterdam: Rodopi, 2001.

Lyman, R. S., V. Maeker, and P. Liang, eds. *Social and Psychological Studies in Neuropsychiatry in China*. Peking: Henri Vetch, 1939.

Lyman, Richard. "Psychiatry in China." *Archives of Neurology and Psychiatry* 37, no. 4 (April 1937): 765–771.

Ma, Zhao. *Runaway Wives, Urban Crimes, and Survival Tactics in Wartime Beijing, 1937–1949*. Cambridge, MA: Harvard University Press, 2015.

Ma, Zhiying. "An 'Iron Cage' of Civilization? Missionary Psychiatry, the Chinese Family, and a Colonial Dialectic of Enlightenment." In Chiang, *Psychiatry and Chinese History*, 91–110.

———. "Psychiatric Subjectivity and Cultural Resistance: Experience and Explanations of Schizophrenia in Contemporary China." In *Chinese Modernity and the Individual Psyche*, edited by Andrew Kipnis, 203–228. New York: Palgrave Macmillan, 2012.

MacCormack, Geoffrey. "The Legal Treatment of Insane Persons in Late Imperial China." *Journal of Legal History* 13, no. 3 (1992): 251–269.

MacDonald, Michael. *Mystical Bedlam: Madness, Anxiety, and Healing in Seventeenth-Century England*. Cambridge: Cambridge University Press, 1981.

MacKinnon, Stephen. *Power and Politics in Late Imperial China*. Berkeley: University of California Press, 1980.

———. "Toward a History of the Chinese Press in the Republican Period." *Modern China* 23, no. 1 (January 1997): 3–32.

Mahone, Sloan, and Megan Vaughan, eds. *Psychiatry and Empire*. New York: Palgrave Macmillan, 2007.

Makari, George. *Revolution in Mind: The Creation of Psychoanalysis*. New York: HarperCollins, 2008.

———. *Soul Machine: The Invention of the Modern Mind*. New York: W. W. Norton, 2015.

Maslow, Abraham. *The Farther Reaches of Human Nature*. New York: Viking Press, 1971.

McCartney, J. Lincoln. "Neuropsychiatry in China." *Archives of Neurology and Psychiatry* 18, no. 1 (1927): 87–95.

McCulloch, Jock. *Colonial Psychiatry and 'the African Mind.'* Cambridge: Cambridge University Press, 1995.

Menghe sijia yi'an yihua ji [Medical case records from the four families of the Menghe lineage]. Shanxi: Shanxi kexue jishu chubanshe, 2009.

Messner, Angelika C. "On 'Translating' Western Psychiatry into the Chinese Context in Republican China." In *Mapping Meanings: The Field of New Learning in Late Qing China*, edited by Michael Lackner and Natascha Vittinghoff, 639–658. Leiden: Brill, 2004.

Micale, Mark, and Roy Porter, eds. *Discovering the History of Psychiatry*. Oxford: Oxford University Press, 1994.

Mills, John. *Control: A History of Behavioral Psychology*. New York: New York University Press, 1998.

Mitchell, Timothy, ed. *Questions of Modernity*. Minneapolis: University of Minnesota Press, 2000.

Mittler, Barbara. "Gendered Advertising in China: What History Do Images Tell?" *European Journal of East Asian Studies* 6, no. 1 (2007): 13–41.

———. *A Newspaper for China? Power, Identity, and Change in Shanghai's News Media, 1872–1912*. Cambridge, MA: Harvard East Asian Monographs, 2004.

Miyasaki, Ichisada. *China's Examination Hell: The Civil Service Examinations of Imperial China*. New Haven, CT: Yale University Press, 1976.

Muir, William Ker, Jr. *Police: Streetcorner Politicians*. Chicago: University of Chicago Press, 1977.

Mülhahn, Klaus. *Criminal Justice in China: A History*. Cambridge, MA: Harvard University Press, 2007.

Munro, Robin. *Dangerous Minds: Political Psychiatry in China Today and Its Origins in the Mao Era*. New York: Human Rights Watch, 2002.

Nakamura, Karen. *A Disability of the Soul: An Ethnography of Schizophrenia and Mental Illness in Contemporary Japan*. Ithaca, NY: Cornell University Press, 2013.

Naquin, Susan. *Peking: Temples and City Life, 1400–1900*. Berkeley: University of California Press, 2000.

Nathan, Andrew. *Peking Politics, 1918–1923: Factionalism and the Failure of Constitutionalism*. Berkeley: University of California Press, 1976.

Nedostup, Rebecca. *Superstitious Regimes: Religion and the Politics of Chinese Modernity*. Cambridge, MA: Harvard University Asia Center, 2009.

Neighbors, Jennifer. "The Long Arm of Qing Law? Qing Dynasty Homicide Rulings in Republican Courts." *Modern China* 35, no. 1 (2009): 3–37.

Nevius, John. *Demon Possession*. Grand Rapids, MI: Kregel Publications, 1968.

Ng, Vivien. *Madness in Imperial China: From Illness to Deviance*. Norman: University of Oklahoma Press, 1990.

"Ni you shenjing bing ma?" [Are you crazy?] *Liangyou huabao*, no. 124 (1937): 36–37.

Norman, Conolly. "The Family Care of the Insane." *Medical Press and Circular* 131 (November 29, 1905): 557–560.

Oppenheim, Janet. *Shattered Nerves: Doctors, Patients, and Depression in Victorian England*. Oxford: Oxford University Press, 1991.

Packard, Elizabeth. *Modern Persecution, or Insane Asylums Unveiled*. New York: Pelletreau and Raynor, 1873.

Pang Jing. *Shiyong cuimian shu* [Applied hypnotism]. Shanghai: Zhonghua shuju, 1923.

Parry-Jones, William. *The Trade in Lunacy: A Study of Private Madhouses in England in the Eighteenth and Nineteenth Centuries*. London: Routledge & Kegan Paul, 1972.

"Patent Medicines in Japan." *British Medical Journal* 1, no. 2455 (January 18, 1908): 161–163.

Payton, Andrew, and Peggy Thoits. "Medicalization, Direct-to-Consumer Advertising, and Mental Illness Stigma." *Society and Mental Health* 1, no. 1 (March 2011): 55–70.

Pearson, Veronica. "The Development of Psychiatric Services in China: Christianity, Communism, and Community." In *Medical Transitions in Twentieth-Century China*, edited by Bridie Andrews and Mary Bullock, 146–172. Bloomington: Indiana University Press, 2014.

Peking Union Medical College. Annual Reports.

Peking Union Medical College. *Dedication Ceremonies and Medical Conference, September 15–22, 1921*. Peking: n.p., 1922.

Peng Hsiao-yen. *Dandyism and Transcultural Modernity: The Dandy, the Flaneur, and the Translator in 1930s Shanghai, Tokyo, and Paris*. London: Routledge, 2010.

———. "A Traveling Disease: The 'Malady of the Heart,' Scientific Jargon, and Neo-Sensation." In *China and Its Others: Knowledge Transfer through Translation, 1829–2010*, edited by James St. André and Peng Hsiao-yen, 95–138. Amsterdam: Rodopi, 2012.

Petzold, Matthias. "The Social History of Chinese Psychology." In *Psychology in Twentieth-Century Thought and Society*, edited by Mitchell Ash and William Woodward, 213–232. Cambridge: Cambridge University Press, 1987.

Phillips, Michael, Hanhui Chen, Kate Diesfeld, Bin Xie, Hui G. Cheng, Graham Mellsop, and Xiehe Liu. "China's New Mental Health Law: Reframing Involuntary Treatment." *American Journal of Psychiatry* 170, no. 6 (June 2013): 588–591.

Phillips, Michael, Jingxuan Zhang, Qichang Shi, Zhiqiang Song, Zhijie Ding, Shutao Pang, Xianyun Li, et al. "Prevalence, Treatment, and Associated Disability of Mental Disorders in Four Provinces in China during 2001–05." *Lancet* 373, no. 9680 (2009): 2041–2053.

Pols, Johannes. "Managing the Mind: The Culture of American Mental Hygiene, 1910–1950." PhD diss., University of Pennsylvania, 1997.

Porter, Roy. "Foucault's Great Confinement." *History of the Human Sciences* 3, no. 1 (February 1990): 47–54.

———. *Health for Sale: Quackery in England, 1660–1850*. Manchester: Manchester University Press, 1989.

———. *Madmen: A Social History of Madhouses, Mad Doctors, and Lunatics*. Stroud, UK: Tempus, 2004.

———. *Mind Forg'd Manacles: A History of Madness in England from the Restoration to the Regency*. Cambridge, MA: Harvard University Press, 1987.

———. *A Social History of Madness: The World through the Eyes of the Insane*. New York: Weidenfeld & Nicolson, 1988.

Porter, Roy, and David Wright, eds. *The Confinement of the Insane: International Perspectives, 1800–1965*. Cambridge: Cambridge University Press, 2003.

"President Li Yuan-Hung on Medical Work in China." *China Medical Missionary Journal* 37, no. 7 (July 1923): 588–589.

Proceedings of the First International Congress on Mental Hygiene. New York: International Committee for Mental Hygiene, 1932.

Pruitt, Ida. "Hospital Social Service in Diagnosis and Treatment." *China Medical Journal* 28 (1928): 432–443.

———. "Medical Social Workers: Their Work and Training," *China Medical Journal* 49 (1935): 909–916.

"Qinghua daxue qu Wu zhenxiang" [Facts of the Expel Wu (Movement) at Qinghua University]. *Zhongguo sheying xuehui huabao* 6, no. 297 (1931): 1.

"Qu Guo xuanyan" [Expel Guo manifesto]. *Guoli Zhejiang daxue xiaokan* 24, no. 203 (December 23, 1935).

Ran, Mao-Sheng, Meng-Ze Xiang, Peggy Simpson, and Cecilia Lai-Wan Chan. *Family-Based Mental Health Care in Rural China.* Hong Kong: Hong Kong University Press, 2005.

Reardon-Anderson, James. *The Study of Change: Chemistry in China, 1840–1949.* Cambridge: Cambridge University Press, 1991.

Richardson, Theresa. *The Century of the Child: The Mental Hygiene Movement and Social Policy in the United States and Canada.* Albany: State University of New York Press, 1989.

Roberts, David. *Victorian Origins of the British Welfare State.* New Haven, CT: Yale University Press, 1960.

Rogaski, Ruth. *Hygienic Modernity: Meanings of Health and Disease in Treaty-Port China.* Berkeley: University of California Press, 2004.

Rose, Anne. "Racial Experiments in Psychiatry's Provinces: Richard S. Lyman and His Colleagues in China and the American South, 1932–51." *History of Psychiatry* 23, no. 4 (2012): 419–436.

Ross, Edward Alsworth. *The Changing Chinese: The Conflict of Oriental and Western Cultures in China.* London: T. Fisher Unwin, 1911.

Ross, Robert. "The Insane in China: Examination Hints." *China Medical Journal* 24 (1920): 514–518.

———. "Mental Hygiene." *China Medical Journal* 15 (1926): 8–13.

Rothman, David. *The Discovery of the Asylum: Social Order and Disorder in the New Republic.* Boston: Little, Brown, 1971.

Rowe, William. *China's Last Empire: The Great Qing.* Cambridge, MA: Harvard University Press, 2009.

Royds, W. M. "Japanese Patent Medicines." *Transactions of the Asiatic Society of Japan* 35–36 (1907).

Sadowsky, Jonathan. *Imperial Bedlam: Institutions of Madness in Colonial Southwest Nigeria.* Berkeley: University of California Press, 1999.

Sammons, Thomas. *Proprietary Medicine and Ointment Trade in China.* Washington, DC: Government Printing Office, 1917.

Savill, Thomas Dixon. *Clinical Lectures on Neurasthenia.* London: Henry J. Glaisher, 1908.

Scheff, Thomas. *Being Mentally Ill: A Sociological Theory.* Chicago: Aldine, 1966.

Scheid, Volker. *Chinese Medicine in Contemporary China: Plurality and Synthesis.* Durham, NC: Duke University Press, 2002.

———. *Currents of Tradition in Chinese Medicine, 1626–2006.* Seattle, WA: Eastland Press, 2007.

Schneck, Jerome. *A History of Psychiatry.* Springfield, IL: Charles C. Thomas, 1960.

Schwarcz, Vera. *The Chinese Enlightenment: Intellectuals and the Legacy of the May Fourth Movement of 1919*. Berkeley: University of California Press, 1986.

Schwartz, Benjamin. "Culture, Modernity, and Nationalism: Further Reflections." *Daedalus* 122, no. 3 (Summer 1993): 207–226.

Scott, James. *Weapons of the Weak: Everyday Forms of Peasant Resistance*. New Haven, CT: Yale University Press, 1985.

Scull, Andrew. *Hysteria: The Disturbing History*. Oxford: Oxford University Press, 2011.

———. *The Insanity of Place/The Place of Insanity*. London: Routledge, 2006.

———. *Madhouse: A Tragic Tale of Megalomania and Modern Medicine*. New Haven, CT: Yale University Press, 2007.

———. *Madness in Civilization: A Cultural History of Insanity from the Bible to Freud, from the Madhouse to Modern Medicine*. London: Thames & Hudson, 2015.

———. *The Most Solitary of Afflictions: Madness and Society in Britain, 1700–1900*. New Haven, CT: Yale University Press, 1993.

———. *Social Order/Mental Disorder: Anglo-American Psychiatry in Historical Perspective*. Berkeley: University of California Press, 1989.

———. "Was Insanity Increasing?" In *Social Order/Mental Disorder*, 239–249.

Scull, Andrew, Charlotte MacKenzie, and Nicholas Hervey. *Masters of Bedlam: The Transformation of the Mad-Doctoring Trade*. Princeton, NJ: Princeton University Press, 1996.

Selden, Charles. "Conditions in South China in Relation to Insanity." *American Journal of Insanity* 70, nos. 2–4 (1913): 411–426.

———. "The Life of John G. Kerr." *Chinese Medical Journal* 49 (1935): 364–376.

———. "Treatment of the Insane II." *China Medical Journal* 23, no. 4 (July 1909): 221–232.

———. "Treatment of the Insane III." *China Medical Journal* 23, no. 6 (November 1909): 373–384.

———. "Work among the Chinese Insane and Some of Its Results." *China Medical Missionary Journal* 19, no. 1 (January 1905): 1–17.

"Shanghai fengdian yiyuan feifa jingu yi jianfu" [Shanghai asylum illegally detains a healthy woman]. *Funü yuebao* 2, no. 3 (1936): 44–47.

Shapiro, Hugh. "How Different Are Chinese and Western Medicine? The Case of Nerves." In *Medicine across Cultures: History and Practice of Medicine in Non-Western Cultures*, edited by Helaine Selin, 351–372. New York: Kluwer, 2003.

———. "Neurasthenia and the Assimilation of Nerves into China." Paper presented at the Symposium on the History of Disease, Academia Sinica, Taiwan, June 16–18, 2000.

———. "Operatic Escapes: Performing Madness in Neuropsychiatric Beijing." In *Science and Technology in Modern China, 1880s–1940s*, edited by Jing Tsu and Benjamin Elman, 297–326. Leiden: Brill, 2014.

———. "Pathologizing Marriage: Neuropsychiatry and the Escape of Women in Early Twentieth-Century China." In Chiang, *Psychiatry and Chinese History*, 129–142.

———. "The Puzzle of Spermatorrhea in Republican China." *positions* 6, no. 3 (1998): 551–595.

———. "The View from a Chinese Asylum: Defining Madness in 1930s Peking." PhD diss., Harvard University, 1995.

"Shehui weisheng jiaoyu: Shiji gongzuo" [Social hygiene education: Practical work]. *Beiping shi weisheng ju di'er weisheng qu shiwu suo nianbao*, no. 2 (1935): 115–118.

Shen Jiaben. *Da Qing xianxing xinglü anyu* [Commentary on the great Qing penal code currently in use]. Beijing: Falü guan, 1909.

Shih, Shu-mei. *The Lure of the Modern: Writing Modernism in Semicolonial China, 1917–1937*. Berkeley: University of California Press, 2001.

Shi Mingzheng. "Beijing Transforms: Urban Infrastructure, Public Works, and Social Change in the Chinese Capital, 1900–1928." PhD diss., Columbia University, 1993.

Shorter, Edward. *A History of Psychiatry: From the Era of the Asylum to the Age of Prozac*. New York: Wiley, 1997.

Showalter, Elaine. *The Female Malady: Women, Madness, and English Culture, 1830–1980*. New York: Penguin, 1987.

Shu Yueyu. "Zhang Yinian: Zhongguo xinli weisheng de kaituo zhe" [Zhang Yinian: Progenitor of Chinese mental hygiene]. *Ziran bianzheng fa tongxun*, no. 6 (2015): 138–146.

Sidel, Ruth. "The Role of Revolutionary Optimism in the Treatment of Mental Illness in the People's Republic of China." *American Journal of Orthopsychiatry* 43, no. 5 (1973): 732–736.

Sidel, Victor, and Ruth Sidel. *Serve the People: Observations on Medicine in the People's Republic of China*. Boston: Beacon Press, 1973.

Simonis, Fabien. "Mad Acts, Mad Speech, and Mad People in Late Imperial Chinese Law and Medicine." PhD diss., Princeton University, 2010.

———. "Medicaments and Persuasion: Medical Therapies for Madness in Nineteenth-Century China." In Chiang, *Psychiatry and Chinese History*, 55–70.

Sivin, Nathan. *Traditional Medicine in Contemporary China*. Ann Arbor: University of Michigan, 1987.

Si Yi. "Jingshen bing yu xiandai shehui" [Mental illness and modern society]. *Qinghua zhoukan* 43, no. 4 (1935): 6–17.

Smith, S. A. "Talking Toads and Chinless Ghosts: The Politics of 'Superstitious Rumor' in the People's Republic of China, 1961–65." *American Historical Review* 111, no. 2 (April 2006): 405–427.

Sommer, Matthew. *Sex, Law, and Society in Late Imperial China*. Stanford, CA: Stanford University Press, 2002.

Song Jiaoren. *Song Jiaoren riji* [The diary of Song Jiaoren]. Changsha: Hunan renmin chubanshe, 1980.

Song Siming. *Jingshen bing zhi shehui de yinsu yu fangzhi* [The social causes and prevention of mental illness]. Shanghai: Zhonghua shuju, 1944.

Spence, Jonathan. *To Change China: Western Advisers in China, 1620–1960*. New York: Penguin, 1969.

Stone, Martin. "Shellshock and the Psychologists." In *The Anatomy of Madness: Essays in the History of Psychiatry*, vol. 2, edited by William Bynum, Roy Porter, and Michael Shepherd, 242–271. London: Routledge, 1985.

Strand, David. *Rickshaw Beijing: City People and Politics in the 1920s*. Berkeley: University of California Press, 1989.

Strauss, Julia. "Creating 'Virtuous and Talented Officials' for the Twentieth Century: Discourse and Practice in *Xinzheng* China." *Modern Asian Studies* 37, no. 4 (October 2003): 831–850.

———. *Strong Institutions in Weak Polities: State Building in Republican China, 1927–1940*. Oxford: Oxford University Press, 1998.

Sun Xiong. *Biantai xingwei* [Abnormal behavior]. Shanghai: Shijie shuju, 1939.

Sun Zhongshan. *Sunwen xueshuo* [Doctrines of Sun Wen]. Shanghai: Minzhi shuzhu, 1925.

———. *Xinli jianshe* [Psychological reconstruction]. Chongqing: Hangkong weiyuan hui, 1940 [1925].

Su Yigong. *Ming Qing lüdian yu tiaoli* [Laws and ordinances in the Ming and Qing]. Beijing: Zhongguo zhengfa daxue chubanshe, 1999.

Suzuki, Akihito. "Global Theory, Local Practice: Shock Therapies in Japanese Psychiatry, 1920–1945." In Ernst and Mueller, *Transnational Psychiatries*, 116–141.

———. *Madness at Home: The Psychiatrist, the Patient, and the Family in England 1820–1860*. Berkeley: University of California Press, 2006.

———. "State, Family, and the Insane in Japan, 1900–1945." In Porter and Wright, *Confinement of the Insane*, 193–225.

Szasz, Thomas. *The Manufacture of Madness: A Comparative Study of the Inquisition and the Mental Health Movement*. New York: Harper & Row, 1970.

———. *The Myth of Mental Illness: Foundations of a Theory of Personal Conduct*. New York: Harper & Row, 1961.

Szto, Peter. "The Accommodation of Insanity in Canton, China: 1857–1935." PhD diss., University of Pennsylvania, 2002.

———. "Psychiatric Space and Design Antecedents: The John G. Kerr Refuge for the Insane." In Chiang, *Psychiatry and Chinese History*, 71–90.

Tai Shuangqiu, ed. *Xinli weisheng* [Mental hygiene]. Shanghai: Jiaoyu bianyi guan chuban, 1935.

Tang Erhe. "Jingshen bing yu qi zhiliao" [Mental illness and its treatment]. *Dongfang zazhi* 21, no. 8 (1924): 92–94.

Tang, Xiaobing. "Lu Xun's 'Diary of a Madman' and a Chinese Modernism." *PMLA* 107, no. 5 (October 1992): 1222–1234.

Thomson, Mathew. "Mental Hygiene as an International Movement." In *International Health Organizations and Movements, 1918–1939*, edited by Paul Weindling, 283–304. Cambridge: Cambridge University Press, 1995.

Tian Tao and Guo Chengwei, eds. *Qingmo Beijing chengshi guanli fagui* [Statutes on the administration of Beijing at the end of the Qing dynasty]. Beijing: Beijing yanshan chubanshe, 1996.

T'ien Ju-k'ang. "Traditional Chinese Beliefs and Attitudes toward Mental Illness." In Tseng and Wu, *Chinese Culture and Mental Health*, 67–81.

Tseng, Wen-shing, and David Wu, eds. *Chinese Culture and Mental Health*. Orlando, FL: Academic Press, 1985.

Unschuld, Paul. *Medicine in China: A History of Ideas*. Berkeley: University of California Press, 2010 [1985].

———. *Nan Jing: The Classic of Difficult Issues*. Berkeley: University of California Press, 2016 [1986].

Unschuld, Paul, and Hermann Tessenow. *Huangdi neijing suwen: An Annotated Translation of Huang Di's Inner Classic—Basic Questions*. Berkeley: University of California Press, 2011.

Vance, Lee J. "Evolution of Patent Medicine." *Popular Science Monthly*, May 1891.

Van Gulik, Robert Hans. *Sexual Life in Ancient China: A Preliminary Survey of Chinese Sex and Society*. Leiden: Brill, 1961.

Veith, Ilza. "Psychiatric Thought in Chinese Medicine." *Journal of the History of Medicine and Allied Sciences* 10 (1955): 261–268.

Von Glahn, Richard. *The Sinister Way: The Divine and the Demonic in Chinese Religious Culture*. Berkeley: University of California Press, 2004.

Wallace, Edwin, and John Gach, eds. *History of Psychiatry and Medical Psychology*. New York: Springer, 2008.

Wang, David Der-Wei. *Fictional Realism in Twentieth-Century China*. New York: Columbia University Press, 1992.

Wang Kangjiu. *Beijing weisheng dashi ji* [Important events in Beijing hygiene]. Beijing: Beijing kexue jishu chubanshe, 1994.

Wang Mengying. *Wang Mengying yi'an yizhu* [Medical case records of Wang Mengying]. Beijing: Xueyuan chubanshe, 2009.

Wang Qiuyuan. "Nao zhi shengli: Xin yu nao zhi yanjiu" [Physiology of the brain: Research on the heart and brain]. *Dazhong yixue yuekan* 1, nos. 9–10 (1934): 4–5.

Wang Runmin. "Zangzao—Xiesideli zhi yanjiu" [Research on zangzao—hysteria]. In Zhou, *Jingshen bing guangyi*, 15–16.

Wang Wenji. "Yufang, shiying yu gaizao: Minguo shiqi de xinli weisheng" [Prevent, conform, and transform: Republican-era mental hygiene]. In *Jiankang yu shehui* [Health and society], edited by Zhu Pingyi, 237–258. Taibei: Lianjing, 2013.

———. "Zhixing weibi heyi: Gu Jiegang yu shenjing shuairuo de ziwo guanli" [Gu Jiegang and the management of neurasthenia in Republican China]. In *Weisheng yu yiliao*, 65–99. Taibei: Zhongyang yanjiu yuan, 2013.

Wang Ziming. "Guangbo jiangyan: Jingshen bing yu shehui" [Broadcast speech: Mental illness and society]. *Weisheng yuekan* 1, nos. 8–9 (1935): 71–74.

Wang Zucheng. "Ji Zhongguo diyi wei nüxing jingshen bing xue jia: Gui Zhiliang jiaoshou" [Remembering China's first female psychiatrist: Professor Gui Zhiliang]. *Jingshen yixue lishi* 23, no. 3 (2011): 191–192.

Watson, John B. *Behaviorism*. Chicago: University of Chicago Press, 1924.

———. "Psychology as the Behaviorist Views It." *Psychological Review* 20 (1913): 158–177.

Wei Hongsheng. *Jingshen duanlian zhiliao shiyan wenda* [Questions and answers on experiments related to the exercise and treatment of the spirit]. Beiping: n.p., 1936.

———. *Jingshen jiankang shiyan lu* [Records of healthy spirit practice]. Beiping: Jingshen xue yanjiu hui faxing, 1937.

Wei Yulin. "Cong yanjiu jingshen bing tandao jingshen weisheng" [Speaking of mental hygiene from the perspective of psychiatric research]. *Weisheng yuekan* 2, nos. 7–8 (1936): 28–31.

———. "Duiyu jingshen bingren ying zhuyi de shixiang" [Matters to which attention should be paid regarding the mentally ill]. *Weisheng yuekan* 2, no. 1 (1936): 8–10.

"Weisheng yaowen" [Important health news]. *Weisheng yuekan* 3, no. 5–6 (1936): 92–93.

Weng Zhilong. "Jingshen bingyuan yingyou de shebei" [The equipment that insane asylums should have]. *Minzhong yibao* 6 (1931): 35–41.

White, Hugh. *Demonism Verified and Analyzed*. Shanghai: Presbyterian Mission Press, 1922.

White, William. "The Origin, Growth, and Significance of the Mental Hygiene Movement." *Science* 72, no. 1856 (July 25, 1930): 77–81.

Will, Pierre-Etienne. *Bureaucracy and Famine in Eighteenth-Century China*. Stanford, CA: Stanford University Press, 1990.

Williams, Frankwood. *Mental Hygiene*. Chicago: American Library Association, 1929.

———. *Russia, Youth, and the Present-Day World: Further Studies in Mental Hygiene*. New York: Farrar & Reinhart, 1934.

Wong, K. C. "A Short History of Psychiatry and Mental Hygiene in China." *Chinese Medical Journal* 68 (1950): 44–48.

Woo, Toh. "An Analysis of 2,330 Case Work Records of the Social Service Department, Peiping Union Medical College." In *Bulletins of the Social Research Department, 1928–1933*. New York: Garland, 1982 [1931].

Woods, Andrew. "The Incidence of Nervous Diseases in China." *China Medical Journal* 40 (1926): 1070–1082.

———. "The Menace of Insanity to Popular Government." *National Medical Journal of China* 7, no. 1 (March 1921): 201–206.

———. "The Nervous Diseases of the Chinese." *Archives of Neurology and Psychiatry* 21 (March 1929): 542–570.

Wu, Huaiting. "The Construction of a Consumer Population in Advertising in 1920s China." *Discourse & Society* 20, no. 1 (January 2009): 147–171.

Wu Jiangleng. "Shenjing bing de shiren" [The nervous poet]. *Shaonian shehui* 2 (1919): 15–16.

Wu Nanxuan. "Guoji xinli weisheng yundong" [The international mental hygiene movement]. *Guoli zhongyang daxue jiaoyu congkan* 2, no. 1 (1934): 1–39.

———. "Shehui kongzhi dineng de zhongyao he fangfa" [The importance and methods of the social control of the feebleminded]. *Guoli zhongyang daxue jiaoyu congkan* 1, no. 1 (1933): 63–97.

———. "Xinli weisheng yiyi fanwei yu zhongyao xing" [The meaning and importance of mental hygiene]. *Guoli zhongyang daxue jiaoyu congkan* 2, no. 1 (1934): 1–11.

Wu, Yi-Li. "Bodily Knowledge and Western Learning in Late Imperial China: The Case of Wang Shixiong (1808–68)." In *Historical Epistemology and the Making of Modern Chinese Medicine*, edited by Howard Chiang, 80–112. Manchester: Manchester University Press, 2012.

Wu Yongmei and Li Peide [Pui-tak Lee]. *Tuxiang yu shangye wenhua: fenxi Zhongguo jindai guanggao* [Graphic images and consumer culture: Analysis of modern advertising culture in China]. Hong Kong: Hong Kong University Press, 2014.

Wu, Yu-chuan. "A Disorder of Ki: Alternative Treatments for Neurasthenia in Japan, 1890–1945." PhD diss., University College London, 2012.

Xiao Xiaorong. "Xinli weisheng zhi jiben yuanze" [Basic principles of mental hygiene]. *Guoli zhongyang daxue jiaoyu congkan* 2, no. 1 (1934): 1–13.

Xie Guan. *Zhongguo yixue da cidian* [Dictionary of Chinese medicine]. Shanghai: Shangwu yinshu guan, 1927.

"Xin Zhonghua minguo xingfa" [New penal code for the Republic of China]. *Zhonghua minguo xingfa xinjiu quanwen duizhao biao* [Comparison chart of the old and new Republican penal codes]. Beiping: 1935.

Xu Ke. *Shiyong Beijing zhinan* [Practical guide to Beijing]. Shanghai: Shangwu yinshuguan, 1920.

Xu, Xiaoqun. "The Fate of Judicial Independence in Republican China, 1912–1937." *China Quarterly* 149 (March 1997): 1–28.

———. "National Essence vs. Science: Chinese Native Physicians' Fight for Legitimacy, 1912–1937." *Modern Asian Studies* 31, no. 4 (October 1997): 847–877.

Xu, Yamin. "Policing Civility on the Streets: Encounters with Litterbugs, 'Nightsoil Lords,' and Street Corner Urinators in Republican Beijing." *Twentieth-Century China* 30, no. 2 (2005): 28–71.

Xu Zhuodai. "Xurong fengzi" [The vain lunatic]. *Hong zazhi* 2, no. 60 (1923): 1–9.

Yang Huanwen. "Kuangdianxian zhi yanjiu" [Research on kuang, dian, and xian]. *Dazhong yixue yuekan* 1, no. 9 (1933): 64–69.

Yang Nianqun. *Zaizao bingren: Zhongxi yi chongtu xia de kongjian zhengzhi, 1832–1985* [Remaking patients: Politics of space in the conflicts between traditional Chinese medicine and Western medicine]. Beijing: Renmin daxue chubanshe, 2006.

Yan Guocai, ed. *Zhongguo xinli xue shi ziliao xuanbian, di si juan* [Collection of materials on the history of Chinese psychology, vol. 4]. Beijing: Renmin jiaoyu chubanshe, 1990.

Yap, P. M. "The Mental Illness of Hung Hsiu-ch'uan, Leader of the Taiping Rebellion." *Far Eastern Quarterly* 13, no. 3 (May 1954): 287–304.

Yee, Frank Ki Chun. "Police in Modern China." PhD diss., University of California, Berkeley, 1942.

Yeh, Wen-hsin. *The Alienated Academy: Culture and Politics in Republican China, 1919–1937.* Cambridge, MA: Harvard University Press, 1990.

———, ed. *Becoming Chinese: Passages to Modernity and Beyond.* Berkeley: University of California Press, 2000.

———. *Shanghai Splendor: Economic Sentiments and the Making of Modern China, 1843–1949.* Berkeley: University of California Press, 2007.

Yip, Ka-che. *Health and National Reconstruction in Nationalist China: The Development of Modern Health Services, 1929–1937.* Ann Arbor, MI: Association of Asian Studies, 1995.

Yoo, Theodore Jun. *It's Madness: The Politics of Mental Health in Colonial Korea.* Berkeley: University of California Press, 2016.

Young, James Harvey. *American Health Quackery.* Princeton, NJ: Princeton University Press, 1992.

———. *The Toadstool Millionaires: A Social History of Patent Medicines in America before Federal Regulation.* Princeton, NJ: Princeton University Press, 1972.

Yu Guojuan. *Qingchao xingbu tongxing tiaoli* [Regulations of the Qing dynasty Board of Punishments]. Zhejiang: Zhejiang guji chubanshe, 2012.

Yu, Ning. *The Chinese HEART in a Cognitive Perspective: Culture, Body, and Language.* Berlin: Mouton de Gruyter, 2009.

Yu Pingke. *Cuimian shu hanshou jiangyi* [Correspondence teaching materials on hypnotism]. Shanghai: Zhongguo xinling yanjiu hui, 1931.

Yu Shenchu. "Diankuang bing zhi yanjiu" [Research on madness]. *Dazhong yixue yuekan* 1, no. 2 (1933): 14–16.

Yuan Xi. *Beijing chengshi fazhan shi, jindai juan* [History of the development of Beijing, modern edition]. Beijing: Beijing yanshan chubanshe, 2008.

Zarrow, Peter. *After Empire: The Conceptual Transformation of the Chinese State, 1885–1924.* Stanford, CA: Stanford University Press, 2012.

Zhang Kan and Zhao Chengjie. *Zhongguo dangdai yixue jia huicui* [Compilation of modern Chinese doctors]. Jilin: Jilin kexue jishu chubanshe, 1991.

Zhang Kecheng. *Nannü shengzhi qixing shenjing shuairuo de yufang ji zhiliao* [Prevention and treatment of sexual neurasthenia in men and women]. Shanghai: Shenghuo yiyuan, 1934.

Zhang Ning. "Nao wei yishen zhi zhu: cong 'Ailuo Bunaozhi' kan jindai Zhongguo shenti guan de bianhua" [From heart to brain: Ailuo brain tonic and the new concept of the body in modern China]. *Zhongyang yanjiuyuan jindaishi yanjiusuo jikan* 74 (December 2011): 1–40.

Zhang, Peiyao, David W. Wong, Billy K. L. So, and Hui Lin. "An Exploratory Spatial Analysis of Western Medical Services in Republican Beijing." *Applied Geography* 32, no. 2 (March 2012): 556–565.

Zhang Shoutao. "Minguo zhongyang daxue danghua jiaoyu yanjiu" [Research into the partification of education at National Central University during the Republican period]. *Dang'an yu jianshe* 3 (2015): 56–58.

Zhang Xianwen and Fang Qingqiu. *Zhonghua minguo shi da cidian* [Dictionary of Republican history]. Jiangsu: Jiangsu guji chubanshe, 2001.

Zhang Yan and Sun Yanjing, eds. *Minguo shiliao congkan* [Historical data from the Republican period], vols. 734 and 766. Zhengzhou: Daxiang chubanshe, 2009.

Zhang, Yanhua. *Transforming Emotions with Chinese Medicine: An Ethnographic Account from Contemporary China.* Albany: State University of New York Press, 2007.

Zhang Yaojie. *Xuan'an bainian: Song Jiaoren an yu Guomindang* [An unsettled case of the century: The case of Song Jiaoren and the Guomindang]. Taibei: Guojia tushuguan chuban, 2010.

Zhang Yinian. *Xinli weisheng gailun* [Introduction to mental hygiene]. Shanghai: Shangwu yinshu guan, 1936.

———. "Xinli weisheng yu ertong xundao" [Mental hygiene and the guidance of children]. In Tai, *Xinli weisheng*, 15–26.

———. "Xinli weisheng zai xuexiao ji jiating zhong de yingyong" [The utility of mental hygiene in the school and at home]. *Xinli jikan* 2, no. 2 (1937): 1–11.

Zhao Han'en. *Jingshen bingxue* [Psychiatry]. Shanghai: Shangwu yinshu guan, 1929.

Zheng Shibin. *Riben jiating yao* [Japanese home medicine]. Taiwan: Pasidun Publishing, 2015.

Zheng Zhong and Liu Jingyu, eds. *Minzhong chuantong zhibing xiao juezhao* [Unique tricks to cure illness in popular tradition]. Beijing: Zhongguo zhongyiyao chubanshe, 2012.

Zhongguo jingshen yanjiu hui, ed. *Zhongguo jingshen yanjiu hui jingshen tekan* [Chinese Spirit Research Association special issue]. Shanghai: Zhongguo jingshen yanjiu hui chubanshe, 1936.

"Zhongguo xinli weisheng xiehui gongzuo baogao" [Work report for the Chinese Association of Mental Hygiene]. *Jianguo jiaoyu*, no. 1 (1938): 39–41.

Zhonghua minguo xingfa [Penal code of the Republic of China]. Nanjing: Sifa bu, 1928.

Zhonghua minguo zanxing xin xinglü [Temporary new penal code of the Republic of China]. Shanghai: Commercial Press, 1927.

Zhou Chuan. *Zhongguo jinxiandai gaodeng jiaoyu renwu cidian* [Dictionary of figures in higher education in modern China]. Fujian: Fujian jiaoyu chubanshe, 2012.

Zhou Lichuan. *Jingshen bing guangyi* [The broad meaning of mental illness]. Shanghai: Siming yiyi shuwu, 1931.

Zhou Shaoyuan. *Zhongguo jindai xingfa de zhaoduan* [The beginnings of modern Chinese criminal law]. Beijing: Shangwu yinshu guan, 2012.

Zhou Xiaonong. *Zhou Xiaonong yi'an, di'er ban* [Medical case records of Zhou Xiaonong, vol. 2]. Shanghai: Shanghai kexue jishu chubanshe, 2008.

Zhou Zuoren. *Jingdian zuopin xuan* [Anthology of classic works]. Beijing: Dangdai shijie chubanshe, 2002.

Zhu Guangqian. *Biantai xinli xue* [Abnormal psychology]. Shanghai: Shangwu yinshu guan, 1933.

Zhu Ziqiang and Gao Zhanxiang. *Zhongguo wenhua da baike quanshu, jiaoyu juan* [Encyclopedia of Chinese culture, education edition]. Changchun: Changchun chubanshe, 1994.

Zong Zihe. "Shuo nao" [Speaking of the brain]. *Dazhong yixue yuekan* 1, no. 7 (1933): 22–23.

Index

Page numbers in italics refer to figures.

STUDIES OF
THE WEATHERHEAD EAST ASIAN INSTITUTE,
COLUMBIA UNIVERSITY

Selected Titles
(Complete list at: http://weai.columbia.edu/publications/studies-weai/)

Making Time: Astronomical Time Measurement in Tokugawa Japan, by Yulia Frumer. University of Chicago Press, 2018.

Resurrecting Nagasaki: Reconstruction and the Formation of Atomic Narratives, by Chad Diehl. Cornell University Press, 2018.

Promiscuous Media: Film and Visual Culture in Imperial Japan, 1926–1945, by Hikari Hori. Cornell University Press, 2018.

The End of Japanese Cinema: Industrial Genres, National Times, and Media Ecologies, by Alexander Zahlten. Duke University Press, 2017.

The Chinese Typewriter: A History, by Thomas S. Mullaney. The MIT Press, 2017.

Mobilizing without the Masses: Control and Contention in China, by Diana Fu. Cambridge University Press, 2017.

Forgotten Disease: Illnesses Transformed in Chinese Medicine, by Hilary A. Smith. Stanford University Press, 2017.

Food of Sinful Demons: Meat, Vegetarianism, and the Limits of Buddhism in Tibet, by Geoffrey Barstow. Columbia University Press, 2017.

Aesthetic Life: Beauty and Art in Modern Japan, by Miya Mizuta Lippit. Harvard University Asia Center, 2017.

Youth for Nation: Culture and Protest in Cold War South Korea, by Charles R. Kim. University of Hawaii Press, 2017.

Socialist Cosmopolitanism: The Chinese Literary Universe, 1945–1965, by Nicolai Volland. Columbia University Press, 2017.

Yokohama and the Silk Trade: How Eastern Japan Became the Primary Economic Region of Japan, 1843–1893, by Yasuhiro Makimura. Lexington Books, 2017.

The Social Life of Inkstones: Artisans and Scholars in Early Qing China, by Dorothy Ko. University of Washington Press, 2017.

Darwin, Dharma, and the Divine: Evolutionary Theory and Religion in Modern Japan, by G. Clinton Godart. University of Hawaii Press, 2017.

Dictators and Their Secret Police: Coercive Institutions and State Violence, by Sheena Chestnut Greitens. Cambridge University Press, 2016.

The Cultural Revolution on Trial: Mao and the Gang of Four, by Alexander C. Cook. Cambridge University Press, 2016.

Inheritance of Loss: China, Japan, and the Political Economy of Redemption after Empire, by Yukiko Koga. University of Chicago Press, 2016.

Homecomings: The Belated Return of Japan's Lost Soldiers, by Yoshikuni Igarashi. Columbia University Press, 2016.

Samurai to Soldier: Remaking Military Service in Nineteenth-Century Japan, by D. Colin Jaundrill. Cornell University Press, 2016.

The Red Guard Generation and Political Activism in China, by Guobin Yang. Columbia University Press, 2016.

Accidental Activists: Victim Movements and Government Accountability in Japan and South Korea, by Celeste L. Arrington. Cornell University Press, 2016.

Ming China and Vietnam: Negotiating Borders in Early Modern Asia, by Kathlene Baldanza. Cambridge University Press, 2016.

Ethnic Conflict and Protest in Tibet and Xinjiang: Unrest in China's West, coedited by Ben Hillman and Gray Tuttle. Columbia University Press, 2016.

One Hundred Million Philosophers: Science of Thought and the Culture of Democracy in Postwar Japan, by Adam Bronson. University of Hawaii Press, 2016.

Conflict and Commerce in Maritime East Asia: The Zheng Family and the Shaping of the Modern World, c. 1620-1720, by Xing Hang. Cambridge University Press, 2016.

Chinese Law in Imperial Eyes: Sovereignty, Justice, and Transcultural Politics, by Li Chen. Columbia University Press, 2016.

Imperial Genus: The Formation and Limits of the Human in Modern Korea and Japan, by Travis Workman. University of California Press, 2015.

Yasukuni Shrine: History, Memory, and Japan's Unending Postwar, by Akiko Takenaka. University of Hawaii Press, 2015.

The Age of Irreverence: A New History of Laughter in China, by Christopher Rea. University of California Press, 2015.

The Knowledge of Nature and the Nature of Knowledge in Early Modern Japan, by Federico Marcon. University of Chicago Press, 2015.

The Fascist Effect: Japan and Italy, 1915–1952, by Reto Hofmann. Cornell University Press, 2015.

The International Minimum: Creativity and Contradiction in Japan's Global Engagement, 1933–1964, by Jessamyn R. Abel. University of Hawaii Press, 2015.

Empires of Coal: Fueling China's Entry into the Modern World Order, 1860–1920, by Shellen Xiao Wu. Stanford University Press, 2015.